Infant Nutrition: A Practical Handbook

Infant Nutrition: A Practical Handbook

Editor: Karol Prosser

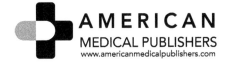

AMERICAN
MEDICAL PUBLISHERS
www.americanmedicalpublishers.com

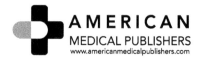

AMERICAN
MEDICAL PUBLISHERS
www.americanmedicalpublishers.com

Cataloging-in-Publication Data

Infant nutrition : a practical handbook / edited by Karol Prosser.
    p. cm.
Includes bibliographical references and index.
ISBN 978-1-63927-697-4
1. Infants--Nutrition. 2. Nutrition disorders in infants. 3. Children--Nutrition.
4. Nutrition disorders in children. I. Prosser, Karol.
RJ216 .I54 2023
649.33--dc23

American Medical Publishers,
41 Flatbush Avenue,
1st Floor, New York,
NY 11217, USA

ISBN 978-1-63927-697-4 (Hardback)

Contents

Preface

In my initial years as a student, I used to run to the library at every possible instance to grab a book and learn something new. Books were my primary source of knowledge and I would not have come such a long way without all that I learnt from them. Thus, when I was approached to edit this book; I became understandably nostalgic. It was an absolute honor to be considered worthy of guiding the current generation as well as those to come. I put all my knowledge and hard work into making this book most beneficial for its readers.

Infant nutrition refers to the study of the nutritional requirements of infants. A diet that lacks in vital minerals, calories, fluids or vitamins is deemed insufficient. Breast milk offers the best nutrition for the crucial early months of growth as compared to infant formula. It has numerous benefits for neonates and infants, including improved immunity, growth and development. Breastfeeding reduces the risk of sudden infant death syndrome, anemia and obesity. Solid foods are often provided to infants after four to six months from their birth. Proper infant nutrition requires the provision of vital nutrients that promote development, appropriate growth, function, and resistance to disorders and infections. An expectant mother can ensure optimal nutrition by choosing whether to bottle-feed or breastfeed the infant after birth. The topics covered in this book offer the readers new insights on infant nutrition. It is a vital tool for all researching and studying this field. This book is a resource guide for experts as well as students.

I wish to thank my publisher for supporting me at every step. I would also like to thank all the authors who have contributed their researches in this book. I hope this book will be a valuable contribution to the progress of the field.

Editor

The Course of IGF-1 Levels and Nutrient Intake in Extremely and Very Preterm Infants during Hospitalisation

Dana F.J. Yumani, Alexandra K. Calor * and Mirjam. M. van Weissenbruch

Amsterdam UMC, Department of Pediatrics, VU University Medical Center,
1081 HV Amsterdam, The Netherlands; d.yumani@amsterdamumc.nl (D.F.J.Y.);
m.vanweissenbruch@amsterdamumc.nl (M.M.v.W.)
* Correspondence: a.k.calor@amsterdamumc.nl

Abstract: Background: Insulin-like growth factor 1 (IGF-1) plays an important role in the complex association between nutrition, growth, and maturation in extremely and very preterm infants. Nevertheless, in this population, research on associations between IGF-1 and nutrition is limited. Therefore this study aimed to evaluate the possible associations between the course of IGF-1 levels and nutrient intake between preterm birth and 36 weeks postmenstrual age (PMA). Methods: 87 infants born between 24 and 32 weeks gestational age were followed up to 36 weeks PMA. Actual daily macronutrient intake was calculated, and growth was assessed weekly. IGF-1 was sampled from umbilical cord blood at birth and every other week thereafter. Results: There was an inverse relationship between the amount of parenteral nutrition in the second week of life and IGF-1. Total protein, fat, and carbohydrate intake, as well as total energy intake, primarily showed a positive association with IGF-1 levels, particularly between 30 and 33 weeks PMA. Gestational age, bronchopulmonary dysplasia (BPD), and weight were significant confounders in the association between nutrient intake and IGF-1 levels. Conclusion: Parenteral nutrition was found to be a negative predictor of IGF-1 levels, and there could potentially be a time frame in which macronutrient intake is unable to impact IGF-1 levels. Future research should aim to narrow down this time frame and to gain more insight into factors enhancing or decreasing the response of IGF-1 to nutrition, e.g., age and inflammatory state, to align nutritional interventions accordingly.

Keywords: preterm infants; insulin-like growth factor; nutrient intake; postnatal growth

1. Introduction

Preterm birth leads to an abrupt disruption of fetal development, leaving preterm infants in a precarious situation where they need to thrive despite an immature gastrointestinal tract and not fully developed immune and endocrine functions. Insulin-like growth factor 1 (IGF-1) stimulates growth and plays a crucial role in the complex association between early nutrient intake, growth, and maturation [1]. In preterm infants, IGF-1 is mainly stimulated by insulin and nutrition [1,2]. However, to what extent various macronutrients impact IGF-1 levels in different phases of postnatal life is yet to be elucidated.

In the few studies relating actual nutrient intake to IGF-1 levels between preterm birth and hospital discharge, protein and energy intake had a positive association with IGF-1 levels [3–5]. Remarkably, one previous study reported that in preterm infants, the positive association between IGF-1 and nutrient intake was only apparent after 30 weeks postmenstrual age (PMA) [4]. This suggests that there might be a limited window of opportunity for nutrition to influence early postnatal growth.

It is to be noted that, to the best of our knowledge, only protein and energy intake have been studied in relation to IGF-1 levels in preterm infants. Interestingly, in adults, studies assessing fat and carbohydrate intake in relation to IGF-1 have been inconclusive. This leaves us with a gap in knowledge concerning the potential impact of dietary fat and carbohydrate intake on IGF-1 levels in preterm infants [6–8].

In addition, the route of nutrient administration is another largely uncharted research area in relation to IGF-1 levels in preterm infants. Animal studies have shown that in a state of inflammation or poor nutrient intake, enteral feeding results in higher IGF-1 levels than parenteral feeding. This is thought to be due to a reduction in inflammatory cytokine levels after enteral feeding [9,10]. These findings suggest that the route of nutrient administration could mediate cytokine production and consequently influence IGF-1 levels. To our knowledge, this is yet to be investigated in preterm infants.

Given the impact of poor growth and subsequent accelerated growth on later health outcomes in infants born preterm [11–13], it is pertinent to gain insight into factors influencing early postnatal growth, in order to obtain potential interventions to avert later adverse outcomes. In this light, the association between nutrition and IGF-1 is of particular interest, because nutrition is a factor which lends itself well for intervention and could lead to changes in clinical practice. Nevertheless, research on the relationship between nutrition and IGF-1 in preterm infants is scarce, and most studies were published over a decade ago. Meanwhile, nutrition and neonatal intensive care have significantly changed. In addition, in previous studies, the infants were either on full enteral feeds or the relationship with the proportion of parenteral feeding was not taken into account. In this explorative observational study, associations between the macronutrient intake, the proportion of parenteral feeding, and IGF-1 were assessed in very and extremely preterm infants between birth and 36 weeks PMA.

2. Methods

2.1. Study Population

This paper describes the results of the "Nutrition in relation to the endocrine regulation of preterm growth" (NUTRIE) study, a longitudinal observational study on nutrition in relation to the endocrine regulation of growth and body composition in preterm infants. Eighty-seven participants were enrolled between September 2015 and July 2018. Infants born between 24 and 32 weeks of gestation were eligible for study participation if they were born without substantial congenital anomalies, and were admitted to the neonatal intensive care unit (NICU) of Amsterdam UMC, location VU University Medical Center in Amsterdam, The Netherlands. Informed consent was obtained in the first week of life. The study was approved by the medical ethics committee of the VU Amsterdam and was registered at the Dutch Trial Register (www.trialregister.nl; NTR5311).

2.2. Nutrition

Infants initially received total parenteral nutrition and minimal enteral feeding. During total parental feeding, clinicians aimed to achieve an energy intake of 85–100 kcal kg^{-1} day^{-1}, a protein intake of 3–4 g kg^{-1} day^{-1}, and a fat intake of 3–3.5 g kg^{-1} day^{-1}. One the first day of life, parenteral glucose administration was targeted at 5.5–7 mg.kg^{-1} min^{-1}, going up to maximum 12 mg kg^{-1} min^{-1} after the first week of life, depending on blood glucose levels. Full enteral feeding (160 mL kg^{-1} day^{-1}) was aimed to be achieved within 7 to 10 days after birth with a total protein intake of 3.5 to 4.5 g kg^{-1} day^{-1} and a total energy intake of 110 to 140 kcal kg^{-1} day^{-1}. Infants were primarily fed human milk. If own mother's milk was insufficient or unavailable, donor human milk was administered up to 32 weeks PMA, followed by preterm starters formula until discharge home. If parents declined the use of donor human milk, infants were fed preterm starters formula from birth, whenever own mother's milk was unavailable.

Clinicians aimed to achieve 15–20 g weight gain kg^{-1} day^{-1}, with a weight SD score above −1 SD. Head circumference growth was targeted at 1 cm per week and length at 1.25 cm per week.

Breast milk fortifier (Nutrilon Nenatal Breast Milk Fortifier, Nutricia, Wageningen, The Netherlands) was added to human milk once an enteral intake of 100 mL kg^{-1} day^{-1} was achieved. In case of poor growth, as assessed by the clinician in charge, intake was increased to a maximum of 180 mL/kg, permitted that the infant's condition allowed for an increased fluid intake. If poor growth persisted, up to 1% protein fortifier (Nutrilon Nenatal Protein Fortifier, Nutricia, Wageningen, The Netherlands) was added to the fortified human milk. Lastly, up to 4% of a high-energy, long-chain triglyceride, fat emulsion (Calogen, Nutricia, Wageningen, The Netherlands) was added if growth remained restricted despite fortification. In case of growth restriction in formula-fed infants, intake was increased to 180 mL kg^{-1} day^{-1} and an additional 1.5 g of preterm starters formula was added per 100 mL formula (Nutrilon Nenatal Start, Nutricia, Wageningen, The Netherlands). In addition, protein fortifier and a fat emulsion could be added to the formula if poor growth persisted.

2.3. Study Procedures

All participants were admitted to the NICU of Amsterdam UMC, location VU University medical center within 24 h from birth. Infants in good clinical condition were discharged to step-down units in other hospitals at a PMA of 30 weeks and a weight of at least 1000 g.

Obstetric data, clinical condition and intake up to 36 weeks PMA were collected from hospital records.

2.4. Growth

Growth was assessed weekly between birth and 36 weeks PMA. Weight was measured on an electronic scale to the nearest gram, length was measured on a length board to the nearest 0.1 cm, and occipital-frontal head circumference was measured with a nonstretchable measuring tape to the nearest 0.1 cm. The measurements were done by the nursing staff.

Standard deviation scores (SDS) of weight, length and head circumferences were calculated according to Fenton [14].

2.5. Intake

Daily macronutrient intake was calculated from actual intake data obtained from hospital records. Own mother's milk composition was based on reference values [15,16] (Table 1). Donor human milk composition was based on analyses of the donor milk batches administered to the first 23 study participants.

Table 1. Reference values used for the nutritional composition of human milk per 100 mL.

Variables	OMM	OMM + BMF (4.4g/100 mL)	DHM	DHM + BMF
Energy (kcal)	68.5	83.8	60	75
Protein (g)	1.5	2.6	0.8	1.9
Protein/energy ratio (g/100 kcal)	2.2/100		1.3/100	
Carbohydrates (g)	7.3	10.0	7.5	10.2
Fat (g)	3.3	3.3	2.9	2.9

BMF: Breast milk fortifier, DHM: donor human milk, OMM: own mother's milk.

2.6. Endocrine Parameters

IGF-1 was sampled from umbilical cord blood at birth and from venipuncture or capillary puncture every other week between birth and 36 weeks PMA. A chemiluminescence immunoassay (LIAISON®, DiaSorin, Saluggia, Italy) was used to analyze IGF-1 (intra-assay percent coefficient of variation (% CV): 8%, inter-assay % CV: 7%). The number of samples per week PMA is depicted below (Table 2).

Table 2. Sample size for IGF-1 analyses per postmenstrual age.

PMA	24	25	26	27	28	29	30	31	32	33	34	35	36
N Total	2	3	7	17	21	33	30	34	25	33	25	26	29
N Postnatal	0	0	1	3	6	12	16	22	25	33	25	26	29

N Total reflects the total number of samples taken. N Postnatal reflects the number of samples excluding umbilical cord blood.

2.7. Potential Confounders

The following comorbidities were assessed as potential confounders in the association between nutrient intake and IGF-1:

- Bronchopulmonary dysplasia (BPD); defined as having had a need for supplemental oxygen for at least 28 days at 36 weeks PMA or discharge home (whichever came first) [17].
- Necrotizing enterocolitis (NEC); classified according to the Modified Bell's staging criteria [18].
- Late-onset sepsis (LOS), defined as sepsis occurring 72 h after birth with a positive blood culture or a full course of antibiotic treatment [19].
- Retinopathy of prematurity (ROP), classified according to the International Classification for Retinopathy of Prematurity [20].
- Intraventricular hemorrhage (IVH), classified according to the Papile grading system [21].
- Patent ductus arteriosus (PDA), which was defined as hemodynamically significant if treatment was prescribed [22].

In addition, gender, gestational age at birth, postmenstrual age at the time of blood sampling, weight and weight SD score were assessed as potential confounders.

2.8. Statistical Analysis

The change in IGF-1 over time was predicted for each individual using mixed models. The associations between nutrient intake, IGF-1, and potential confounders were assessed with regression analyses. Analyses were conducted using IBM® SPSS® Statistics 26 for Windows (IBM Corp., Armonk, NY, USA). Two-sided statistical significance was assumed at p-values less than 0.05.

3. Results

Eighty-seven infants were included in primary analysis (Figure 1). Baseline characteristics are shown in Table 3.

3.1. Changes in IGF-1 During Hospitalisation

Between birth and the second week of life, IGF-1 levels dropped from 4.8 nmol/L to 3.2 nmol/L in extremely preterm infants (mean decrease −1.5, 95% CI −5.2–2.2, $p = 0.314$). In very preterm infants, IGF-1 showed a mean decrease of 0.3 nmol/L (95% CI −2.1–1.4, $p = 0.675$) between birth and the second week of life. From the second week of life, IGF-1 showed a mean (SD) increase of 0.6 (0.2) nmol/L per week in very preterm infants and 0.7 (0.1) nmol/L per week in extremely preterm infants (mean difference 0.1, 95% CI 0.0–0.2, $p = 0.143$) (Figure 2).

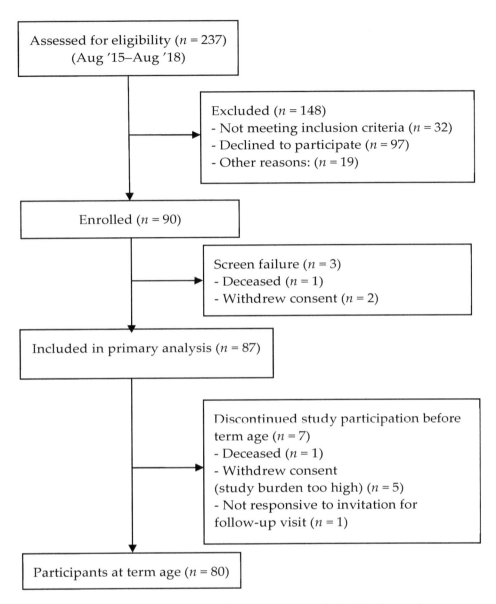

Figure 1. Flow diagram of participants included in the study.

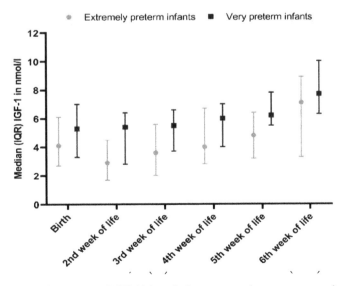

Figure 2. Insulin-like growth factor 1 (IGF-1) levels in extremely preterm and very preterm infants.

Table 3. Characteristics of the study population.

Variables	($n = 87$)
Gender, n (%)	
Male	44 (50.6)
Female	43 (49.4)
Ethnicity, n (%)	
White	66 (75.9)
Other	21 (24.1)
Gestational age (weeks), mean (SD)	29.0 (1.8)
Extremely preterm, n (%)	25 (28.7)
Very preterm, n (%)	62 (71.3)
Birthweight (g), mean (SD)	1210 (216)
Birthweight SDS, mean (SD)	0.0 (0.7)
Birthweight SDS < -1.3, n (%)	3 (3.4)
BPD, n (%)	30 (34.5)
NEC, n (%)	8 (9.2)
LOS, n (%)	30 (34.5)
PDA, n (%)	
Hemodynamically Insignificant PDA	11 (12.6)
Hemodynamically Significant PDA	8 (9.2)
ROP, n (%)	
ROP stage I	4 (4.6)
ROP stage III	1 (1.1)
IVH, n (%)	
IVH grade I	8 (9.2)
IVH grade II	11 (12.6)
IVH grade III	4 (4.6)

BPD: Bronchopulmonary dysplasia, IVH: intraventricular hemorrhage, LOS: Late-onset sepsis; NEC: Necrotizing enterocolitis; PDA: patent ductus arteriosus, ROP: retinopathy of prematurity.

Compared to boys, at birth, IGF-1 levels were lower in girls. In addition, IGF-1 levels had an inverse relationship with gestational age at birth and PMA at the time of sampling. Postnatal age in days at the time of sampling did not predict IGF-1 levels. After correcting for weight, IGF-1 levels were no longer predicted by gender, gestational age at birth, and postmenstrual age at the time of blood sampling either, and weight remained the only significant predictor of IGF-1 levels.

3.2. IGF-1 Levels in Relation to Growth

Mean birth weight SDS was 0.04, with three out of 87 infants being small for gestational age (weight SDS < -1.3) (Figure 3). At 36 weeks PMA 17 out of 80 infants had a weight SDS below -1.3 SDS. Between the second week of life and 36 weeks PMA, five out of 80 infants showed catch-up growth (increase in weight SDS > 0.67). IGF-1 positively correlated with previous, concurrent, and subsequent weight and weight SDS. When weight SDS was corrected for absolute weight in grams, only weight remained a significant predictor of IGF-1 levels. Compared to infants with a weight of 1000 g or more, infants with a weight below 1000 g had a 2.5 nmol/L lower IGF-1 at two weeks postnatal age (95% CI $-3.7--1.3$, $p < 0.001$).

3.3. IGF-1 Levels and Route of Administration

On the fourteenth day of life, 80% of infants received full enteral feeding. Figure 4 displays the ratio between parenteral and enteral intake in the first two weeks of life. At two weeks postnatal age, 73 out of 87 infants were fed more than 90% own mother's milk, 10 were fed donor human milk, and 4 were formula-fed. From the second week of life, mean nutrient intake was within the references of our local protocol (Figure 5). The percentage of parenteral intake from the eighth through to the twelfth day of life, expressed as $\frac{\text{parenteral energy intake}}{\text{total energy intake}}$, was associated with lower IGF-1 levels at two weeks postnatal age. Gestational age, weight, BPD, and hemodynamically significant PDA were confounders in the relationship between parenteral intake and IGF-1 levels. Based on the F-change, the best predictive model included weight, BPD, and hemodynamically significant PDA. After correcting for these confounders, the association between the percentage of parenteral nutrition and IGF-1 levels remained significant (Table 4).

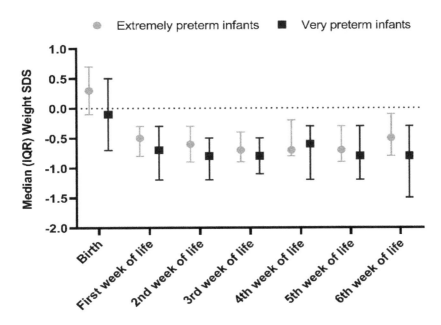

Figure 3. Weight SD score in extremely and very preterm infants.

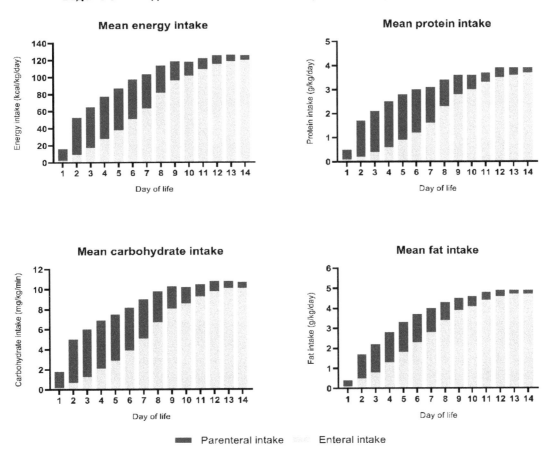

Figure 4. Parenteral and enteral nutrient intake in preterm infants in the first two weeks of life.

Table 4. Regression analyses of parenteral nutrition as a predictor of IGF-1 levels at 2 weeks postnatal age.

Variables	B (SE)	β	*p*-Value
Included variables			
Constant	1.482 (1.359)		0.281
Percentage parenteral intake on day 8	−0.027 (0.011)	−0.234	0.019
Weight on day 8 (grams)	0.004 (0.001)	0.478	<0.001
BPD	−1.134 (0.516)	−0.233	0.032
Hemodynamic significant PDA	−1.350 (0.793)	−0.159	0.095

$R^2 = 0.574$, $p < 0.001$; percentage parenteral intake: $\frac{\text{parenteral energy intake}}{\text{total energy intake}}$, BPD: bronchopulmonary dysplasia, PDA: persistent ductus arteriosus, IGF-1: insulin-like growth factor 1.

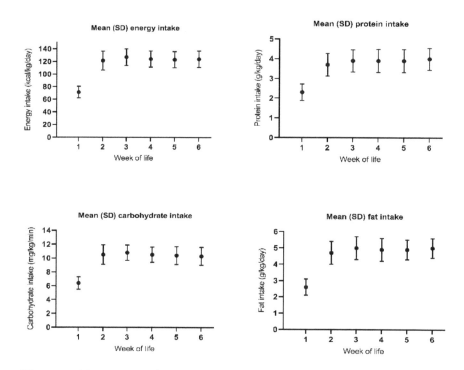

Figure 5. Nutrient intake in preterm infants in the first six weeks of life.

Day 1 is not equal to 24 h for all study subjects.

3.4. Nutrient Intake in Relation to Concurrent IGF-1 Levels

Positive associations were found between energy intake and IGF-1 levels at 30 to 33 weeks PMA (Table 5). BPD was a significant confounder from 32 weeks PMA. Protein, carbohydrate, and fat intake showed a similar pattern (Table 5). In addition, however, protein intake showed a positive association with IGF-1 levels at 28 weeks PMA: per gram increase in protein intake IGF-1 levels showed an increase of 1.1 nmol/L, $R^2 = 0.506$, $p = 0.032$. This is in contrast to a lack of associations at 29 weeks PMA with a larger sample size ($n = 12$) than the sample size at 28 weeks PMA. At 28 weeks PMA, IGF-1 was measured in six infants, of whom five had a recent history of sepsis and required an erythrocyte transfusion within 24 h of the blood sampling. Nutrient intake per kg body weight was not associated with IGF-1 levels at any point in time. After correcting for weight in multivariate analysis, the associations between total nutrient intake and IGF-1 lost their significance (Table 5). In univariate analysis at 30 weeks PMA, weight explained 45% of the variance in IGF-1 levels, compared to 33% of the variance that was explained by nutrient intake. By 33 weeks PMA, these numbers declined to respectively 17% and 15%.

Table 5. Regression analyses of intake as a predictor of IGF-1 levels at 30 weeks postmenstrual age.

Variables	Model R^2	Model p-Value	B (SE)	β	p-Value
Energy intake model 1:	0.605	0.006			
Constant			11.8 (6.7)		0.106
Energy intake (kcal/day)			0.05 (0.02)	0.6	0.015
Gestational age (weeks)			−0.6 (0.2)	−0.5	0.029
Energy intake model 2:	0.640	0.014			
Constant			9.4 (7.1)		0.215
Energy intake (kcal/day)			0.03 (0.03)	0.3	0.395
Gestational age (weeks)			−0.5 (0.2)	−0.4	0.073
Weight (grams)			0.003 (0.003)	0.36	0.348
Protein intake model 1:	0.578	0.009			
Constant			14.5 (6.7)		0.053
Protein intake (g/day)			1.2 (0.4)	0.6	0.013
Gestational age (weeks)			−0.6 (0.2)	−0.5	0.025
Protein intake model 2:	0.625	0.017			
Constant			10.2 (7.6)		0.209
Protein intake (g/day)			0.5 (0.8)	0.2	0.561
Gestational age (weeks)			−0.5 (0.2)	−0.4	0.089
Weight (grams)			0.004 (0.003)	0.4	0.289
Carbohydrate intake model 1:	0.593	0.014			
Constant			9.1 (7.8)		0.268
Carbohydrate intake (g/day)			0.3 (0.1)	0.6	0.022
Gestational age (weeks)			−0.4 (0.3)	−0.4	0.111
Carbohydrate intake model 2:	0.690	0.007			
Constant			5.5 (6.9)		0.444
Carbohydrate intake (g/day)			0.2 (0.1)	0.3	0.144
Gestational age (weeks)			−0.4 (0.2)	−0.3	0.113
Weight (grams)			0.004 (0.002)	0.5	0.052
Fat intake model 1:	0.581	0.008			
Constant			12.3 (6.9)		0.102
Fat intake (g/day)			1.1 (0.4)	0.6	0.012
Gestational age (weeks)			−0.6 (0.2)	−0.5	0.034
Fat intake model 2:	0.631	0.015			
Constant			9.4 (7.2)		0.225
Fat intake (g/day)			0.5 (0.7)	0.3	0.494
Gestational age (weeks)			−0.5 (0.3)	−0.4	0.083
Weight (grams)			0.003 (0.003)	0.4	0.273

IGF-1: Insulin-like growth factor 1.

3.5. Nutrition in Relation to Changes in IGF-1 According to Postnatal Age

The change in IGF-1 levels in the first four weeks of life was positively associated with protein, carbohydrate, fat, and total energy intake (after correction for gestational age). IGF-1 levels increased with 0.01 nmol/L per 10 kcal, $R^2 = 0.266$, $p < 0.001$. Comorbidities were not a significant confounder. After correcting for weight, total nutrient intake was no longer a significant predictor of change in IGF-1.

3.6. Nutrition in Relation to Changes in IGF-1 According to Postmenstrual Age

Looking at postmenstrual age, there was a positive association between total nutrient intake from 28 through 31 weeks PMA and the change in IGF-1 between birth and 32 weeks PMA (after correcting for gestational age). IGF-1 levels increased with 0.2 nmol/L per 10 kcal, $R^2 = 0.287$, $p = 0.002$. Comorbidities were not a significant confounder. However, after correcting for weight, energy intake could no longer predict the change in IGF-1. All macronutrients showed a similar pattern.

4. Discussion

This study shows that the proportion of parenteral nutrition is negatively associated with IGF-1 levels in extremely and very preterm infants. Gestational age, BPD, and weight were significant confounders in the association between nutrient intake and IGF-1 levels. Total protein, fat, and carbohydrate intake, as well as total energy intake, showed a positive association with IGF-1 levels, particularly between 30 and 33 weeks PMA.

4.1. The Effect of the Various Macronutrients on IGF-1 Levels

Studies in preterm infants consistently show that protein intake is positively associated with IGF-1 levels [3–5]. However, not all studies could show that energy intake was a predictor of IGF-1 after correction for confounders [3]. In our study, higher total protein intake and higher total energy intake were associated with higher IGF-1 levels. In contrast to previous studies, our study did not find an association between nutrient intake per kg bodyweight and IGF-1 levels. Weight explained more of the variance in IGF-1 than nutrient intake. However, it should be noted that the variance in nutrient intake per kg bodyweight may have been too small to show significant differences in IGF-1 levels in our population. This is due to the univocal application of our local nutrition protocol. For example, from 33 weeks PMA the interquartile range in protein intake was between 3.7 and 4.1 g kg^{-1} day^{-1}. This range was notably smaller compared to previous research [4] and could have limited the statistical power.

To our knowledge, the impact of fat and carbohydrate intake on IGF-1 levels in preterm infants has not been studied previously. Meanwhile, studies in adults have been inconclusive, with some finding positive associations [7], while others found negative associations [6] or no association at all [8]. In our study, total fat and total carbohydrate intake showed a positive association with IGF-1 levels. Interestingly, both carbohydrate and fat intake had a comparable impact on IGF-1 when compared to protein intake—a one SD change in any of the macronutrients led to a change of 0.6 SD in IGF-1 levels at 30 weeks PMA. Although it has been suggested that the role of proteins is more important than that of carbohydrates and fat in stimulating IGF-1 [3,6], like dietary proteins, dietary fat and carbohydrates have been found to increase hepatic IGF-1 expression in animal studies [23]. Moreover, fat and carbohydrates provide the majority of the total energy intake, which has repeatedly been shown to have a positive association with IGF-1 levels and thus supports our findings.

4.2. The Route of Nutrient Administration

Parenteral feeding was found to be negatively associated with IGF-1 levels. It could be hypothesized that less exposure of the gastrointestinal tract to nutrition enhances a pro-inflammatory state in the immature gut, which in turn could lead to lower IGF-1 levels. Indeed, a pro-inflammatory state in preterm infants has been associated with decreased IGF-1 levels [24]. It has also been demonstrated that colostrum and maternal milk contain high concentrations of anti-inflammatory cytokines [25]. These anti-inflammatory cytokines could potentially lower the relatively pro-inflammatory state in the immature gut and consequentially increase IGF-1 levels. In one study, preterm infants who received own mother's milk from birth were shown to have higher levels of IGF-1 at term equivalent age compared to those who were formula fed from birth [26]. Moreover, animal studies found that in a state of inflammation or nutrient deprivation, parenteral feeding was associated with lower IGF-1 levels compared to enteral feeding. This appears to be due to a decrease in pro-inflammatory cytokines after enteral feeding [9,10]. This leads us to believe that the neutralizing effect of anti-inflammatory cytokines, which are particularly abundant in colostrum and breast milk, is diminished and results in lower IGF-1 levels when parenteral nutrition is increased.

It could also be suggested that infants who received relatively higher proportions of parenteral nutrition were the more vulnerable, smaller, younger, and iller infants, and thus the association with lower IGF-1 levels. However, after correcting for gestational age, weight, and comorbidities, parenteral nutrition remained a significant predictor of IGF-1 levels.

4.3. Window of Effect of Nutrient Intake on IGF-1 Levels

In our population, the influence of nutrition on IGF-1 levels seemed to be most apparent between 30 and 33 weeks PMA. Hypothesizing, preterm infants may have to reach a certain level of maturity before an impact of nutrition on the IGF-1 axis can be noted. In support of this, Smith and colleagues found that the magnitude of the rise in IGF-1 levels per gram protein increased with increasing gestational and postnatal age. Hansen-Pupp and colleagues also found nutrient intake not to influence IGF-1 levels at lower postmenstrual ages, but only from 32 weeks PMA onwards. Speculatively, other factors than maturity could influence when IGF-1 levels start to respond to nutrient intake. Of note, in our study, in a set of infants who were ill, a positive association between total protein intake and IGF-1 levels was already found at 28 weeks PMA. This was in contrast to the other macronutrients and total energy intake, which only showed positive associations with IGF-1 levels from 30 weeks PMA onwards. Among the set of infants of whom blood was sampled at 28 weeks, all but one had a recent history of sepsis and anemia requiring erythrocyte transfusion. It could be speculated that the state of inflammation triggered a higher sensibility of the IGF-1 axis to protein uptake. Despite their IGF-1 levels still being low, 1 g of protein might have triggered more increase in IGF-1 compared to infants who were not ill.

It is noteworthy that in our population, no associations between nutrient intake and IGF-1 levels were found at 34 and 35 weeks PMA, in contrast to other studies [3–5]. However, Ëngstrom and colleagues found that in infants with a weight of less than 2000 g, protein supplementation had a stronger association with IGF-1 levels compared to infants over 2000 g. Perhaps this can explain why the positive trend our study found at 34 and 35 weeks PMA was not statistically significant.

In contrast to the relationship between nutrient intake and concurrent IGF-1 levels described above, our results showed nutrient intake to influence the change in IGF-1 at a younger PMA. For every macronutrient, intake from 28 weeks PMA was associated with the change in IGF-1 levels between birth and 32 weeks PMA. Hypothesizing, total macronutrient intake before 30 weeks may not reach the threshold to increase concurrent IGF-1 levels, but it might stimulate the IGF-1 axis to mature more rapidly and in this way cause a more rapid increase in IGF-1 levels over time.

4.4. Strengths and Limitations

This is the first study to evaluate the contribution of all macronutrients in relation to circulatory IGF-1 levels in preterm infants from birth until 36 weeks of gestation. In addition, to the best of our knowledge, the proportion of parenteral nutrition has not been investigated previously in relation to IGF-1 levels. In line with previous research, our results demonstrate a slow increase in IGF-1 levels in the first weeks of life [4]. However, our results failed to support previous findings on nutrient intake per kg body weight. As previously mentioned, our population had little variation in nutrient intake per kg body weight. This could potentially explain the lack of statistically significant findings. In addition, despite the considerable overall sample size, this study had a relatively small sample size per week. This was due to the low sample frequency (on alternating weeks) and the relatively small number of extremely preterm infants, which resulted in a sample size ranging from 1 infant at 26 weeks PMA to 33 infants at 33 weeks PMA. This may have contributed to our findings. Moreover, it is important to note that this was an exploratory observational study. Therefore, the findings should be interpreted with caution and strong conclusions on potential causative relationships cannot be made.

5. Conclusions

Our findings further illustrate the complex association of maturation, concurrent comorbidities, and nutrition in relation to IGF-1 levels. The proportion of parenteral nutrition was found to be a negative predictor of IGF-1 levels, affirming the importance of stimulating enteral nutrition and limiting parenteral nutrition as much as possible in clinical practice. Our findings point towards a potential time frame in which nutrition is unable to impact IGF-1 levels. Future research should aim to narrow down this time frame and to gain more insight into factors enhancing or decreasing the response of IGF-1 to nutrition, e.g., age and inflammatory state, to align nutritional interventions accordingly.

Author Contributions: D.F.J.Y.: Conception and design, acquisition of data, analysis and interpretation of data, drafting article, and final approval of the version to be published. A.K.C.: Conception and design, acquisition of data, analysis and interpretation of data, drafting article, and final approval of the version to be published. M.M.v.W.: Conception and design, interpretation of data, revision of article, and final approval of the version to be published. All authors have read and agree to the published version of the manuscript.

Acknowledgments: The authors would like to express their gratitude to all the infants and their families who participated in this study. We thank Femke Maingay, Sophie van der Schoor, and Dianne Maingay for their contribution to the data collection.

Abbreviations

IGF-1: insulin-like growth factor 1, PMA: postmenstrual age, NICU: neonatal intensive care unit, SDS: standard deviation score, BPD: bronchopulmonary dysplasia, NEC: necrotizing enterocolitis, LOS: late onset sepsis, IVH: intraventricular hemorrhage, ROP: retinopathy of prematurity, PDA: patent ductus arteriosus

References

1. Larnkjaer, A.; Molgaard, C.; Michaelsen, K.F. Early nutrition impact on the insulin-like growth factor axis and later health consequences. *Curr. Opin. Clin. Nutr. Metab. Care* **2012**, *15*, 285–292. [CrossRef]

2. Yumani, D.F.; Lafeber, H.N.; van Weissenbruch, M.M. Dietary proteins and IGF I levels in preterm infants: Determinants of growth, body composition, and neurodevelopment. *Pediatric Res.* **2015**, *77*, 156–163. [CrossRef]

3. Engstrom, E.; Niklasson, A.; Wikland, K.A.; Ewald, U.; Hellstrom, A. The role of maternal factors, postnatal nutrition, weight gain, and gender in regulation of serum IGF-I among preterm infants. *Pediatric Res.* **2005**, *57*, 605–610. [CrossRef]

4. Hansen-Pupp, I.; Löfqvist, C.; Polberger, S.; Niklasson, A.; Fellman, V.; Hellström, A.; Ley, D. Influence of insulin-like growth factor I and nutrition during phases of postnatal growth in very preterm infants. *Pediatric Res.* **2011**, *69*, 448–453. [CrossRef] [PubMed]

5. Smith, W.J.; Underwood, L.E.; Keyes, L.; Clemmons, D.R. Use of insulin-like growth factor I (IGF-I) and IGF-binding protein measurements to monitor feeding of premature infants. *J. Clin. Endocrinol. Metab.* **1997**, *82*, 3982–3988. [CrossRef] [PubMed]

6. Giovannucci, E.; Pollak, M.; Liu, Y.; Platz, E.A.; Majeed, N.; Rimm, E.B.; Willett, W.C. Nutritional predictors of insulin-like growth factor I and their relationships to cancer in men. *Cancer Epidemiol. Biomark. Prev.* **2003**, *12*, 84–89.

7. Kaklamani, V.G.; Linos, A.; Kaklamani, E.; Markaki, I.; Koumantaki, Y.; Mantzoros, C.S. Dietary fat and carbohydrates are independently associated with circulating insulin-like growth factor 1 and insulin-like growth factor-binding protein 3 concentrations in healthy adults. *J. Clin. Oncol.* **1999**, *17*, 3291–3298. [CrossRef] [PubMed]

8. Norat, T.; Dossus, L.; Rinaldi, S.; Overvad, K.; Grønbæk, H.; Tjønneland, A.; Olsen, A.; Clavel-Chapelon, F.; Boutron-Ruault, M.C.; Boeing, H.; et al. Diet, serum insulin-like growth factor-I and IGF-binding protein-3 in European women. *Eur. J. Clin. Nutr.* **2007**, *61*, 91–98. [CrossRef] [PubMed]

9. O'Leary, M.J.; Xue, A.; Scarlett, C.J.; Sevette, A.; Kee, A.J.; Smith, R.C. Parenteral versus enteral nutrition: Effect on serum cytokines and the hepatic expression of mRNA of suppressor of cytokine signaling proteins, insulin-like growth factor-1 and the growth hormone receptor in rodent sepsis. *Crit. Care (Lond. Engl.)* **2007**, *11*, R79. [CrossRef]

10. Wojnar, M.M.; Fan, J.; Li, Y.H.; Lang, C.H. Endotoxin-induced changes in IGF-I differ in rats provided enteral vs. parenteral nutrition. *Am. J. Physiol.* **1999**, *276*, E455–E464. [CrossRef]

11. Cormack, B.E.; Harding, J.E.; Miller, S.P.; Bloomfield, F.H. The Influence of Early Nutrition on Brain Growth and Neurodevelopment in Extremely Preterm Babies: A Narrative Review. *Nutrients* **2019**, *11*, 2029. [CrossRef] [PubMed]

12. Embleton, N.D.; Korada, M.; Wood, C.L.; Pearce, M.S.; Swamy, R.; Cheetham, T.D. Catch-up growth and metabolic outcomes in adolescents born preterm. *Arch. Dis. Child.* **2016**, *101*, 1026–1031. [CrossRef] [PubMed]

13. Lapillonne, A.; Griffin, I.J. Feeding preterm infants today for later metabolic and cardiovascular outcomes. *J. Pediatr.* **2013**, *162*, S7–S16. [CrossRef] [PubMed]

14. Fenton, T.R.; Kim, J.H. A systematic review and meta-analysis to revise the Fenton growth chart for preterm infants. *BMC Pediatr.* **2013**, *13*, 59. [CrossRef]

15. Boyce, C.; Watson, M.; Lazidis, G.; Reeve, S.; Dods, K.; Simmer, K.; McLeod, G. Preterm human milk composition: A systematic literature review. *Br. J. Nutr.* **2016**, *116*, 1033–1045. [CrossRef]

16. Gidrewicz, D.A.; Fenton, T.R. A systematic review and meta-analysis of the nutrient content of preterm and term breast milk. *BMC Pediatr.* **2014**, *14*, 216. [CrossRef]

17. Jobe, A.H.; Bancalari, E. Bronchopulmonary dysplasia. *Am. J. Respir. Crit. Care Med.* **2001**, *163*, 1723–1729. [CrossRef]

18. Kliegman, R.M.; Walsh, M.C. Neonatal necrotizing enterocolitis: Pathogenesis, classification, and spectrum of illness. *Curr. Probl. Pediatr.* **1987**, *17*, 213–288. [CrossRef]

19. Bekhof, J.; Reitsma, J.B.; Kok, J.H.; Van Straaten, I.H. Clinical signs to identify late-onset sepsis in preterm infants. *Eur. J. Pediatr.* **2013**, *172*, 501–508. [CrossRef]

20. International Committee for the Classification of Retinopathy of P. The International Classification of Retinopathy of Prematurity revisited. *Arch. Ophthalmol.* **2005**, *123*, 991–999. [CrossRef]

21. Papile, L.A.; Burstein, J.; Burstein, R.; Koffler, H. Incidence and evolution of subependymal and intraventricular hemorrhage: A study of infants with birth weights less than 1500 gm. *J Pediatr.* **1978**, *92*, 529–534. [CrossRef]

22. Jain, A.; Shah, P.S. Diagnosis, Evaluation, and Management of Patent Ductus Arteriosus in Preterm Neonates. *JAMA Pediatr.* **2015**, *169*, 863–872. [CrossRef] [PubMed]

23. Bertucci, J.I.; Blanco, A.M.; Canosa, L.F.; Unniappan, S. Direct actions of macronutrient components on goldfish hepatopancreas in vitro to modulate the expression of ghr-I, ghr-II, igf-I and igf-II mRNAs. *Gen. Comp. Endocrinol.* **2017**, *250*, 1–8. [CrossRef] [PubMed]

24. Hansen-Pupp, I.; Hellstrom-Westas, L.; Cilio, C.M.; Andersson, S.; Fellman, V.; Ley, D. Inflammation at birth and the insulin-like growth factor system in very preterm infants. *Acta Paediatr.* **2007**, *96*, 830–836. [CrossRef]

25. MohanKumar, K.; Namachivayam, K.; Ho, T.T.; Torres, B.A.; Ohls, R.K.; Maheshwari, A. Cytokines and growth factors in the developing intestine and during necrotizing enterocolitis. *Semin. Perinatol.* **2017**, *41*, 52–60. [CrossRef]

26. Alzaree, F.A.; AbuShady, M.M.; Atti, M.A.; Fathy, G.A.; Galal, E.M.; Ali, A.; Elias, T.R. Effect of Early Breast Milk Nutrition on Serum Insulin-Like Growth Factor-1 in Preterm Infants. *Open Access Maced. J. Med Sci.* **2019**, *7*, 77–81. [CrossRef]

2

Lactobacillus Acidophilus/Bifidobacterium Infantis Probiotics are Beneficial to Extremely Low Gestational Age Infants Fed Human Milk

Ingmar Fortmann [1,*](iD), Janina Marißen [1], Bastian Siller [1], Juliane Spiegler [1](iD),
Alexander Humberg [1], Kathrin Hanke [1], Kirstin Faust [1], Julia Pagel [1,2], Leila Eyvazzadeh [1],
Kim Brenner [1], Claudia Roll [3], Sabine Pirr [4], Dorothee Viemann [4], Dimitra Stavropoulou [5],
Philipp Henneke [5,6], Birte Tröger [7], Thorsten Körner [7], Anja Stein [8], Christoph Derouet [9],
Michael Zemlin [9](iD), Christian Wieg [10], Jan Rupp [2,11], Egbert Herting [1], Wolfgang Göpel [1] and
Christoph Härtel [1,2]

[1] Department of Pediatrics, University of Lübeck, 23562 Lübeck, Germany; janina.marissen@uksh.de (J.M.);
    bastian.siller@uksh.de (B.S.); uni@dr-spiegler.de (J.S.); alexander.humberg@uksh.de (A.H.);
    kathrin.hanke@uksh.de (K.H.); kirstin.faust@uksh.de (K.F.); julia.pagel@uksh.de (J.P.);
    leila.eyvazzadeh@gmail.com (L.E.); kim.brenner@uksh.de (K.B.); Egbert.Herting@uksh.de (E.H.);
    wolfgang.goepel@uksh.de (W.G.); christoph.haertel@uksh.de (C.H.)
[2] German Center for Infection Research (DZIF), Partner Site Hamburg-Lübeck-Borstel-Riems,
    38124 Braunschweig, Germany; jan.rupp@uksh.de
[3] Department of Pediatrics, Vestische Children's Hospital Datteln, 45711 Datteln, Germany;
    c.roll@kinderklinik-datteln.de
[4] Department of Neonatology, Hannover Medical School, 30159 Hannover, Germany;
    pirr.sabine@mh-hannover.de (S.P.); viemann.dorothee@mh-hannover.de (D.V.)
[5] Center for Pediatrics and Adolescent Medicine, Medical Center and Medical Faculty, University of Freiburg,
    79098 Freiburg, Germany; dimitra.stavropoulou@uniklinik-freiburg.de (D.S.);
    philipp.henneke@uniklinikum-freiburg.de (P.H.)
[6] Institute for Immunodeficiency, Medical Center and Medical Faculty, University of Freiburg,
    79098 Freiburg, Germany
[7] Children's Hospital Links der Weser Bremen, 28277 Bremen, Germany;
    birte.troeger@gesundheitnord.de (B.T.); thorsten.koerner@klinikum-bremen-ldw.de (T.K.)
[8] Department of Neonatology and General Pediatrics, University of Essen, 45147 Essen, Germany;
    anja.stein@uk-essen.de
[9] Department of Neonatology and General Pediatrics, Saar University of Homburg, 66424 Homburg,
    Germany; christoph.derouet@uks.eu (C.D.); michael.zemlin@uks.eu (M.Z.)
[10] Children's Hospital Aschaffenburg-Alzenau, 63739 Aschaffenburg, Germany;
    christian.wieg@klinikum-ab-alz.de
[11] Department of Infectious Diseases and Medical Microbiology, University of Lübeck, 23562 Lübeck, Germany
*   Correspondence: Matsingmar.Fortmann@uksh.de

Abstract: Objective: To evaluate the nutrition-related effects of prophylactic *Lactobacillus acidophilus/ Bifidobacterium infantis* probiotics on the outcomes of preterm infants <29 weeks of gestation that receive human milk and/or formula nutrition. We hypothesize that human-milk-fed infants benefit from probiotics in terms of sepsis prevention and growth. Methods: We performed an observational study of the German Neonatal Network (GNN) over a period of six years, between 1 January, 2013 and 31 December, 2018. Prophylactic probiotic use of *L. acidophilus/B. infantis* was evaluated in preterm infants <29 weeks of gestation ($n = 7516$) in subgroups stratified to feeding type: (I) Exclusively human milk (HM) of own mother and/or donors (HM group, $n = 1568$), (II) HM of own mother and/or donor and formula (Mix group, $n = 5221$), and (III) exclusive exposure to formula (F group, $n = 727$). The effect of probiotics on general outcomes and growth was tested in univariate models and adjusted in linear/logistic regression models. Results: 5954 (76.5%) infants received *L. acidophilus/B. infantis* prophylactically for the prevention of necrotizing enterocolitis (NEC). Probiotic use was associated with improved growth measures in the HM group (e.g., weight gain velocity in g/day: effect size B = 0.224; 95% CI: 2.82–4.35; $p < 0.001$) but not in the F group (effect size B = −0.06; 95% CI: −3.05–0.28; $p = 0.103$). The HM group had the lowest incidence of clinical sepsis (34.0%) as compared to the Mix group (35.5%) and the F group (40.0%). Only in the Mix group, probiotic supplementation proved to be protective against clinical sepsis (OR 0.69; 95% CI: 0.59–0.79; $p < 0.001$). Conclusion: Our observational data indicate that the exposure to *L. acidophilus/B. infantis* probiotics may promote growth in exclusively HM-fed infants as compared to formula-fed infants. To exert a sepsis-preventive effect, probiotics seem to require human milk.

Keywords: probiotic prophylaxis; human milk; prematurity; sepsis; growth failure

1. Introduction

Probiotics that act as gut colonizers of human-milk-fed infants [1] have a high potential to foster the early microbiome development [2]. Thus, they might prevent dysbiosis-associated complications such as necrotizing enterocolitis (NEC) and sepsis [3,4]. Numerous studies on the therapeutic effects of probiotics in preterm infants have been performed [4]. However, the results remain inconclusive due to a high variability in study protocols, target populations and endpoints, probiotic formulations (e.g., strain composition and inclusion of single vs. multiple strains), and the context of nutrition [5]. After the publication of several meta-analyses proposing a benefit for preterm infants' short-term outcomes, prophylaxis with *Bifidobacterium longum* and *Bifidobacterium infantis/Lactobacillus acidophilus* has been adopted into clinical routine by many European neonatal intensive care units (NICUs), for example in Austria [6], the Netherlands [7], and Germany [8]. In hospitals of the German Neonatal Network (GNN), the implementation of probiotic use in 2009/2010 led to a decrease in NEC incidence in infants discharged in 2011 and 2012 after the change of strategy [8]. Despite the use of probiotics in >80% of extremely low-birth-weight infants (ELBWI), however, NEC and sepsis still remain significant causes of morbidity and mortality in this vulnerable population [9]. To promote a more personalized medical approach to preterm babies, there is an urgent need to define those populations who would benefit most from probiotic prophylaxis. Recent data suggest that the type of enteral feeding (breastmilk or bovine-based formula) modifies the effects of probiotics in preterm infants [6,7]. In line with this, the nutritional content of human milk oligosaccharides (HMOs)—a major metabolic source for bifidobacteria—was found to be predictive for the NEC risk [10]. Human milk contains numerous immune-related compounds such as leukocytes, lysozymes, nucleotides, and cytokines [11], whereas HMOs were found to directly mediate the prebiotic effect of bifidobacterial growth [12].

Herein we hypothesize that human milk as a nutritional source is required for probiotics to provide a sepsis-preventive and growth-promoting effect. Accordingly, we performed an observational study in a large GNN cohort of extremely preterm infants <29 weeks of gestation discharged after the year 2012 and evaluated the impact of probiotics in the context of feeding strategies.

2. Methods

2.1. The German Neonatal Network

The German Neonatal Network (GNN; www.vlbw.de) is a population-based observational multicenter cohort study enrolling Very low birth weight infants (VLBWI) at 64 neonatal intensive care units (NICUs) in Germany. Within the study period, data were collected from infants discharged between 1 January, 2013 and 31 December, 2018. Preterm infants of a birth weight <1500 g and/or a gestational age between 22 + 0 and 28 + 6 weeks, who were actively managed with intensive care, met the inclusion criteria. Infants with lethal malformations or those treated with comfort (palliative) care were excluded from the study. In the analysis of this study, only cases with complete documentation for feeding type were included.

After obtaining written informed parental consent, predefined data on general neonatal characteristics and antenatal and postnatal treatment and outcome were recorded for each patient on clinical record files at the participating centers. After discharge, data sheets were sent to the study center (University of Lübeck). Data quality was evaluated by a physician trained in neonatology via annual on-site monitoring of completed record files. After monitoring, data were coded and evaluated.

2.2. Prophylactic Probiotic Supplementation

The probiotic formulation consisting of *B. infantis.* and *L. acidophilus* corresponds to the formulation that has been most commonly used among the participating study sites in the past [8]. Probiotics were provided once or twice daily in capsules beginning from day 1 to 3 of life until day 28 of life. The recommended daily dose contained $1–3 \times 10^9$ CFU (Colony forming units) *L. acidophilus* and $1–1.5 \times 10^9$ *B. infantis*.

2.3. Subgroups Stratified to Type of Milk Feeding

The preparation (pasteurization, freezing, storage) of human milk (own mother's and donor's milk) before use was carried out according to local standards (e.g., cytomegalovirus sero-prevalence of mother) at the study site. In all centers providing donor milk, the samples were pasteurized before use for feeding. Three "human milk feeding" strata were applied:

I HM (HM group): Infants who were exclusively fed with own mother's and/or donor's milk.

II Mix (Mix group): Infants who were fed with HM and formula at any time during the primary stay in hospital.

III Formula (F group): Infants who were exclusively fed with formula.

2.4. Definitions

Gestational age was calculated from the "best obstetric estimate". This is defined as the estimate of the infant's gestation based on the birth attendant's final estimate by using early prenatal ultrasound and obstetric examination [13].

Small-for-gestational age (SGA) was defined as a birth weight less than the 10th percentile for gestational age according to gender-specific standards for birth weight by gestational age in Germany [14].

Full enteral feeding was defined as enteral nutrition at a minimum of 150 mL/kg body weight per day.

Weight gain velocity was defined as gain in body weight, calculated as g/day (difference of the parameter at birth and at discharge/number of days in hospital). Growth velocity of body length was defined as gain in body length, calculated as mm/day (difference of the parameter at birth and at discharge/number of days in hospital). Head growth velocity was defined as gain in head circumference, calculated as mm/day (difference of the parameter at birth and at discharge/number of days in hospital). Z-scores are numerical measurements of the value's relationship to the mean of the group values measured in terms of standard deviations from the mean (between −3.0 and 3.0). Z-scores were calculated for birth weight according to the 2003 Fenton preterm growth chart [15,16].

Clinical sepsis was defined as condition with at least two signs of systemic inflammatory response (temperature >38 °C or <36.5 °C, tachycardia >200/min, new onset or increased frequency of bradycardias or apneas, hyperglycemia >140 mg/dL, base excess <−10 mval/L, changed skin color, increased oxygen requirements), one laboratory sign (e.g., C-reactive protein >20 mg/L, immature/total neutrophil ratio >0.2, white blood cell count <5/nL), and the neonatologist's decision to treat with anti-infective drugs for at least 5 days but no proof of causative agent in blood culture [17]. Blood culture confirmed sepsis was defined as clinical sepsis with proof of causative agent in the blood culture.

If coagulase-negative *Staphylococcus* (CoNS) was isolated as a single pathogen in one peripheral blood culture, two clinical signs and one laboratory sign were required for classification of CoNS sepsis [17].

Bronchopulmonary dysplasia (BPD) was diagnosed when needing supplemental oxygen or ventilatory support at 36 weeks of postmenstrual age. Necrotizing enterocolitis (NEC) was defined as necrotizing intestinal inflammation requiring surgery, and focal intestinal perforation (FIP) was FIP requiring surgical treatment classified by the attending surgeon. Retinopathy of prematurity (ROP) was defined as typical retinal changes (ophthalmoscopy) requiring interventions such as laser therapy, cryotherapy, or intraocular vascular endothelial growth factor inhibitors.

2.5. Statistical Analyses

Data analyses were performed using the SPSS 24.0 data analysis package (Munich, Germany). Hypotheses in the univariate analysis were evaluated with Fisher's exact test and Mann–Whitney U test. Only two-sided tests were used. A *p*-value of <0.05 was considered as statistically significant for single tests.

Subsequent to univariate analyses, we included parameters with a *p*-value < 0.1 in multivariate logistic regression models and known confounders as independent variables: gestational age per week, gender, multiples, and SGA status. Odd ratios and 95% confidence intervals were calculated in order to identify the influence of probiotic prophylaxis on outcomes independent of the abovementioned confounders. The following outcome parameters were tested in multivariate models: necrotizing enterocolitis, retinopathy of prematurity requiring intervention, bronchopulmonary dysplasia, clinical sepsis, and blood culture confirmed sepsis. To address the problem of multiple comparisons, we performed Bonferroni corrections for multivariate analyses in order to protect from statistical Type I errors. Additional information derived from Bonferroni correction is indicated in Tables 1 and 2 accordingly. In addition, we tested nested models for our analyses by calculating the Akaike information criterion (AIC) for all multivariate calculations in order to estimate relative quality for each model.

Table 1. Effect of probiotic treatment on short-term outcomes in the context of feeding types.

	I HM	II Mix	III Formula
Surgery for NEC	OR 1.37 (95% CI: 0.69–2.73) $p = 0.38$	OR 0.84 (95% CI: 0.59–1.15) $p = 0.26$	OR 0.89 (95% CI: 0.5–2.0) $p = 0.9$
Clinical sepsis	OR 0.95 (95% CI: 0.73–1.22) $p = 0.67$	OR 0.69 (95% CI: 0.59–0.79) $p < 0.001$ *	OR 1.20 (95% CI: 0.9–1.7) $p = 0.243$
Sepsis (BC positive)	OR 1.09 (95% CI: 0.78–1.53) $p = 0.60$	OR 0.89 (95% CI: 0.74–1.06) $p = 0.19$	1.10 (95% CI: 0.7–1.8) $p = 0.662$
ROP	OR 1.51 (95% CI: 0.73–3.10) $p = 0.27$	OR 1.04 (95% CI: 0.72–1.51) $p = 0.83$	OR 1.35 (95% CI: 0.63–2.94) $p = 0.44$
BPD	OR 0.86 (95% CI: 0.65–1.14) $p = 0.31$	OR 0.90 (95% CI: 0.77–1.05) $p = 0.19$	1.31 (95% CI: 0.87–1.96) $p= 0.19$

HM, human milk, NEC, necrotizing enterocolitis, ROP, retinopathy of prematurity, BPD, bronchopulmonary dysplasia; NEC, necrotizing enterocolitis. Logistic regression analyses were performed by using the following independent variables: gestational age, multiple birth, gender, SGA, and treatment with probiotics. * Bonferroni correction did not change significance of the *p*-value.

Table 2. Effect of probiotics on growth parameters of the GNN cohort during their primary stay in hospital.

	I HM	II Mix	III Formula
Body weight at discharge (z-score, Fenton)	B = 0.261 95% CI: 0.48–0.71 p <0.001 *	B = 0.026 95% CI: 0.01–0.1 p = 0.029 #	B = 0.015 95% CI: −0.12–0.18 p = 0.72
Weight gain (z-score, Fenton)	B = 0.23 95% CI: 0.42–0.62 p < 0.001 *	B= 0.022 95% CI: −0.01–0.1 p = 0.078	B= 0.06 95% CI: −0.04–0.26 p = 0.14
Growth velocity (g/day)	B = 0.224 95% CI: 2.82–4.35 p < 0.001 *	B = 0.00 95% CI: −0.61–0.62 p = 0.98	B = −0.06 95% CI: −2.90–−0.45 p = 0.15
Growth velocity of body length (mm/day)	B = 0.179 95% CI: 0.13–0.24 p < 0.001 *	B = 0.019 95% CI: −0.01–0.04 p = 0.184	B = −0.012 95% CI: −0.11–0.08 p = 0.761
Head growth velocity (mm/day)	B = 0.117 95% CI: 0.05–0.12 p < 0.001*	B = 0.03 95% CI: 0.003–0.04 p = 0.023 #	B = -0.002 95% CI: −0.08–0.07 p = 0.966

HM, human milk. Growth velocity, weight gain, and growth of body length and head circumference were calculated by differences between parameters at birth and respective measures at discharge/number of days (duration of stay). Linear regression analyses were performed by using the following independent variables: gestational age, birth weight, multiple birth, gender, maternal descent, and exposure to probiotic prophylaxis within the three subgroups. * Bonferroni correction did not change significance of the p-value. # Not significant after Bonferroni correction.

In order to evaluate the influence of probiotic prophylaxis on growth parameters, we conducted linear regression models using known/probable confounders as independent variables: gestational age per week, birth weight, gender, multiple birth, and maternal descent. Effect size and 95% confidence intervals (CI) were calculated. The following outcome parameters were tested in linear models: Z-score-based body weight at discharge according the 2003 Fenton growth chart for preterm infants, z-score-based weight gain, growth velocity of body weight (g/day), body length (mm/day) and head circumference (mm/day). A p-value of <0.05 was considered statistically significant. For primary and subgroup analyses, we used a uniform dataset with available data for all metric parameters. Infants with incomplete data for variables that were used in our analyses were not included.

Graphical analysis was carried out using GraphPad Prism (Version 6.00, GraphPad Software, La Jolla, CA, USA).

2.6. Ethical Approval

All study parts were ethically approved by the University of Lübeck Ethical Committee and the committees of the participating centers (vote no. 08-022). Informed consent was obtained from all subjects. All methods were carried out in accordance with relevant guidelines and regulations, specifically: the Declaration of Helsinki, the current revision of ICH (The International Council for Harmonisation) Topic E6, the Guidelines for Good Clinical Practice, and the Guidelines of the Council for International Organization of Medical Sciences, the WHO (World Health Organization) ("Proposed International Guidelines for Biomedical Research Involving Human Subjects").

3. Results

From 1 January, 2013 until 31 December, 2018, 7516 extremely low gestational age neonates (ELGANs) were discharged in 64 GNN centers. The study cohort had a mean gestational age at birth of 26.5 weeks (median 26.7 weeks; SD 1.6 weeks) and a mean birth weight of 855 g (median 845 g; SD 248 g, Table 3). Patients were hospitalized for a median of 85 days. Moreover, 1568 infants (20.9%) were exclusively fed with human milk (HM) during their primary stay, 5221 infants (69.5%) received both HM of mothers/donors and formula (Mix group), and 727 infants (9.6%) were fed exclusively formula nutrition (F group).

Table 3. Clinical characteristics of the GNN cohort stratified to type of milk feeding.

	I HM	II Mix	III Formula	*p*-Value (HM vs. Formula)	Total
Number of infants *n*, (%)	1568, (20.9)	5221, (69.5)	727, (9.6)		7516, (100)
Gestational age (weeks)	26.4/1.68 (26.57)	26.52/1.61 (26.7)	26.6/1.95 (26.9)	0.024 [#]	26.5/1.63 (26.7)
Birth weight (g)	841/257 (830)	861/245 (850)	858/243 (850)	0.067 [#]	855/248 (845)
Z–score (birth weight)	−0.25/0.98 (−0.15)	−0.20/−0.92 (0.13)	−0.25/−0.16 (0.03)	0.661 [#]	−0.22/0.93 (−0.14)
Gender, male (%)	54.4	52.9	52.4	0.380	53.2
Multiples (%)	30.9	34.4	26.1	0.020	33.1
SGA (%)	14.6	12.1	13.6	0.526	12.9
Caesarean section (%)	88.4	90.8	87.3	0.471	89.9
Vaginal delivery (%)	11.6	9.2	12.7	0.471	10.1
Hospitalization (days)	83/39 (79)	87/38 (81)	85/45 (80)	0.372 [#]	85/40 (80)
Time to full enteral feeds (days)	18.5/14.6 (14.0)	17.7/14.3 (14.0)	19.8/1 (17.8)	0.341 [#]	18.2/15.1 (14.0)
Duration of intravenous line (days)	26.0/23.7 (18.0)	26.2/25.1(18.0)	28.1/27.6 (18.0)	0.779 [#]	26.4/25.3 (18.0)

HM, human milk; SGA, small-for-gestational-age (<10th Voigt percentile); *p*-values were derived from chi-square test, if not otherwise indicated ([#], Mann–Whitney-U test). Continuous variables and z-scores are shown as mean/SD (median).

3.1. Human Milk Feeding Has Increased in GNN Centers from 2013 to 2018

To account for time trends in enteral feeding practices and current developments in human milk banks, we evaluated the proportion of infants receiving human milk (own-mother; donor milk), mix, or exclusively formula according to the year of the infant's discharge. There has been an increasing rate of ELGANs that receive HM (72.8% in 2013 versus 91.3% in 2018; Figure 1) during primary stay in hospital and at discharge (47.2% in 2013 versus 66.6% in 2018). The administration of donor milk started in 2013 in 3.1% of infants and increased to 22.7% in 2018.

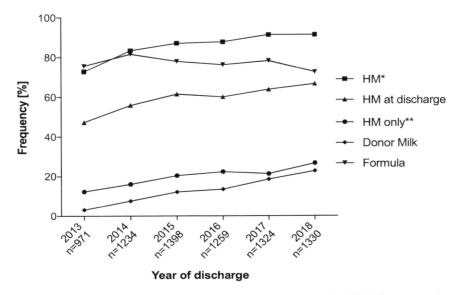

Figure 1. Changes in enteral feeding on German Neonatal Network (GNN) neonatal intensive care units (NICUs) between 2013 and 2018. HM, human milk; * includes all infants that were exposed to HM; ** includes all infants that were fed exclusively HM (own mother and/or donor).

3.2. Formula-Fed Infants Have an Increased Risk for Adverse Short-Term Outcomes

In Table 3, the clinical characteristics of the groups are described with no major differences between the groups. *L. acidophilus/B. infantis* probiotics were administered prophylactically to 5682 ELGAN (76.5%) infants, with a frequency of 74.8% for infants receiving HM (HM group) and 74.9% for those with formula (F group; *p* = 0.935). Notably univariate analyses revealed that the F group had significantly higher rates of NEC (6.2% vs. 3.1%; $p < 0.001$), clinical sepsis (40.2% vs. 34.0%; $p = 0.004$), and severe ROP (6.5% vs. 3.2%; $p = 0.004$) as compared to the HM group. Exclusively formula-fed infants (F group) had a higher body weight at discharge and weight gain/day, head circumference, and body length than infants receiving HM in univariate analyses ($p < 0.001$, Table 4).

Table 4. Treatment, outcomes, and growth parameters of the GNN cohort stratified to type of milk feeding.

	I HM	II Mix	III Formula	p-Value (HM vs. Formula)	Total
Number of infants n, (%)	1568 (20.9)	5221 (69.5)	727 (9.6)		7516 (100)
Antibiotic treatment (%)	94.3	93.5	95.3	0.323	93.7
Probiotic prophylaxis (%)	74.8	78.3	74.9	0.935	76.5
Surgery for NEC (%)	3.1	3.8	6.2	<0.001 [#]	3.9
BC-confirmed sepsis (%)	14.6	16.8	15.7	0.506	16.3
Clinical sepsis (%)	34.0	35.5	40.2	0.004	35.6
BPD (%)	26.4	28.5	28.7	0.240	28.0
Severe ROP (%)	3.2	3.6	6.5	0.004	3.9
Weight (g) at discharge	2460/750 (2460)	2711/733 (2650)	2752/1020 (2731)	<0.001 [#]	2653/818 (2615)
Z-score (birth weight)	−1.73/−1.63 (0.03)	−1.35/−1.32 (0.85)	−1.22/−1.22 (0.79)	<0.001 [#]	−1.40/0.88 (−1.36)
Weight gain velocity (g/day)	19.1/ 6.3 (19.7)	21.5/ 9.3 (21.6)	22.2/ 10.1 (22.4)	<0.001 [#]	21.1/9.09 (21.4)
Weight at discharge (z-scores, Fenton)	−1.53/1.42 (0.03)	−1.16/−1.12 (0.83)	−1.03/−0.99 (0.79)	<0.001 [#]	−1.2/0.86 (−1.15)
Growth velocity of body length (mm/day)	1.36/0.44 (1.37)	1.43/0.39 (1.42)	1.49/0.48 (1.45)	<0.001 [#]	1.42/0.41 (1.41)
Head growth velocity (mm/day)	0.98/0.37 (0.98)	1.03/0.28 (1.03)	1.06/0.40 (1.02)	<0.001 [#]	1.02/0.31 (1.02)

HM, human milk; BPD, bronchopulmonary dysplasia; NEC, necrotizing enterocolitis; ROP, retinopathy of prematurity; BC, blood culture. Growth velocity and weight gain were calculated by differences between parameters at birth and respective measures at discharge/number of days (duration of stay). Continuous variables and z-scores are shown as mean/SD (median); p-values were derived from Fisher's exact test or Mann–Whitney-U test if indicated with [#].

3.3. Probiotics Reduce the Risk for Clinical Sepsis in Infants with Human Milk and Formula Exposure

In the HM group, probiotics were not associated with reduced risk for adverse outcomes such as sepsis or BPD. In the Mix group, probiotics were associated with a risk reduction for clinical sepsis compared to untreated infants (univariate: 33.9% vs. 41.3%, $p < 0.001$; logistic regression: OR 0.69; 95% CI: 0.59–0.79, $p < 0.001$; Tables 1 and 5). There were no significant effects of probiotics on the risk of NEC, ROP, sepsis, and BPD in the F group.

Table 5. Outcomes of the GNN cohort stratified to type of milk feeding and treatment with probiotics.

	I HM		p	II Mix		p	III Formula		p
	No Probiotics	Probiotics		No Probiotics	Probiotics		No Probiotics	Probiotics	
Number of infants n, (%)	395 (25.2)	1173 (74.8)		1135 (21.7)	4086 (78.3)		182 (25.1)	545 (74.9)	
NEC (%)	2.8	3.3	0.65	4.4	3.6	0.21	7.2	5.9	0.54
Clinical sepsis (%)	36.6	33.2	0.02	41.3	33.9	<0.001[#]	37.0	41.0	0.35
BC-confirmed sepsis (%)	14.6	14.6	0.98	18.2	16.5	0.17	15.0	15.8	0.79
Severe ROP (%)	2.7	3.5	0.45	3.8	3.6	0.76	2.9	7.4	0.34
BPD	30.5	25.0	0.003	29.5	28.2	0.38	26.5	29.3	0.48

HM, human milk; BPD, bronchopulmonary dysplasia; NEC, necrotizing enterocolitis; ROP, retinopathy of prematurity; BC, blood culture. Continuous variables and z-scores are shown as mean/SD (median). Categorical variables are shown as percent. p-values were derived from Fisher's exact test or Mann–Whitney-U test if indicated with [#].

3.4. Probiotics Have a Growth-Promoting Effect in Exclusively Human-Milk-Fed Infants

A major effect of probiotic administration on growth was only observed in the HM group, i.e., higher body weight at discharge including Fenton z-scores (-1.49 vs. -2.13; $p < 0.001$), z-score-based weight gain (-1.30 vs. -1.83; $p < 0.001$), and growth rates of body weight, body length, and head circumference (Table 6). Weight gain velocity of HM infants (20.7 g/day) almost reached levels of mix (21.5 g/day), and formula-fed infants (21.9 g/day). In order to address confounding factors such as gestational age (catch-up growth of smaller infants), we performed a linear regression model including gestational age, birth weight, gender, multiple birth, and maternal descent (Table 2). In HM infants, probiotics were associated with higher bodyweight at discharge (effect size B = 0.261; 95% CI: 0.48–0.71; $p < 0.001$) and z-score-based weight gain. Notably probiotic treatment was associated with increased weight gain velocity (effect size B = 0.224; 95% CI: 2.82–4.35; $p < 0.001$), body length, and head circumference. This (probiotic) effect was observed to a lesser extent in the Mix group (body weight at discharge, head growth velocity), while Formula infants were not affected by probiotics in that aspect (Table 2).

Table 6. Growth parameters of the GNN cohort stratified to type of milk feeding and treatment with probiotics.

	I HM		p	II Mix		p	III Formula		p
	No Probiotics	Probiotics		No Probiotics	Probiotics		No Probiotics	Probiotics	
Weight (g) at discharge [#]	2213/782 (2190)	2542/721 (2535)	<0.001	2692/833 (2670)	2716/756 (2640)	0.99	2455/1128 (2540)	2844/958 (2800)	<0.001
Weight at discharge; z-score, Fenton [#]	−2.13/1.13 (−2.11)	1.49/0.87 (−1.43)	<0.001	−1.36/0.91 (−1.31)	−1.35/0.83 (−1,33)	0.79	−1.29/0.83 (−1.19)	−1.21/.78 (−1.23)	0.64
Weight gain (z-scores, Fenton)	−1.83/1.16 (−1.72)	−1.30/0.83 (−1.27)	<0.001	−1.23/0.91 (−1.13)	−1.14/0.80 (−1.12)	0.05	−1.12/0.82 (−1.06)	−1.01/0.78 (−0.99)	0.51
Growth velocity (g/day) [#]	18.81/7.37 (16.19)	20.69/6.63 (20.87)	<0.001	21.48/13.10 (21.60)	21.49/7.97 (21.62)	0.32	22.80/16.01 (22.00)	21.91/7.12 (22.47)	0.36
Head growth velocity (mm/day)	0.930/0.502 (0.89)	0.996/0.320 (1.0)	<0.001	1.012/0.332 (1.008)	1.11/0.261 (1.028)	0.017	1.058/0.389 (1.036)	1.056/0.400 (1.017)	0.89
Growth velocity (body length; mm/day)	1.210/0.442 (1.216)	1.403/0.429 (1.4)	<0.001	1.413/0.407 (1.406)	1.432/0.380 (1.422)	0.139	1.511/0.654 (1.451)	1.49/0.43 (1.452)	0.775

HM, human milk. Growth velocity, weight gain, and growth of body length and head circumference were calculated by differences between parameters at birth and respective measures at discharge/number of days (duration of stay). Continuous variables and z-scores are shown as mean/SD (median), p-values were derived from Mann–Whitney-U test if indicated with [#].

4. Discussion

Our large-scale population-based data support the hypothesis that the source of enteral feeding has an impact on the effects of *L. acidophilus/B. infantis* probiotics in highly vulnerable preterm infants. In this context, human milk exposure is required for probiotics to provide a sepsis-preventive and growth-promoting effect. Exclusively formula-fed infants did not benefit from the administration of probiotics in terms of sepsis, NEC, or BPD risk.

The feeding of preterm infants with human milk has been previously associated with reduced morbidity and mortality [18–21]. The stabilization of the early host–microbiome interaction has been proposed as a crucial underlying mechanism for this beneficial effect [12]. On the other hand, human milk might not fully meet the nutritional requirements of preterm infants [22], which results in less weight gain in human-milk-fed preterm babies as compared to formula-fed infants [23]. Bovine multicomponent fortification of human milk has been proposed to cause inflammation [24], and there is a lack of scientific evidence about whether or not its routine use can impact growth and other short- and long-term outcomes [25]. Furthermore, there is uncertainty on whether pasteurized donated human milk should be preferred to preterm formula [26]. In clinical reality, most babies in participating GNN units receive a mix of human milk and formula while donor human milk availabilities are increasingly being established but still limited. We noted a temporal trend to higher rates of human milk feeding, which approached 90% in 2018. In such a setting with low NEC rates <4% in babies <29 weeks and 75%

exposure to probiotics, we expected no further risk reduction for NEC by probiotics as compared to our previous findings before/after the introduction of probiotics into clinical routine [8]. In the current cohort study, we noted a promoting effect of probiotics on weight gain and growth velocities in HM-fed infants. Previous studies revealed inconsistent results that were not necessarily adjusted for the type of feeding [27–30]. A meta-analysis of 15 studies including 3751 infants <32 weeks and <1500 g birth weight demonstrated no significant effects of probiotics on weight gain [31]. In comparison to our cohort, the gestational age in this pooled study cohort analysis was higher while mean weight gain/day was lower (16 g/day vs. 21 g/day) indicating that the effects of probiotics are context sensitive. While the huge variability in study designs has been acknowledged, the authors conclude that probiotics are more effective in reducing morbidity when taken in human milk or human milk plus formula form, consumed for <6 weeks, administered at a dosage of $<10^9$ CFU/d, and include multiple strains. We assume that promoted weight gain in HM-fed infants is correlated with the dynamics of the establishing intestinal microbiota, nutrient utilization, and immune–metabolome interaction [4,32]. *L. acidophilus/B. infantis* may require the complex composition of human milk to exert a growth-promoting effect and to stabilize gut immunity in order to prevent translocation sepsis [6,7,33]. Human milk includes endogenous probiotics, prebiotic carbohydrates, stem cells, and a concert of bioactive human milk factors (e.g., S100 A8/9 [34]) that have direct or indirect effects on the vulnerable host–gut microbiota interplay [11]. Hence, the sepsis-preventive effect of human milk may not be additionally increased by probiotics in exclusively HM-fed infants. Infants who are exposed to human milk and formula benefit from probiotics, which would compensate for the reduced abundance of bifidobacteria and lactobacilli in their gut microbiota composition [20,35]. Both, human milk feeding and probiotics might also be able to "reverse" antibiotic-induced gut dysbiosis [36], which needs to be subject to further long-term studies of extremely preterm infants.

Strengths and Limitations

The major strengths of our study design are the large sample size and high quality of the clinical data that are monitored on-site by a study team trained in neonatology. The main limitations are the observational design, the lack of information on the daily type of feeding in the Mix group, indication for supplementation, and timing with bovine and individual fortification of human milk or formula. Furthermore, we did not have exact data on the timing of probiotics, the number of pasteurized milk portions, and the bacterial load of human own-mother milk (if not pasteurized) in the individual infants. Whether probiotics or the probiotic/prebiotic load of human milk is causal for the observed effects, needs to be addressed in future studies including extensive sequencing of human milk microbiome and the gut microbiome of the milk (+probiotic)-fed infants.

5. Conclusions

Evidence of nutrition-related effects of probiotic prophylaxis in preterm infants is scarce. In a large cohort of VLBWI, we conclude that supplementation of *L. acidophilus/B. infantis* and feeding strategies interact and have the potential of improving outcomes and growth in preterm infants. Our data demonstrates sepsis-preventive and growth-promoting effects exclusively in infants receiving human milk, supporting usage of human milk (including human milk from donors) in preterm infants whenever possible. Randomized, placebo-controlled trials as the PRIMAL clinical study [37] are pending to test hypothesis generating observational studies and to evaluate long-term effects of probiotics.

Author Contributions: Conceptualization, I.F., E.H., W.G., and C.H.; data curation, I.F., C.R., P.H., W.G., and C.H.; formal analysis, I.F., J.M., B.S., J.S., A.H., K.H., K.F., J.P., L.E., K.B., C.R., S.P., D.V., D.S., P.H., B.T., T.K., A.S., C.D., M.Z., C.W., J.R., E.H., W.G., and C.H.; funding acquisition, E.H., W.G., and C.H.; investigation, I.F., J.M., C.R., S.P., D.V., P.H., B.T., T.K., A.S., E.H., W.G., and C.H.; methodology, I.F., J.S., K.H., C.R., P.H., A.S., E.H., W.G., and C.H.; project administration, W.G. and C.H.; resources, E.H., W.G., and C.H.; supervision, J.S., E.H., W.G., and C.H.; visualization, I.F.; writing—original draft, I.F. and C.H.; writing—review and editing, J.M., B.S., J.S., A.H., K.H., K.F., J.P., L.E., K.B., C.R., S.P., D.V., D.S., P.H., B.T., T.K., A.S., C.D., M.Z., C.W., J.R., E.H., and W.G. All authors have read and agreed to the published version of the manuscript.

Acknowledgments: The authors are indebted to all parents and their infants. We thank all nurses and doctors and study centers who participate in the GNN. The participants of the German Neonatal Network (GNN) are: Wolfgang Göpel, Department of Pediatrics, University of Lübeck; Meike Bendiks, Children's Hospital, University of Kiel; Martin Andree Berghäuser, Department of Pediatrics, Florence Nightingale Hospital Düsseldorf; Corinna Gebauer, Department of Pediatrics, University of Leipzig, Kai Bockenholt, Children's Hospital Cologne, Amsterdamer Strasse; Ralf Boettger, Perinatal Centre, University of Magdeburg; Bettina Bohnhorst, Department of Neonatology, Hannover Medical School; Thomas Brune, Children's Hospital Lippe; Kristin Dawczynski, Department of Neonatology, University of Jena; Michael Dördelmann, Diakonissenhospital Flensburg; Silke Ehlers, Bürgerhospital Frankfurt; Joachim G. Eichhorn, Children's Hospital Leverkusen; Ursula-Felderhoff-Müser, Department of Pediatrics, University of Essen; Axel Franz, Department of Neonatology, University of Tübingen; Hubert Gerleve, Children's Hospital Coesfeld; Ludwig Gortner, Department of Pediatrics, University of Homburg; Florian Guthmann, Children's Hospital Auf der Bult, Hannover; Roland Haase, Department of Pediatrics, University of Halle; Friedhelm Heitmann, Children's Hospital Dortmund; Michael Heldmann, Department of Neonatology, Helios Hospital Wuppertal; Nico Hepping, St. Marienhospital, Bonn; Roland Hentschel, Department of Pediatrics and Neonatology, University of Freiburg; Georg Hillebrand, MD, Children's Hospital Itzehoe; Thomas Hoehn, Department of Pediatrics, University of Düsseldorf; Mechthild Hubert, Children's Hospital Siegen; Helmut Hummler, Department of Neonatology, University of Ulm; Reinhard Jensen, Children's Hospital Heide; Olaf Kannt, Children's Hospital Schwerin; Thorsten Koerner, Department of Neonatology, Hospital Links der Weser, Bremen; Helmut Küster, Department of Pediatrics, University of Göttingen; Angela Kribs, Department of Pediatrics, University of Cologne, Knud Linnemann, Department of Pediatrics, Ernst-Moritz-Arndt-University of Greifswald; Jens Möller, Children's Hospital Saarbrücken; Dirk Mueller, Children's Hospital Kassel; Dirk Olbertz, Department of Neonatology, Hospital Suedstadt Rostock; Thorsten Orlikowsky, Department of Neonatology, University of Aachen; Jochen Reese, Children's Hospital Eutin; Claudia Roll, Department of Pediatrics, University Witten-Herdecke, Vestische Children's Hospital Datteln; Rainer Rossi, Children's Hospital Berlin-Neukoelln, Berlin; Mario Rüdiger, Department of Neonatology, University of Dresden; Stefan Schaefer, Department of Neonatology, Hospital Nürnberg Süd; Thomas Schaible, Department of Pediatrics, University of Mannheim; Susanne Schmidtke, Department of Neonatology, Asklepios Hospital Hamburg-Barmbek; Stefan Seeliger, Children's Hospital Neuburg/ Ingolstadt; Hugo Segerer, Children's Hospital St. Hedwig, Regensburg; Norbert Teig, Department of Pediatrics, University of Bochum; Hans-Georg Topf, Department of Neonatology, University of Erlangen; Florian Urlichs, Department of Pediatrics, St. Franziskus-Hospital Muenster; Matthias Vochem, Olgahospital Stuttgart; Ursula Weller, Children's Hospital Bielefeld; Axel von der Wense, Children's Hospital Altona e.V.; Claudius Werner, Children's Hospital, Westfälische Wilhelms-Universitiy of Muenster; Christian Wieg, Children's Hospital Aschaffenburg-Alzenau; Jürgen Wintgens, Children's Hospital Mönchengladbach; Welfhard Schneider, Vivantes Hospital Friedrichshain; Esther Rieger-Fackeldey, Department of Neonatology, Klinikum rechts der Isar, Technical University, Munich; Friedrich Ebinger, St. Vincent Hospital Paderborn; Gernot Sinnecker, Department of Pediatrics Wolfsburg; Volkmar Kunde, Christian Children's Hospital Osnabrück and Thomas Völkl, Department of Pediatrics Josefinum Augsburg. We thank Anja Kaufmann, Birgit Schröder, Tim Röntgendorf, Liane Triebwasser, and Sabine Lorenz for data documentation. The participants of the PRIMAL Consortium are Philipp Henneke, Center for Pediatrics and Adolescent Medicine and Institute for Immunodeficiency, University of Freiburg, Germany; Christoph Härtel, Department of Pediatrics, University of Lübeck, Germany; Peer Bork, Structural and Computational Biology Unit, European Molecular Biology Laboratory, Heidelberg, Germany; Stephan Gehring, Department of Pediatrics, University Medical Centre, Mainz, Germany; David Frommhold, Children's Hospital Memmingen, Memmingen, Germany; Michael Zemlin, Department of General Pediatrics and Neonatology, Saarland University, Homburg, Germany; Christian Gille, Department of Neonatology, University of Tübingen, Tübingen, Germany; Dorothee Viemann, Department of Pediatric Pneumology, Allergology, and Neonatology, Hannover Medical School, Hannover, Germany.

Abbreviations

BPD	bronchopulmonary dysplasia
HM	human milk
ELGAN	extremely low gestational age neonates
FIP	focal intestinal perforation
GNN	German Neonatal Network

NEC   necrotizing enterocolitis
NICU   neonatal intensive care unit
ROP   retinopathy of prematurity
SGA   small for gestational age

References

1. Underwood, M.A.; Kalanetra, K.M.; Bokulich, N.A.; Lewis, Z.T.; Mirmiran, M.; Tancredi, D.J.; Mills, D.A. A comparison of two probiotic strains of bifidobacteria in premature infants. *J. Pediatr.* **2013**, *163*, 1585–1591. [CrossRef]

2. Warner, B.B.; Tarr, P.I. Necrotizing enterocolitis and preterm infant gut bacteria. *Semin. Fetal Neonatal Med.* **2016**, *21*, 394–399. [CrossRef]

3. Olsen, R.; Greisen, G.; Schrøder, M.; Brok, J. Prophylactic probiotics for preterm infants: A systematic review and meta-analysis of observational studies. *Neonatology* **2016**, *109*, 105–112. [CrossRef]

4. Graspeuntner, S.; Waschina, S.; Kunzel, S.; Twisselmann, N.; Rausch, T.K.; Cloppenborg-Schmidt, K.; Viemann, D.; Herting, E.; Göpel, W.; Baines, J.F. Gut dysbiosis with Bacilli dominance and accumulation of fermentation products precedes late-onset sepsis in preterm infants. *Clin. Infect. Dis.* **2019**, *69*, 268–277. [CrossRef]

5. Costeloe, K.; Hardy, P.; Juszczak, E.; Wilks, M.; Millar, M.R. Study PPI. Bifidobacterium breve BBG-001 in very preterm infants: A randomised controlled phase 3 trial. *Lancet* **2016**, *387*, 649–660. [CrossRef]

6. Repa, A.; Thanhaeuser, M.; Endress, D.; Weber, M.; Kreissl, A.; Binder, C.; Berger, A.; Haiden, N. Probiotics (Lactobacillus acidophilus and Bifidobacterium infantis) prevent NEC in VLBW infants fed breast milk but not formula. *Pediatr. Res.* **2015**, *77*, 381–388. [CrossRef]

7. Samuels, N.; van de Graaf, R.; Been, J.V.; de Jonge, R.C.J.; Hanff, L.M.; Wijnen, R.M.H.; Kornelisse, R.F.; Reiss, I.K.M.; Vermeulen, M.J. Necrotising enterocolitis and mortality in preterm infants after introduction of probiotics: A quasi-experimental study. *Sci. Rep.* **2016**, *6*, 31643. [CrossRef]

8. Härtel, C.; Pagel, J.; Rupp, J.; Bendiks, M.; Guthmann, F.; Rieger-Fackeldey, E.; Heckmann, M.; Franz, A.; Schiffmann, J.H.; Zimmermann, B. Prophylactic Use of Lactobacillus acidophilus/Bifidobacterium infantis Probiotics and Outcome in Very Low Birth Weight Infants. *J. Pediatr.* **2014**, *165*, 285–289.e1. [CrossRef] [PubMed]

9. Humberg, A.; Härtel, C.; Rausch, T.K.; Stichtenoth, G.; Jung, P.; Wieg, C.; Kribs, A.; von der Wense, A.; Weller, U.; Höhn, T.; et al. German Neonatal Network. Active perinatal care of preterm infants in the German Neonatal Network. *Arch. Dis. Child Fetal Neonatal Ed.* **2020**, *105*, 190–195. [CrossRef] [PubMed]

10. Autran, C.A.; Kellman, B.P.; Kim, J.H.; Asztalos, E.; Blood, A.B.; Spence, E.C.H.; Patel, A.L.; Hou, J.; Lewis, N.E. Human milk oligosaccharide composition predicts risk of necrotising enterocolitis in preterm infants. *Gut* **2018**, *67*, 1064–1070. [CrossRef] [PubMed]

11. Narayan, N.R.; Méndez-Lagares, G.; Ardeshir, A.; Lu, D.; Van Rompay, K.K.; Hartigan-O'Connor, D.J. Persistent effects of early infant diet and associated microbiota on the juvenile immune system. *Gut Microbes* **2015**, *6*, 284–289. [CrossRef] [PubMed]

12. Zivkovic, A.M.; German, J.B.; Lebrilla, C.B.; Mills, D.A. Human milk glycobiome and its impact on the infant gastrointestinal microbiota. *Proc. Natl. Acad. Sci. USA* **2011**, *108* (Suppl. 1), 4653–4658. [CrossRef] [PubMed]

13. Methods for estimating the due date. Committee Opinion No 700. American College of Obstetricians and Gynecologists. *Obstet Gynecol.* **2017**, *129*, 2150–2154.

14. Voigt, M.; Rochow, N.; Straube, S.; Olbertz, D.M.; Jorch, G. Birth weight percentile charts based on daily measurements for very preterm male and female infants at the age of 154-223 days. *J. Perinat Med.* **2010**, *38*, 289–295. [CrossRef] [PubMed]

15. Fenton, T.R.; Kim, J.H. A systematic review and meta-analysis to revise the Fenton growth chart for preterm infants. *BMC Pediatrics* **2013**, *13*, 59. [CrossRef] [PubMed]

16. Fenton, T.R. A new growth chart for preterm babies: Babson and Benda's chart updated with recent data and a new format. *BMC Pediatr.* **2003**, *3*, 13. [CrossRef]

17. Geffers, C.; Baerwolff, S.; Schwab, F.; Gastmeier, P. Incidence of healthcare- associated infections in high-risk neonates: Results from the German surveillance system for very-low-birthweight infants. *J. Hosp. Infect.* **2008**, *68*, 214–221. [CrossRef]

18. Daniels, M.C.; Adair, L.S. Breast-Feeding Influences Cognitive Development in Filipino Children. *J. Nutr.* **2005**, *135*, 2589–2595. [CrossRef]

19. Meinzen-Derr, J.; Poindexter, B.; Wrage, L.; Morrow, A.L.; Stoll, B.; Donovan, E.F. Role of human milk in extremely low birth weight infants' risk of necrotizing enterocolitis or death. *J. Perinatol.* **2009**, *29*, 57–62. [CrossRef]

20. Sisk, P.M.; Lovelady, C.A.; Dillard, R.G.; Gruber, K.J.; O'Shea, T.M. Early human milk feeding is associated with a lower risk of necrotizing enterocolitis in very low birth weight infants. *J. Perinatol.* **2007**, *27*, 428–433. [CrossRef]

21. Corpeleijn, W.E.; Kouwenhoven, S.M.; Paap, M.C.; Van Vliet, I.; Scheerder, I.; Muizer, Y.; Helder, O.K.; van Goudoever, J.B.; Vermeulen, M.J. Intake of own mother's milk during the first days of life is associated with decreased morbidity and mortality in very low birth weight infants during the first 60 days of life. *Neonatology* **2012**, *102*, 276–281. [CrossRef] [PubMed]

22. Dewey, K.G. Growth Characteristics of Breast-Fed Compared to Formula-Fed Infants. *Biol. Neonate* **1998**, *74*, 94–105. [CrossRef] [PubMed]

23. Spiegler, J.; Preuss, M.; Gebauer, C.; Bendiks, M.; Herting, E.; Goepel, W. Does breastmilk influence the development of bronchopulmonary dysplasia? *J. Pediatr.* **2016**, *169*, 76–80 e4. [CrossRef] [PubMed]

24. Battersby, C.; Statnikov, Y.; Santhakumaran, S.; Gray, D.; Modi, N.; Costeloe, K.; UK Neonatal Collaborative and Medicines for Neonates Investigator Group. The United Kingdom National Neonatal Research Database: A validation study. *PLoS ONE* **2018**, *13*, e0201815. [CrossRef]

25. Rochow, N.; Landau-Crangle, E.; Fusch, C. Challenges in breast milk fortification for preterm infants. *Curr. Opin. Clin. Nutr. Metab. Care* **2015**, *18*, 276–284. [CrossRef]

26. Mills, L.; Modi, N. Clinician enteral feeding preferences for very preterm babies in the UK. *Arch. Dis. Child Fetal Neonatal Ed.* **2015**, *100*, F372–F373. [CrossRef]

27. Steenhout, P.; Rochat, F.; Hager, C. The effect of Bifidobacterium lactis on the growth of infants: A pooled analysis of randomized controlled studies. *Ann. Nutr. Metab.* **2009**, *55*, 334–340. [CrossRef]

28. Kitajima, H.; Sumida, Y.; Tanaka, R. Early administration of Bifidobacterium breve to preterm infants: Randomized controlled trial. *Arch. Dis. Child Fetal Neonatal Ed.* **1997**, *76*, F101–F107. [CrossRef]

29. Sari, F.N.; Eras, Z.; Dizdar, E.A.; Erdeve, O.; Uras, N.; Dilmen, U. Do oral probiotics affect growth and neurodevelopmental outcomes in very low-birth-weight preterm infants? *Am. J. Perinatol.* **2012**, *29*, 579–586. [CrossRef]

30. Aceti, A.; Gori, D.; Barone, G.; Callegari, M.L.; Fantini, M.P.; Indrio, F.; Maggio, L.; Meneghin, F.; Morelli, L.; Zuccotti, G.; et al. Probiotics and time to achieve full enteral feeding in human milk-fed and formula-fed preterm infants: Systematic review and meta-analysis. *Nutrients* **2016**, *8*, 471. [CrossRef]

31. Sun, J.; Marwah, G.; Westgarth, M.; Buys, N.; Ellwood, D.; Gray, P.H. Effects of Probiotics on Necrotizing Enterocolitis, Sepsis, Intraventricular Hemorrhage, Mortality, Length of Hospital Stay, and Weight Gain in Very Preterm Infants: A Meta-Analysis. *Adv. Nutr.* **2017**, *8*, 749–763. [CrossRef] [PubMed]

32. Jacquot, A.; Neveu, D.; Aujoulat, F.; Mercier, G.; Marchandin, H.; Jumas-Bilak, E.; Picaud, J.C. Dynamics and clinical evolution of bacterial gut microflora in extremely premature patients. *J. Pediatr.* **2011**, *158*, 390–396. [CrossRef] [PubMed]

33. Aceti, A.; Maggio, L.; Beghetti, I.; Gori, D.; Barone, G.; Callegari, M.; Fantini, M.P.; Indrio, F.; Meneghin, F.; Morelli, L.; et al. Probiotics Prevent Late-Onset Sepsis in Human Milk-Fed, Very Low Birth Weight Preterm Infants: Systematic Review and Meta-Analysis. *Nutrients* **2017**, *9*, 904. [CrossRef] [PubMed]

34. Heinemann, A.S.; Pirr, S.; Fehlhaber, B.; Mellinger, L.; Burgmann, J.; Busse, M.; Ginzel, M.; Friesenhagen, J.; von Köckritz-Blickwede, M.; Ulas, T.; et al. In neonates S100A8/S100A9 alarmins prevent the expansion of a specific inflammatory monocyte population promoting septic shock. *FASEB J.* **2017**, *31*, 1153–1164. [CrossRef] [PubMed]

35. Underwood, M.A.; German, J.B.; Lebrilla, C.B.; Mills, D.A. Bifidobacterium longum subspecies infantis: Champion colonizer of the infant gut. *Pediatr. Res.* **2015**, *77*, 229–235. [CrossRef] [PubMed]

36. Härtel, C.; Pagel, J.; Spiegler, J.; Buma, J.; Henneke, P.; Zemlin, M.; Viemann, D.; Gille, C.; Gehring, S.; Frommhold, D.; et al. Lactobacillus acidophilus/Bifidobacterium infantis probiotics are associated with increased growth of VLBWI among those exposed to antibiotics. *Sci. Rep.* **2017**, *7*, 5633. [CrossRef]
37. Marißen, J.; Haiß, A.; Meyer, C.; Van Rossum, T.; Bünte, L.M.; Frommhold, D.; Gille, C.; Goedicke-Fritz, S.; Göpel, W.; Hudalla, H. Efficacy of Bifidobacterium longum, B. infantis and Lactobacillus acidophilus probiotics to prevent gut dysbiosis in preterm infants of 28+0-32+6 weeks of gestation: A randomised, placebo-controlled, double-blind, multicentre trial: The PRIMAL Clinical Study protocol. *BMJ Open* **2019**, *9*, e032617. [CrossRef]

3

Amino Acid Composition of Breast Milk from Urban Chinese Mothers

Clara L. Garcia-Rodenas [1,*], **Michael Affolter** [1], **Gerard Vinyes-Pares** [2], **Carlos A. De Castro** [1], **Leonidas G. Karagounis** [1], **Yumei Zhang** [3], **Peiyu Wang** [4] **and Sagar K. Thakkar** [1]

[1] Nestlé Research Center, Nestec Ltd., Lausanne 1000, Switzerland; michael.affolter@rdls.nestle.com (M.A.); carlosantonio.decastro@rdls.nestle.com (C.A.D.C.); leonidas.karagounis@rdls.nestle.com (L.G.K.); sagar.thakkar@rdls.nestle.com (S.K.T.)
[2] Nestlé Health Sciences, Nestec Ltd., Epalinges 1066, Switzerland; gerard.vinyespares@nestle.com
[3] Department of Nutrition and Food Hygiene, School of Public Health, Peking University, Beijing 100191, China; zhangyumei@hsc.pku.edu.cn
[4] Department of Social Medicine and Health Education, School of Public Health, Peking University, Beijing 100191, China; wpeiyu@bjmu.edu.cn
* Correspondence: clara.garcia@rdls.nestle.com

Abstract: Human breast milk (BM) amino acid (AA) composition may be impacted by lactation stage or factors related to geographical location. The present cross-sectional study is aimed at assessing the temporal changes of BMAA over lactation stages in a large cohort of urban mothers in China. Four hundred fifty BM samples, collected in three Chinese cities covering eight months of lactation were analyzed for free (FAA) and total (TAA) AA by o-phthalaldehyde/ fluorenylmethylchloroformate (OPA/FMOC) derivatization. Concentrations and changes over lactation were aligned with previous reports. Both the sum and the individual TAA values significantly decreased during the first periods of lactation and then generally leveled off. Leucine and methionine were respectively the most and the least abundant indispensable amino acids across all the lactation stages, whereas glutamic acid + glutamine (Glx) was the most and cystine the least abundant dispensable AA. The contribution of FAA to TAA levels was less than 2%, except for free Glx, which was the most abundant FAA. In conclusion, the AA composition of the milk from our cohort of urban Chinese mothers was comparable to previous studies conducted in other parts of the world, suggesting that this is an evolutionary conserved trait largely independent of geographical, ethnic, or dietary factors.

Keywords: breast milk; amino acids; lactation period; cross-sectional study

1. Introduction

Evolution has shaped the composition of breast milk to ensure optimal development of healthy term offspring. However, breast milk composition is not constant and appears to be affected by multiple factors, including lactation stage, mothers' genetic background and diet, gestational age at delivery, or geographical location [1].

Breast milk protein is a key nutrient supporting body growth and organ development during the first few months of life by providing nitrogen and indispensable amino acids (IAA) required for body protein building and by stimulating the secretion of growth-promoting hormones (i.e., insulin, insulin-like growth factor (1-IGF1)). Potent insulinotropic amino acids such as the branched chain amino acids—Leucine, Lysine, and Threonine—can be particularly important in this context. However, emerging evidence suggests that the relatively low levels of protein and insulinotropic amino acids in breast milk may be protective against the development of metabolic disorders later in infant life [2]. Because body weight, body composition, growth rate, and volume of milk intake are known to change with an infant's age [3,4], infant requirements in terms of both protein and individual amino acid composition also varies along the different stages of lactation [3].

Most amino acids in breast milk are found as constituents of protein chains, but there is also a certain amount of free amino acids (FAA), which usually account for less than 10% of the total amino acid (TAA) levels [5,6]. Although still poorly explored, emerging evidence suggests specific physiological roles of the FAA fraction, such as appetite control [7]. Many studies have analyzed the TAA content in human milk, but they often characterize a limited number of samples, do not account for the important lactation-stage associated changes, or both. The number of studies on FAA is even more limited. In their systematic review of breast milk amino acid composition studies from different continents, Zhang et al. [8] report geographical differences in the content of some TAA and FAA, although data from some regions of the world is relatively limited. In particular, studies looking at breast milk protein quality in China are scarce, with only two small studies reporting on the average TAA composition of one to six months [9] and 7–180 days [10] postpartum milk. To our knowledge, no data on TAA and FAA content in milk from Chinese mothers along lactation is available to date.

The objective of this cross-sectional study was to assess the temporal changes of FAA and TAA in milk secreted during the different stages of lactation in a large cohort of Chinese mothers from three different cities in urban China.

2. Materials and Methods

2.1. Subjects

This study was part of the Maternal, Infant and Nutrition Growth study (MING), a cross-sectional study designed to investigate the dietary and nutritional status of pregnant women, lactating mothers, and young children aged from birth up to three years living in urban areas of China [11]. In addition, the human milk composition of the lactating mothers was characterized. The study was conducted between October 2011 and February 2012. A multi-stage milk sampling from lactating mothers in three cities (Beijing, Suzhou, and Guangzhou) was performed for breast milk characterization. In each city, two hospitals with maternal and child care units were randomly selected; at each site, mothers at lactation periods from 0 to 240 days were randomly selected based on child registration information. Subjects included in the 0–5-day period were recruited at the hospital, whereas the other subjects were invited by telephone to join the study; if participation was dismissed, a replacement was found. Response rate was 52%. Recruitment, milk collection, and baseline data collection were completed on separate days.

Stratified milk sampling of 540 lactating mothers in six lactation periods of 0 to 4, 5 to 11, and 12 to 30 days, and 1–2, 2–4, and 4–8 months, was obtained in the MING study. Nevertheless, only 450 milk samples were analyzed in the amino acid study, as the 0- to 4-day stage could not be included due to the limited volume of milk collected during this period.

Eligibility criteria included women between 18 and 45 years of age giving birth to a single, healthy, full-term infant and exclusively breastfeeding until at least 4 months after birth. Exclusion criteria included gestational diabetes, hypertension, cardiac diseases, acute communicable diseases, and postpartum depression. Lactating women who had nipple or lacteal gland diseases, who had been receiving hormonal therapy during the three months preceding recruitment, or who had insufficient skills to understand study questionnaires were also excluded.

The study was conducted according to the guidelines in the Declaration of Helsinki. All of the procedures involving human subjects were approved by the Medical Ethics Research Board of Peking University (No. IRB00001052-11042). Written informed consent was obtained from all subjects participating in the study. The study was registered at ClinicalTrials.gov (NCT01971671)

2.2. Data Collection

All subjects responded to a general questionnaire including socio-economic and lifestyle aspects of the mother. The self-reported weight at delivery, the number of gestational weeks at delivery, and the delivery method were also recorded. Additionally, a physical examination (height, weight, mid-arm circumference, blood pressure, and hemoglobin levels) was also carried out.

Data collection was done through face-to-face interviews on the day of milk sample collection. The infant's date of birth and gender information was collected retrospectively by phone interview.

2.3. Sample Collection

Breast milk sampling was standardized for all subjects and performed with an electric pump (Horigen HNR/X-2108ZB, Xinhe Electrical Apparatuses Co., Ltd., Beijing, China). Samples were collected at the second feeding in the morning (9–11 a.m.) to avoid circadian influence on the outcomes. Single full breast was emptied, and an aliquot of 40 mL was secured for characterization purposes. The rest of the milk was returned to the mother for infant feeding. One-milliliter aliquots of each sample were transported on dry ice to a laboratory and stored at $-80\ ^{\circ}C$ until further analysis.

2.4. Amino Acid Analysis

All samples were analyzed by Eurofins Technology Service (Suzhou) Co. Ltd., Suzhou, China.

TAA content was determined according to a validated o-phthalaldehyde/ fluorenylmethylchloroformate (OPA/FMOC) derivatization procedure described by Blankenship et al. [12]. Briefly, protein-bound amino acids were converted to the free state by acid hydrolysis in 6 M of hydrochloric acid at 110 $^{\circ}C$ for 22 h with a phenol antioxidant in the absence of oxygen. The digests were derivatized with ortho-phthalaldehyde (OPA), mecaptopropionic acid (MCP), and 9-fluorenylmethyl chloroformate (FMOC-Cl) under alkaline conditions prior to injection. Separation and quantification of the amino acid derivatives were performed by high-performance liquid chromatography HPLC with a UV/diode array and fluorescence detection. The limit of detection (LOD) was 1 mg/100 g and the limit of quantification (LOQ) was 5 mg/100 g. Average repeatability was 12%, and reproducibility between duplicate determinations was 18% for the 18 measured amino acids with recoveries ranging from 64.9% to 129.6%.

FAA content was determined according to the same OPA/FMOC method, but without the acid hydrolysis step. All samples were analyzed in duplicate.

2.5. Statistical Analysis

Multiple linear regression was applied to analyze the effect of the lactation period on the levels of TAA and FAA. This model was adjusted for the effects of maternal age and body mass index (BMI), infant gender, mode of delivery, and geographical location. Comparisons were made regarding each subsequent lactation period (5–11 days vs. 12–30 days, 12–30 days vs. 1–2 months, 1–2 months vs. 2–4 months, and 2–4 months vs. 4–8 months) by calculating contrast estimates produced by the model.

For the socio-demographic and anthropometric data, analysis of variance was applied for the continuous variable in question and the lactation period in order to check if there was at least 1 period that was different than the others. For factor variables, an independence test was performed in order to detect differences in distribution among the different period.

All statistical analyses were performed with the statistical software R (version 3.0.1; R Foundation, Vienna, Austria).

3. Results

3.1. Subject Characteristics

In this cross-sectional study, TAA and FAA were quantified in 450 breast milk samples collected at different stages from early to late lactation in healthy urban Chinese women. The recruitment flowchart from eligibility to sample analysis is illustrated in Figure 1.

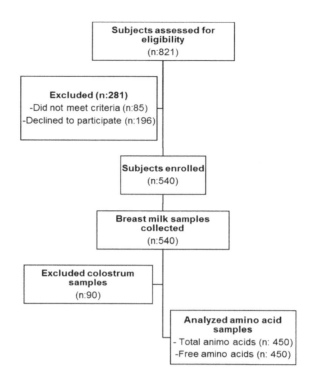

Figure 1. Study flow chart.

Subject demographics and anthropometry are described in Table 1. Maternal age, weight, BMI, and mode of delivery were significantly different among the lactation stage cohorts. No other significant differences were observed in maternal and infant characteristics analyzed.

Table 1. Maternal and infant characteristics.

	Lactation Period					
	5–11 Days	12–30 Days	1–2 Months	2–4 Months	4–8 Months	
	($n = 90$)	($n = 90$)	($n = 90$)	($n = 90$)	($n = 90$)	p Value
MOTHER						
Age (years), Mean (SD)	27 (4)	27 (3)	28 (4)	27 (4)	26 (4)	0.005
Height (cm), Mean (SD)	160 (4)	160 (5)	161 (5)	161 (5)	159 (5)	0.102
Weight (kg), Mean (SD)	60.7 (8.7)	60.8 (7.9)	61.9 (8.9)	58.4 (8.3)	56.2 (8.1)	<0.001
BMI (kg/m^2), Mean (SD)	23.7 (3.2)	23.7 (3.0)	23.9 (3.1)	22.5 (2.9)	22.2 (3.1)	<0.001
Gestational weight gain (kg), Mean (SD)	16.7 (7.4)	16.2 (6.0)	15.9 (5.7)	15.9 (5.9)	14.9 (7.6)	0.419
Postpartum weight loss (kg), Mean (SD)	9.1 (6.1)	8.6 (5.3)	9.8 (4.0)	10.0 (6.2)	10.6 (5.9)	0.119
Non-Smoker, n (%)	90 (100)	89 (99)	90 (100)	86 (98)	89 (100)	0.176
Cesarean delivery, n (%)	39 (42)	43 (48)	53 (59)	35 (39)	35 (38)	0.004
Household income (RMB/month)						
<2000 RMB, n (%)	20 (22)	17 (19)	24 (27)	26 (29)	31 (34)	
2000–4000 RMB, n (%)	37 (41)	45 (50)	41 (46)	40 (44)	41 (46)	
>4000 RMB, n (%)	30 (33)	22 (24)	23 (26)	22 (24)	18 (20)	
Unknown, n (%)	1 (1)	6 (7)	2 (2)	0 (0)	0 (0)	0.206
INFANT						
Males, n (%)	51 (57)	48 (53)	48 (53)	54 (60)	43 (48)	0.865
Gestational age at birth (weeks), Mean (SD)	39.3 (1.2)	39.2 (1.3)	39.2 (1.6)	39.4 (1.3)	39.5 (1.5)	0.684

3.2. Total Amino Acids

The levels of TAA were compared across different lactation stages after adjusting for maternal age and BMI as well as for mode of delivery, infant gender, and geographical location.

The sum of TAA in milk samples significantly decreased with increasing lactation stage until the 2–4-month milk, which did not differ significantly from that at 4–8 months (Figure 2A). Median values ranged between 1608 mg/100 g and 1053 mg/100 g in the 5–11-day and the 2–4-month samples, respectively.

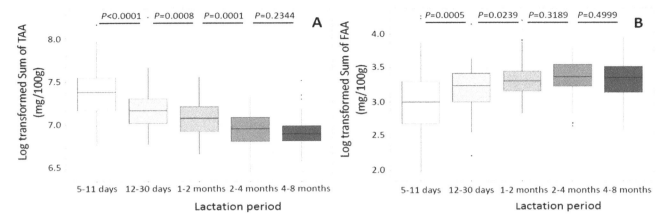

Figure 2. Box plot of the log-transformed sum of total (TAA, (**A**)) and of free (FAA, (**B**)) amino acids in milk from the different lactation periods. n = 90 milk samples per lactation period. Statistically significant differences between two periods were set at $p < 0.05$.

Concentrations of total IAA are reported in Table 2. Leucine and methionine were respectively the most and the least abundant IAA in our sample set across all the lactation stages. The levels of all IAA were highest in the early milk samples and then decreased with increasing lactation period until 2–4 months. Some differences of lower magnitude were still perceived between the two latest lactation stages; in particular, the levels of Leucine, lysine, and methionine were higher and the levels of histidine and phenylalanine were lower in 2–4-month than in 4–8-month milk.

Table 2. Total amino acid content (mg/100 g) of milk from the different lactation periods.

	5–11 Days	**12–30 Days**	**1–2 Months**	**2–4 Months**	**4–8 Months**
			Lactation Period		
IAA [†]					
Histidine	51.2 (19.9)	44.5 [§] (14.1)	36.5 [§] (12.6)	34.9 [§] (7.2)	25.0 [§] (6.8)
Isoleucine	81.0 (23.4)	71.6 [§] (15.4)	64.6 [§] (16.8)	54.0 [§] (11.6)	53.8 (10.7)
Leucine	153.7 (63.2)	133.7 [§] (35.1)	130.3 (33.5)	108.1 [§] (24.9)	122.6 [§] (38.8)
Lysine	112.0 (31.0)	93.8 [§] (23.1)	78.8 [§] (18.9)	63.4 [§] (13.1)	67.9 [§] (13.1)
Methionine	21.8 (11.7)	16.7 [§] (6.6)	13.0 [§] (9.0)	9.2 [§] (6.1)	11.8 [§] (7.1)
Phenylalanine	64.4 (35.9)	52.4 [§] (18.3)	40.4 [§] (13.6)	37.6 [§] (10.8)	28.4 [§] (9.0)
Threonine	85.1 (28.1)	66.9 [§] (14.6)	58.0 [§] (13.3)	50.0 [§] (8.7)	48.6 (11.3)
Valine	97.9 (34.3)	81.1 [§] (16.7)	72.1 [§] (21.0)	59.7 [§] (16.0)	60.9 (12.7)
DAA [†]					
Alanine	70.9 (23.0)	55.9 [§] (14.3)	45.9 [§] (15.7)	38.7 [§] (10.9)	38.6 (9.1)
Arginine	106.5 (36.6)	90.8 [§] (22.8)	77.0 [§] (24.5)	64.6 [§] (21.3)	65.3 (16.7)
Asx [‡]	132.9 (84.1)	115.5 [§] (54.4)	106.9 (40.0)	97.2 (56.8)	83.8 [§] (24.6)
Cystine	25.4 (12.5)	17.7 [§] (6.3)	12.5 [§] (5.2)	12.3 (3.4)	9.9 [§] (5.5)
Glx [‡]	248.1 (193.7)	220.1 [§] (92.4)	216.3 (59.3)	188.6 (105.2)	182.8 [§] (30.8)
Glycine	46.3 (15.2)	34.5 [§] (9.7)	27.6 [§] (10.5)	23.6 [§] (7.0)	23.5 (6.8)
Proline	140.2 (42.4)	117.7 [§] (26.5)	110.6 [§] (25.4)	95.3 [§] (20.9)	94.5 (17.2)
Serine	77.8 (27.0)	59.0 [§] (14.1)	47.9 [§] (9.8)	42.9 [§] (8.1)	41.7 (8.0)
Tyrosine	72.5 (30.4)	57.7 [§] (14.1)	44.1 [§] (19.5)	41.4 (13.9)	37.1 [§] (10.3)
SUM	1608.3 (589.5)	1296.5 [§] (368.4)	1188.1 [§] (341.7)	1053.2 [§] (291.9)	992.4 (175.9)

[†] IAA = indispensable amino acids; DAA = dispensable amino acid; [‡] Asx = sum of aspartic acid + asparagine; Glx = sum of glutamic acid + glutamine. Medians (inter-quartile ranges) of n = 90 samples per lactation period are shown. A median with a "§" superscript is significantly different from the median of the previous lactation period ($p < 0.05$).

Regarding dispensable amino acids (DAA) (Table 2) Glx (sum of glutamic acid + glutamine) was the most and cystine the least abundant amino acids. Again, the highest concentration for all DAA was recorded in the earliest milk (i.e., 5–11 days), and a subsequent decrease was observed in most DAA across the intermediate time points until reaching similar levels at the two latest lactation stages. In contrast, stable levels were observed for Glx and Asx (sum of aspartic acid + asparagine) between the 12–30-day and 2–4-month milk. A further decrease occurred in the 4–8-month samples.

3.3. Free Amino Acids

The levels of FAA were compared across the different lactation stages after adjusting for maternal age and BMI as well as for mode of delivery, infant gender, and geographical location.

In contrast to TAA, the sum of the individual FAA content was lower in the first compared with the latest lactation stages, with median values ranging between 20.1 mg/100 g of milk at 5–11 days and 29.0 mg/100 g of milk at 2–4 months (Figure 2B).

Concentrations of the individual FAA are reported in Table 3. Glx was the most abundant in FAA across the data set, and its concentration was higher in mature milk than in early-stage milk. In the latest lactation stages, it contributed up to more than 70% of the FAA mass. Similarly to Glx, levels of alanine, cystine, glycine, and serine were lowest in the early-stage milk. Opposite changes were observed in free IAA, of which highest concentrations were generally found in early-stage samples. The only exception was threonine, which remained stable across the lactation periods.

Table 3. Free AA content (mg/100 g) of milk from the different lactation periods.

	Lactation Period				
	5–11 Days	**12–30 Days**	**1–2 Months**	**2–4 Months**	**4–8 Months**
IAA [†]					
Histidine	0.29 (0.21)	0.42 [§] (0.23)	0.33 [§] (0.15)	0.33 (0.19)	0.28 (0.10)
Isoleucine	0.17 (0.11)	0.19 (0.13)	0.13 [§] (0.10)	0.13 (0.07)	0.15 [§] (0.07)
Leucine	0.33 (0.20)	0.4 (0.2)	0.34 [§] (0.14)	0.33 (0.14)	0.34 (0.15)
Lysine	0.61 (0.51)	0.56 [§] (0.28)	0.46 [§] (0.20)	0.42 [§] (0.23)	0.54 [§] (0.28)
Methionine	0.11 (0.07)	0.13 (0.13)	0.10 [§] (0.07)	0.07 [§] (0.06)	0.12 [§] (0.05)
Phenylalanine	0.31 (0.17)	0.40 (0.17)	0.32 [§] (0.17)	0.33 (0.17)	0.30 (0.12)
Threonine	0.69 (0.38)	0.69 (0.36)	0.70 (0.36)	0.78 (0.34)	0.85 (0.38)
Valine	0.58 (0.27)	0.70 [§] (0.30)	0.61 [§] (0.21)	0.59 (0.21)	0.59 (0.18)
DAA [†]					
Alanine	1.26 (0.81)	1.75 [§] (0.79)	2.07 [§] (0.67)	1.93 (0.68)	1.85 (0.46)
Arginine	0.46 (0.49)	0.42 [§] (0.28)	0.25 [§] (0.22)	0.25 (0.19)	0.25 (0.13)
Asx [‡]	0.47 (0.36)	0.52 (0.30)	0.54 (0.35)	0.55 (0.38)	0.58 (0.40)
Cystine	0.32 (0.13)	0.49 [§] (0.21)	0.46 (0.17)	0.49 (0.21)	0.50 (0.15)
Glx [‡]	10.89 (9.89)	15.09 [§] (8.74)	18.03 [§] (7.17)	20.22 [§] (7.28)	19.36 (8.07)
Glycine	0.51 (0.29)	0.62 [§] (0.23)	0.68 [§] (0.25)	0.64 (0.28)	0.76 [§] (0.28)
Proline	0.56 (0.33)	0.40 [§] (0.28)	0.54 (0.29)	0.40 (0.31)	0.45 [§] (0.44)
Serine	0.72 (0.43)	0.85 [§] (0.36)	0.91 [§] (0.40)	1.11 [§] (0.63)	1.11 (0.43)
Taurine	2.26 (2.65)	1.91 (1.78)	1.94 (1.31)	1.87 (1.42)	2.03 (1.12)
Tyrosine	0.38 (0.26)	0.40 (0.20)	0.28 [§] (0.17)	0.25 (0.14)	0.28 [§] (0.13)
SUM	20.1 (12.5)	25.5 [§] (10.4)	27.4 [§] (8.0)	29.0 (9.7)	28.6 (10.7)

[†] IAA = indispensable amino acids; DAA = dispensable amino acid; [‡] Asx = sum of aspartic acid + asparagine; Glx = sum of glutamic acid + glutamine. Medians (inter-quartile ranges) of n = 90 samples per lactation period are shown. A median with a "[§]" superscript is significantly different from the median of the previous lactation period ($p < 0.05$).

The contribution of FAA to TAA levels was less than 2% for most amino acids studied. A major exception was free Glx, which, on average, contributed to around 8% of the total Glx concentration. The ratio of free to total Glx gradually increased across the increasing lactation stages, from less than 5% at 5–11 days up to more than 10% at 4–8 months.

Of note is that compared with the TAA (Table 2) inter-individual variability in FAA values was very high (Table 3).

4. Discussion

Amino acids are an essential component in infant nutrition, and their levels in breast milk are believed to be optimal to support healthy growth during the first months of life. Because of this, the amino acid intake from human milk is considered to match infant requirements, and the breast milk amino acid content is used to estimate the protein quality and quantity in breast milk substitutes [3]. Therefore, a reliable evaluation of the amino acid composition in breast milk is important.

The concentration of the sum of TAA—a good proxy of the true protein content—at the different lactation stages was, in our samples, remarkably similar to that reported in transitional, mature, and late milk in a recent systematic review of studies from Africa, Asia, Europe, and North America [8]. A limitation in our study, however, is the lack of colostrum samples. This said, although colostrum is important for the protection of the neonate, the amount of amino acids provided by the colostrum protein is likely limited due to the low secreted volumes as well as to the relatively low digestibility of the major colostrum proteins [13]. Similar to the results reported in the systematic review by Zhang et al. [8], the sum of TAA was greater in the early stage of lactation, slowly declining in concentration as lactation progressed, reaching generally stable levels after 2–4 months. These changes are consistent with the protein content results of the MING study reported elsewhere [11] and with the well-known evolution of the protein content in breast milk, i.e., high during the early lactation stages, and sharply decreasing during the transitional milk period to level off in mature milk [13]. It has been proposed that these changes in the amino acid content of the milk match the infant requirements for growth, which is fast during the neonatal period sharply decreasing during the first months of life [14]. Declining protein concentrations may also prevent amino acid overfeeding as milk volume intake per unit body weight increases along lactation [3,4]. Of note, protein concentration in human milk is remarkably low compared with that from most other mammals. Low protein intake during infancy is believed to protect the individual against obesity and metabolic disease later in life, possibly related to optimal appetite and hormonal programming [15].

The levels of individual TAA's in the different lactation stages of the MING cohort were also close to those reported by Zhang et al. [8]. The only amino acid showing a consistently lower value in our samples was cystine. However, cystine is known to be particularly sensitive to the acid treatment used for protein hydrolysis in our samples [16], and the cystine levels that we report here may underestimate the real values.

Globally, the individual TAA levels showed similar temporal patterns as the sum of TAA. However, whereas a strong decrease between early, transitional, and mature milk was observed for some amino acids such as methionine, cystine, and glycine, this drop was less substantial for Glx levels, which were comparable in transitional and mature milk. This observation is consistent with the fact that besides the variations in protein content, changes in the quality of the protein occur along lactation. Specifically, a significant decline in the concentration of the sulfur amino acid-rich and glycine-rich whey proteins but stable levels of the Glx-rich casein were found in our milk samples [17] and are usually reported [18], resulting in a whey to casein ratio that increases throughout lactation [13] and, as observed in our samples, in an evolving amino acid profile.

As expected from previous reports [6], the contribution of FAA to the TAA mass was less than 3% in all lactation periods. Because of this, the contribution of the FAA to the nutritional requirements of the infant is expected to be low. The physiological importance of FAA for infants is not yet well understood. It has been proposed that FAA are more rapidly absorbed, leading to accelerated appearance in the systemic circulation and thus reaching the peripheral organs faster than the protein-bound amino acids [6,8]. However, to our knowledge, the absorption kinetics of free and protein-bound amino acids in breast milk has never been compared, and the physiological relevance of a potentially faster delivery to the peripheral tissue of the small FAA load delivered by milk remains speculative.

Free Glx was very abundant in our samples, contributing to around 70% of the FAA mass and reaching up to 10% of the total Glx levels in the later lactation periods. Similar observations have also previously been reported where both glutamic acid and glutamine were shown to be the most abundant FAA in human milk throughout the first trimester of lactation [19]. Specifically, the authors of [19] reported a 2.5- and 20-fold increase in glutamic acid and glutamine FAA concentrations, respectively, with progressing lactation. It should be noted that, similar to our findings, these FAAs represented more than 50% of total FAAs at three months [19]. Total Glx was also the most concentrated TAA in our samples, suggesting an important role of this amino acid on the mammary gland metabolism, on infant nutrition, or both, despite the fact that glutamic acid and glutamine are considered DAA that can be synthesized by the body [20]. More specifically, the transamination of glutamic acid by the mucosal intestinal cells yields alanine, which enters the gluconeogenic pathway. In addition, both glutamic acid and glutamine from the lumen act as major energy substrates for the intestinal cells [21,22]. In the neonatal pig for instance, the gastrointestinal tract uses dietary glutamine and glutamate as its key respiratory fuel. In humans, trials with very low birth weight infants and critically ill adult patients highlight the central role of glutamic acid and glutamine in protecting intestinal growth and integrity [23–25], therefore suggesting glutamic acid and glutamine as important molecules in milk for the immature infant gut. More recent results from Ventura et al. [7] also suggest a role of Glutamate on the satiety status of the lactating infant.

Similar to Glx, free alanine, cystine, glycine, and serine also increased along the lactation periods in our samples. Intriguingly, similar findings were reported in the systematic review by Zhang et al. [8], indicating a consistent pattern in stage-associated changes independent of ethnic or geographic factors. This consistency is outstanding in light of the important inter-individual FAA variability in our study, the inter-study variability observed in the report by Zhang et al., and even the intra-individual changes reported by others in transitional and mature breast milk [26]. However, the physiological significance of the concentration rise of these DAA through lactation is not clear. Furthermore, understanding the physiological relevance of the increased inter-individual variability observed in FAA needs to be elucidated.

An important limitation in our study is that our analytical method did not permit to quantify the concentration of tryptophan. Yet the IAA tryptophan is usually the limiting amino acid in infant formula; thus, its concentration in breast milk is often used to estimate the protein quality and to adjust the level of the protein in the formula. Another limitation is the cross-sectional nature of the study that weakens the conclusions related to the stage-driven changes, which would have been best assessed by a longitudinal design. However, our statistical model adjusted for the maternal and infant baseline factors that were known or suspected to impact milk nutrient composition [1], including maternal weight and mode of delivery, which differed between the lactation period cohorts. Our results are also reinforced by the fact that they were remarkably consistent with those previously published.

5. Conclusions

In conclusion, the amino acid composition of the milk from our cohort of urban Chinese mothers was comparable to human milk data from previously reported studies carried out in other parts of the world, suggesting that amino acid composition in breast milk is an evolutionary conserved trait largely independent of geographical, ethnical, or dietary factors.

Acknowledgments: The authors would like to thank the funding sources of this work and Nestec Ltd. for covering the costs for publishing open access. Special acknowledgment to the participants who volunteered for this study: Lawrence Li for project support and guidance, Celia Ning for project management, Qiaoji Li for clinical project management, and Emilie Ba for data management. Special acknowledgment to Jiaji Wang at Guangzhou Medical University, Liqiang Qin at Soochow University School of Public Health and their teams, as well as the project staff at Peking University School of Public Health for their tasks in recruitment and data collection. The Nestlé Research Center and the Nestlé Nutrition Institute China sponsored the study.

Author Contributions: C.L.G.R., L.G.K., and M.A. interpreted the results, drafted, reviewed, and revised the initial manuscript. G.V.P. contributed to the study design, drafted, reviewed, and revised the initial manuscript. S.K.T. contributed to the study design, the breast milk sampling protocol, and the interpretation of the results. Y.Z. and P.W. contributed to study design and performed field collection. C.D.C. performed the statistical analysis and reviewed and revised the initial manuscript. All authors read and approved the final manuscript.

References

1. Stam, J.; Sauer, P.J.; Boehm, G. Can we define an infant's need from the composition of human milk? *Am. J. Clin. Nutr.* **2013**, *98*, 521S–528S. [CrossRef] [PubMed]

2. Michaelsen, K.F.; Greer, F.R. Protein needs early in life and long-term health. *Am. J. Clin. Nutr.* **2014**, *99*, 718S–722S. [CrossRef] [PubMed]

3. World Health Organization; Food and Agriculture Organization of the United Nations; United Nations University. *Joint FAO/WHO/UNU Expert Consultation on Protein and Amino Acid Requirements in Human Nutrition*; WHO technical report series; WHO Press: Geneva, Switzerland, 2007; Volume 935, pp. 1–265.

4. Da Costa, T.H.; Haisma, H.; Wells, J.C.; Mander, A.P.; Whitehead, R.G.; Bluck, L.J. How much human milk do infants consume? Data from 12 countries using a standardized stable isotope methodology. *J. Nutr.* **2010**, *140*, 2227–2232. [CrossRef] [PubMed]

5. Svanberg, U.; Gebre-Medhin, M.; Ljungqvist, B.; Olsson, M. Breast milk composition in Ethiopian and Swedish mothers. III. Amino acids and other nitrogenous substances. *Am. J. Clin. Nutr.* **1977**, *30*, 499–507. [PubMed]

6. Carratu, B.; Boniglia, C.; Scalise, F.; Ambruzzib, A.M.; Sanzinia, E. Nitrogenous components of human milk: Non-protein nitrogen, true protein and free amino acids. *Food Chem.* **2003**, *81*, 357–362. [CrossRef]

7. Ventura, A.K.; Beauchamp, G.K.; Mennella, J.A. Infant regulation of intake: The effect of free glutamate content in infant formulas. *Am. J. Clin. Nutr.* **2012**, *95*, 875–881. [CrossRef] [PubMed]

8. Zhang, Z.; Adelman, A.S.; Rai, D.; Boettcher, J.; Lőnnerdal, B. Amino acid profiles in term and preterm human milk through lactation: A systematic review. *Nutrients* **2013**, *5*, 4800–4821. [CrossRef] [PubMed]

9. Zhao, X.; Xu, Z.; Wang, Y.; Sun, Y. Studies of the relation between the nutritional status of lactating mothers and milk composition as well as the milk intake and growth of their infants in Beijing. Pt. 4. The protein and amino acid content of breast milk. *Acta Nutr. Sin.* **1989**, *11*, 227–232.

10. Ding, M.; Li, W.; Zhang, Y.; Wang, X.; Zhao, A.; Zhao, X.; Wang, P.; Sheng, Q.H. Amino acid composition of lactating mothers' milk and confinement diet in rural North China. *Asia Pac. J. Clin. Nutr.* **2010**, *19*, 344–349. [PubMed]

11. Yang, T.; Zhang, Y.; Ning, Y.; You, L.; Ma, D.; Zheng, Y.; Yang, X.; Li, W.; Wang, J.; Wang, P. Breast milk macronutrient composition and the associated factors in urban Chinese mothers. *Chin. Med. J. (Engl.)* **2014**, *127*, 1721–1725. [PubMed]

12. Blankenship, D.T.; Krivanek, M.A.; Ackermann, B.L.; Cardin, A.D. High-sensitivity amino acid analysis by derivatization with O-phthalaldehyde and 9-fluorenylmethyl chloroformate using fluorescence detection: Applications in protein structure determination. *Anal. Biochem.* **1989**, *178*, 227–232. [CrossRef]

13. Lonnerdal, B. Nutritional and physiologic significance of human milk proteins. *Am. J. Clin. Nutr.* **2003**, *77*, 1537S–1543S. [PubMed]

14. Dupont, C. Protein requirements during the first year of life. *Am. J. Clin. Nutr.* **2003**, *77*, 1544S–1549S. [PubMed]

15. Hassiotou, F.; Geddes, D.T. Programming of appetite control during breastfeeding as a preventative strategy against the obesity epidemic. *J. Hum. Lac.* **2014**, *30*, 136–142. [CrossRef] [PubMed]

16. Peace, R.W.; Gilani, G.S. Chromatographic determination of amino acids in foods. *J. AOAC Int.* **2005**, *88*, 877–887. [PubMed]

17. Affolter, M.; Garcia-Rodenas, C.L.; Vinyes-Pares, G.; Jenni, R.; Roggero, I.; Avanti-Nigro, O.; de Castro, C.A.; Zhao, A.; Zhang, Y.; Wang, P.; et al. Temporal Changes of Protein Composition in Breast Milk of Chinese Urban Mothers and Impact of Caesarean Section Delivery. *Nutrients* **2016**, *8*, E504. [CrossRef] [PubMed]

18. Sindayikengera, S.; Xia, W.S. Nutritional evaluation of caseins and whey proteins and their hydrolysates from Protamex. *J. Zhejiang Univ. Sci. B* **2006**, *7*, 90–98. [CrossRef] [PubMed]

19. Agostoni, C.; Carratu, B.; Boniglia, C.; Lammardo, A.M.; Riva, E.; Sanzini, E. Free glutamine and glutamic acid increase in human milk through a three-month lactation period. *J. Pediatr. Gastroenterol. Nutr.* **2000**, *31*, 508–512. [CrossRef] [PubMed]
20. Reeds, P.J. Dispensable and indispensable amino acids for humans. *J. Nutr.* **2000**, *130*, 1835S–1840S. [PubMed]
21. Reeds, P.J.; Burrin, D.G. Glutamine and the bowel. *J. Nutr.* **2001**, *131*, 2505S–2508S. [PubMed]
22. Rezaei, R.; Wang, W.; Wu, Z.; Dai, Z.; Wang, J.; Wu, G. Biochemical and physiological bases for utilization of dietary amino acids by young pigs. *J. Anim. Sci. Biotechnol.* **2013**, *4*, 7. [CrossRef] [PubMed]
23. Van der Hulst, R.R.; van Kreel, B.K.; von Meyenfeldt, M.F.; Brummer, R.J.; Arends, J.W.; Deutz, N.E.; Soeters, P.B. Glutamine and the preservation of gut integrity. *Lancet* **1993**, *341*, 1363–1365. [CrossRef]
24. Roig, J.C.; Meetze, W.H.; Auestad, N.; Jasionowski, T.; Veerman, M.; McMurray, C.A.; Neu, J. Enteral glutamine supplementation for the very low birthweight infant: Plasma amino acid concentrations. *J. Nutr.* **1996**, *126*, 1115S–1120S. [PubMed]
25. Burrin, D.G.; Stoll, B. Key nutrients and growth factors for the neonatal gastrointestinal tract. *Clin. Perinatol.* **2002**, *29*, 65–96. [CrossRef]
26. Sánchez, C.L.; Cubero, J.; Sánchez, J.; Franco, L.; Rodríguez, A.B.; Rivero, M.; Barriga, C. Evolution of the circadian profile of human milk amino acids during breastfeeding. *J. Appl. Biomed.* **2013**, *11*, 59–70. [CrossRef]

4

On the Importance of Processing Conditions for the Nutritional Characteristics of Homogenized Composite Meals Intended for Infants

Elin Östman *, Anna Forslund, Eden Tareke and Inger Björck

Food for Health Science Centre, Lund University, P.O. Box 124, 221 00 Lund, Sweden;
anna.k.forslund@gmail.com (A.F.); eden.tareke@food-health-science.lu.se (E.T.);
inger.bjorck@food-health-science.lu.se (I.B.)
* Correspondence: elin.ostman@food-health-science.lu.se

Abstract: The nutritional quality of infant food is an important consideration in the effort to prevent a further increase in the rate of childhood obesity. We hypothesized that the canning of composite infant meals would lead to elevated contents of carboxymethyl-lysine (CML) and favor high glycemic and insulinemic responses compared with milder heat treatment conditions. We have compared composite infant pasta Bolognese meals that were either conventionally canned (CANPBol), or prepared by microwave cooking (MWPBol). A meal where the pasta and Bolognese sauce were separate during microwave cooking (MWP_CANBol) was also included. The infant meals were tested at breakfast in healthy adults using white wheat bread (WWB) as reference. A standardized lunch meal was served at 240 min and blood was collected from fasting to 360 min after breakfast. The 2-h glucose response (iAUC) was lower following the test meals than with WWB. The insulin response was lower after the MWP_CANBol (-47%, $p = 0.0000$) but markedly higher after CANPBol ($+40\%$, $p = 0.0019$), compared with WWB. A combined measure of the glucose and insulin responses ($ISI_{composite}$) revealed that MWP_CANBol resulted in 94% better insulin sensitivity than CANPBol. Additionally, the separate processing of the meal components in MWP_CANBol resulted in 39% lower CML levels than the CANPBol. It was therefore concluded that intake of commercially canned composite infant meals leads to reduced postprandial insulin sensitivity and increased exposure to oxidative stress promoting agents.

Keywords: infant food; glycemia; insulinemia; human; advanced glycation end products; carboxymethyl-lysine; early protein hypothesis; protein quality; carbohydrate digestibility; glycemic index

1. Introduction

In the development of infant formulas, weaning food, and composite infant meals, the main aim has traditionally been to ensure the provision of adequate amounts of essential nutrients. Great interest has therefore been devoted to the availability of certain nutrients, such as protein and selected minerals. Two nutritional quality characteristics that are emphasized in food for adults are the availability of carbohydrates affecting the glycemic response, and the presence of process-induced advanced glycation end products (AGEs), which affect the biological value of the protein. Carbohydrate-rich foods with low glycemic impact were recently classified as relevant for the prevention and treatment of type 2 diabetes, coronary heart disease, and probably obesity [1]. High-glycemic meals have been associated with the increased activation of inflammatory markers in the postprandial phase [2]. Elevated intakes of AGEs are of interest due to their association with cardiometabolic risk markers and pathological conditions such as diabetes [3–5]. In the case of powder-based weaning foods, considerable and varying amounts of AGEs were recently reported in milk powder, infant formulas, and gruel [6,7]. Furthermore, high intakes of ultra-processed food products were recently positively and independently associated with increased prevalence of excess weight gain and obesity in different age groups in Brazil [8]. It is interesting to note that composite canned meals intended for small children are subjected to high-temperature treatment. Excessive heat treatment is known to affect the availability of the carbohydrate component [9], and the homogenization of composite infant meals prior to canning is likely to further increase the availability of the carbohydrate components for digestion and absorption [10]. Additionally, homogenization of the meal components could be expected to boost AGE formation by enhancing the accessibility of the necessary precursors.

Based on the above, we hypothesized that the canning of homogenized composite infant meals may render carbohydrates and protein rapidly available for digestion and absorption, leading to high blood glucose and insulin responses. Furthermore, it was hypothesized that the increased availability of carbohydrates and proteins would result in the formation of higher levels of AGEs than in less harshly processed composite meals. The objectives of the present work were to establish some of the nutritional quality characteristics of canned homogenized composite meals intended for infants, and to compare them with more gently processed alternatives.

2. Methods

Two studies were performed, the first of which involved a commercially canned pasta Bolognese meal and a canned composite meal with beef and white beans (Study 1). In the second study, a commercially canned pasta Bolognese meal (purée with some intact soft pieces) was again used and compared with a similar but microwave heat-treated meal (cracked spaghetti with minced meat and vegetables). Separately boiled cracked spaghetti served with a commercially canned meat sauce was also included. White wheat bread (WWB) was used as a reference [11] in both studies to allow the determination of the glycemic index (GI) and the insulinemic index (II). The GI is defined as the incremental area under the blood glucose curve (iAUC) following the intake of a test meal, expressed as a percentage of an equi-carbohydrate reference meal, eaten by the same subject. The II is calculated similarly, based on the corresponding insulin responses. WWB is a starch-rich product considered to be a more physiologically relevant reference product than pure glucose, due to its more complex food matrix. The meal studies were performed in healthy adults to investigate the postprandial effects on glucose and insulin. In Study 2, non-esterified fatty acids (NEFAs) and triglycerides (TGs) were also analyzed. N-carboxymethyl-lysine (CML) was used as a marker of AGEs. The CML contents in some commercially canned composite infant meals and relevant composite frozen meals intended for adults were included for comparison. All test products were heated to eating temperature prior to the analysis of CML, determination of rate of *in vitro* starch hydrolysis, or being served as a test meal.

2.1. General Study Design

Healthy adult volunteers were recruited for the studies. All test subjects gave their informed consent, and were aware that they could withdraw from the study at any time. The studies were approved by the Regional Ethical Review Board in Lund (LU 558-01 and 2012/615). The test meals and the reference meal were served as breakfast in a random order, after overnight fasting. The tests were performed approximately one week apart and commenced at the same time in the morning. Subjects were instructed to maintain their regular lifestyle throughout the period of the study. The day prior to a test they were told to avoid alcohol, excessive physical activity, and food rich in dietary fiber. On the evening (21.00–22.00) before each test, the subjects were instructed to eat a standardized meal consisting of white wheat bread with spread and drink of their own choice. However, the subjects were instructed to have the same evening meal before each test.

2.2. Study 1

Five men and four women aged 24–41 years, with normal body mass indices (23.1 $\pm$ 2.7 kg/m^2; mean $\pm$ SD), normal fasting blood glucose (4.4 $\pm$ 0.05 mmol/L; mean $\pm$ SEM), and who were not taking any medication, participated in the study. The test subjects were recruited and the study performed between October 1999 and February 2000. Test subjects were recruited by advertising on notice boards around the Lund University (LU) campus, and by contacting former volunteers. Two commercially available canned composite meals, "canned Meat&Pasta" and "canned Meat&Beans", intended for infants aged 12 months, were studied. The meals were microwave heated according to the manufacturer's instructions before serving. Both test meals and the reference WWB meal contained 30 g of potentially available carbohydrates [12]. Both the test meals and the reference meal were served with 250 mL water and followed by 150 mL coffee or tea. Finger-prick capillary blood samples were taken repeatedly up to 120 min after ingesting the meal for the analysis of blood glucose concentrations (glucose oxidase-peroxidase reagent) and serum insulin (Insulin ELISA, Mercodia AB, Uppsala, Sweden).

Product Characterization

Levels of CML were determined in freeze-dried samples of selected canned composite infant meals and corresponding frozen ready-to-eat meals intended for adults using gas chromatography mass spectrometry (GC-MS) according to Birlouez-Aragon [3]. The results are presented in Table 1. The *in vitro* rate of starch hydrolysis (hydrolysis index, HI) was analyzed for the meals using the method described by Granfeldt *et al.* [13]. Before HI-analysis, samples of the composite meals were rinsed in a strainer using tap water to obtain the intact pieces of the carbohydrate sources (beans and pasta).

2.3. Study 2

2.3.1. Recipes and Processing Conditions

Canned pasta Bolognese (CANPBol) for infants aged 12 months was bought in the local supermarket, and two other test meals were prepared in the laboratory. In order to investigate the possible advantages of minimal processing of a composite meal, an in-pack pasteurization method was used (MicVac AB, Mölndal, Sweden). The microwave cooked test meal (MWPBol) was based on a recipe resembling that of the CANPBol meal, and contained: 60 g water, 50 g crushed tomatoes (ICA, Solna, Sweden), 17 g carrots, 17 g yellow onions, 16 g minced beef, 13 g manually cracked spaghetti (ICA Italia, Solna, Sweden), 10 g tomato purée (ICA), 10 g celery root, 2 g corn starch (Maizena, Unilever, Solna, Sweden), 2 g rapeseed oil (ICA), 0.15 g iodized salt (Falksalt, Ab Hanson & Möhring, Halmstad, Sweden), 0.2 g dry oregano (Santa Maria, Mölndal, Sweden), 0.1 g dry basil (Santa Maria), and 0.07 g white pepper (Santa Maria). A test meal consisting of separately microwave-cooked pieces of spaghetti (ICA Italia) and canned Bolognese sauce (Felix Köttfärsås Original, Orkla Foods, Eslöv, Sweden) was used to study the effect of preparing the meal components separately (MWP_CANBol). All pasta and canned Bolognese sauce were bought from one batch. In the case of the MWPBol meal, all dried/canned ingredients and minced beef was bought from one batch, but vegetables were bought fresh every week. The minced beef was frozen in portions and thawed prior to the preparation of each serving. Each MWPBol portion was prepared the evening before the test by combining the minced meat with small pieces of the vegetables, crushed tomatoes, spices, and cracked spaghetti. After sealing the tray with plastic film, the portion was cooked in a microwave oven for 8 min, chilled on ice and then stored overnight in a refrigerator. Just before serving, MWPBol meal was reheated in microwave oven for 1.5 min. In the case of the MWP_CANBol meal, cracked spaghetti was boiled in water for 7.5 min using a similar tray sealed with plastic film in microwave oven and stored in the refrigerator overnight. In the morning, the pasta was heated separately for 2 min, and the canned Bolognese sauce was heated separately for 2.5 min, in the microwave oven. The pasta and Bolognese sauce were then mixed on the plate before serving. Each CANPBol portion was weighed on a plate just before serving, and microwave heated for 2.5 min, with breaks for stirring after 1 and 2 min.

2.3.2. Product Characterization

All test and reference meals in Study 2 were standardized so as to contain 35 g available starch, according to Holm et al. [12]. The CANPBol meal and the canned Bolognese sauce were analyzed as bought, without preparation. The microwave-cooked spaghetti was re-heated before analysis, and the starch content converted to dry matter basis. The protein contents in the test meals were determined using an elemental analyzer (FlashEA 1112, Thermo Fischer Scientific Inc., Waltham, MA, USA). The fat contents in the commercial products were estimated from the manufacturers' declarations. In the case of WWB, estimates of the protein and fat contents were based on a previous analysis of a similar product [14]. CML was determined using high-pressure liquid chromatography mass spectrometry (HPLC-MS/MS), with an Accela UHPLC pump with an autoinjector coupled to an LTQ VelosPro Orbitrap mass spectrometer (Thermo Scientific, Waltham, MA, USA). The MS/MS was run in positive electrospray ionization ion trap mode, detecting two selected reaction monitoring (SRM) transitions for CML and two for the internal standard. Xcalibur software (ver. 2.2, Thermo Scientific) was used for both data acquisition and evaluation. Samples were prepared by hydrolyzing 0.3 g sample for 12 h at 110 °C, using 6 M HCl, together with isotope-labelled d4-CML (Larodan Fine Chemicals AB, Malmö, Sweden) as internal standard. CML was extracted after hydrolysis using solid phase extraction (TelosneoPCX, Teknolab Sorbent AB, Västra Frölunda, Sweden). All the dried samples were reconstituted in 0.01% (v/v) nonafluoropentanoic acid (Sigma-Aldrich, Steinheim, Germany) and centrifuged before analysis. Solid phase extraction, chromatographic parameters, ion source parameters, and the SRM transitions were the same as described by Tareke et al. [6,7]. CML analyses were performed on three different days. To check any instrumental inconsistency, duplicates of each sample were analyzed on one occasion. The portion sizes, macronutrient and energy compositions, and the CML contents are presented in Table 2.

2.3.3. Subjects

The inclusion criteria were being a healthy, non-smoker with normal weight (body mass index, BMI, 19–25 kg/m^2), aged 18–40 years, with a stable body weight over the previous two months. Exclusion criteria were being a vegetarian/vegan and/or having food allergies, lactose intolerance, having any disease or taking any medication that might affect the study, as well as being pregnant or lactating.

2.3.4. Sample Collection and Protocol

The subjects arrived at the laboratory at 7:45 a.m. after overnight fasting. A peripheral venous catheter (BD Venflon Dickinson, Helsingborg, Sweden) was inserted into an antecubital vein. Capillary plasma glucose and venous blood samples were collected, after which the individually assigned test meal was served, together with 250 g of tap water (time 0). All meals were tolerated and finished within 10–15 min, except for one test person who needed 20 min to finish eating the CANPBol meal. Blood samples were taken at 15, 30, 45, 60, 90, 120, 240, 270, 300, 330, and 360 min after the beginning of the meal. One hundred and thirty-five minutes after the meal, each subject was given 200 g water to be drunk within 15 min. Two hundred and forty-five minutes after the start of the meal, a standardized lunch, consisting of a ready-to-eat dish of 400 g (2320 kJ) pasta with tomatoes, basil, and mozzarella cheese (Pasta al Pomodoro, Gooh, Lantmännen, Sweden) was served. The lunch meal was served with 250 g tap water, and was to be consumed within 20 min.

2.3.5. Blood Analysis

Blood glucose was analyzed in capillary blood (HemoCue®B-glucose, HemoCue AB, Ängelholm, Sweden). Serum was obtained from venous blood collected in CAT tubes (BD Vacutainer, ref. 368492) and left to clot for 60 min before being centrifuged at 3500 rpm for 10 min at 4 °C. Plasma was obtained in EDTA tubes (BD Vacutainer, ref 368274) and put on ice for a maximum of 30 min until centrifuged at 3500 rpm for 10 min at 4 °C. Samples were then aliquoted in Eppendorf tubes and stored immediately at −20 °C until analysis. Serum insulin and serum TGs were analyzed by a lab at Skåne University Hospital (Clinical Chemistry, Region Skåne, Sweden), whereas NEFAs were analyzed at the department using a colorimetric assay (NEFA C, ACS-ACOD method, WAKO Chemicals GmbH, Neuss, Germany).

3. Statistical Calculations

The least number of subjects required to detect a difference in the GI with a power of 80% at a level of $p < 0.05$, is ten [15]. The sample size in Study 1 was nine, and in order to improve the power of Study 2, twenty-one subjects were included. The iAUCs for glucose and insulin were calculated using GraphPad Prism (GraphPad Software, San Diego, CA, USA) and the trapezoid model. All areas below the baseline were excluded from the calculations. The results are expressed as means ± SEM. Differences resulting in $p < 0.05$ were considered statistically significant.

3.1. Study 1

The 120 min blood glucose and insulin iAUCs were used to determine GI and II, respectively. The statistical differences were evaluated using the general linear model (ANOVA) followed by Tukey's multiple comparisons test using Minitab software (ver. 13, Minitab Inc., State College, PA, USA).

3.2. Study 2

Differences in CML content between the test meals and the reference meal were evaluated with one-way ANOVA using GraphPad Prism (as described above). The composite insulin sensitivity index ($ISI_{composite}$), also called the Matsuda index, was calculated for both the test meals and the reference meal in order to assess the insulin sensitivity.

$ISI_{composite}$ = 10,000/$\sqrt{}$[fasting glucose (mmol/L) × fasting insulin (nmol/L) × glucose iAUC 0–120 min (mmol· min/L) × insulin iAUC 0–120 min (nmol· min/L)] [16,17].

The effects of the test meals and reference meal on glucose and insulin responses, as well as on the NEFA and TG levels, were evaluated using the PROC MIXED SAS procedure. The subject was treated as a random effect and the test meal as a fixed effect. The fixed effect of corresponding baseline (fasting) values was included as a covariate, and time × meal interactions were tested. All models were tested for the normality of residuals. To adjust for multiple comparisons of significant effects, the Tukey–Kramer *post hoc* significance test was performed. Statistical analyses of metabolic outcomes were performed using SAS 9.2 (SAS Institute Inc., Cary, NC, USA) and Minitab software (ver. 16). The data are presented as iAUC values or least-square means (LSMs) ± SEM. The data were also tested for outliers. The fasting level of insulin was found to be an outlier for one subject, and the result was therefore not included in the insulin analyses. In addition, insulin data were lacking for one subject 30 min after the CANPBol meal and for another 240 min after the MWP_CANBol meal. Due to the missing values, those two test meals were excluded from the calculations for insulin. Another subject missed the CANPBol meal, resulting in $n = 20$ for the CANPBol meal for all blood tests except insulin, where $n = 18$.

4. Results

4.1. Study 1

The canned meals intended for infants contained three to four times higher levels of CML (expressed as mg CML/g protein) than frozen meals with similar ingredients but intended for adults (Table 1). The HI for canned beans was 44, which was significantly lower ($p < 0.05$) than the HI of both the canned pasta (109) and WWB reference (100).

The glycemic response to canned Meat&Beans (GI = 48 ± 11) was significantly lower ($p < 0.05$) than that after the reference WWB meal (GI = 100). The GI of canned Meat&Pasta (79 ± 12) did not differ from either of the other two meals. No significant differences were found in the insulin responses, and the II values were 100, 91 ± 13, and 140 ± 30 for WWB, canned Meat&Beans, and canned Meat&Pasta, respectively.

Table 1. *N*-carboxymethyl-lysine (CML) content in canned and homogenized meals intended for infants and in frozen ready-to-eat meals intended for adults.

Meal	CML (mg/g Protein)
Beef stew "Kalops"	
Canned, homogenized	0.33
Frozen	0.08
Hash "Pytt i panna"	
Canned, homogenized	0.45
Frozen	0.14

Results are presented as the mean of two duplicates.

4.2. Study 2

Twenty-one healthy volunteers (14 men and 7 women) participated in Study 2. All female subjects were taking birth control medication. The mean BMI was 21.8 ± 0.3 kg/m² and mean age 24.3 ± 0.9 years (±SEM). All subjects had normal fasting blood glucose levels (5.4 ± 0.06 mmol/L). The recruitment of test subjects and the study were performed from November 2012 to March 2013. Recruitment was performed by advertising on notice boards at and around the LU campus as well as by contacting former volunteers. The macronutrient composition and CML content of the various foods are presented in Table 2. All test and reference meals were similar in content of available carbohydrates and the protein and fat levels as well as energy contents were within the same range for all composite test meals. CANPBol and MWPBol contained significantly higher levels of CML compared with MWP_CANBol. The CML-content of WWB was significantly lower than in all test meals.

Table 2. Portion sizes and contents of macronutrients, energy, and CML in the test meals and reference meal in Study 2.

Meal	Portion g	Starch g/Port	Protein g/Port	Fat [1] g/Port	Energy kJ/Port	CML [2,3] mg/Port
WWB	83	35	4.9	0.7	704	0.41 ± 0.04 [a]
CANPBol	467	34	13	11.7	1232	9.75 ± 0.89 [b]
MWPBol	479	36	15	11.5	1292	8.98 ± 0.13 [b]
MWP_CANBol of which:	309	35	12	9.3	1143	5.94 ± 0.64 [c]
Canned Bolognese sauce	130	3.3	7.3	8.9	-	5.94 ± 0.64 [c]
Pasta, uncooked	42	30	4.4	0.4	-	n.a.
Maize starch (Maizena)	2	1.7	-	-	-	n.a.

[1] Estimated from a previous study (WWB) and manufacturers' declarations (commercial products/ingredients). WWB, white wheat bread; CANPBol, canned mixed meal; MWP_CANBol, canned Bolognese sauce served with microwave-cooked spaghetti; MWPBol, microwave-cooked mixed meal; n.a., not analyzed; [2] Values are presented as mean ± SEM, n = 4; [3] Values within the row not sharing a superscript letter are significantly different, $p < 0.05$.

4.2.1. Blood Glucose Responses

No differences were observed in fasting glucose levels. There was a significant time × meal interaction ($p < 0.0001$) over the 360 min follow-up (Figure 1). Incremental glucose responses (0–120 min) were significantly lower (31%–63%) following all the test meals than after the WWB meal (Table 3). Furthermore, the glucose response (iAUC and GI) after the MWP_CANBol meal was significantly lower than those after the two other test meals, during the same time period. After the standardized lunch meal (iAUC 240–360) the glucose response following the MWP_CANBol breakfast was significantly lower compared to WWB and CANPBol. The cumulative glucose response over the entire test period (iAUC 0–360 min) showed that overall glycemia following the MWPBol and MWP_CANBol meals was lower than following the CANPBol meal and WWB reference meal.

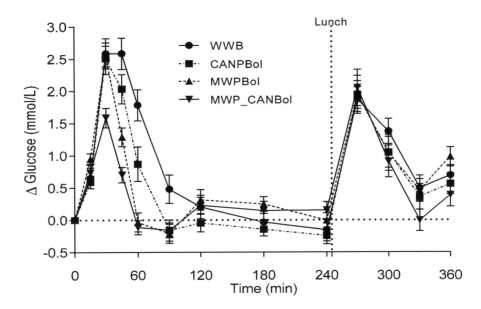

Figure 1. Mean (±SEM) changes in glucose response after the test meals and reference meal and the subsequent standardized lunch (Study 2).

Table 3. Glucose and insulin responses [1], together with a measure of insulin sensitivity after the test meals and the reference meal (Study 2).

	WWB [2]	CANPBol [2]	Δ %	MWPBol [2]	Δ %	MWP_CANBol [2]	Δ %
Glucose							
GI 0–120 min	100 [a]	79 ± 13 [b]	−21	61 ± 5.4 [b]	−39	38 ± 3.6 [c]	−62
iAUC 0–45 min	68.4 ± 6.13 [a]	61.8 ± 5.30 [a]	−10	62.0 ± 3.40 [a]	−9	40.6 ± 4.31 [b]	−41
iAUC 0–120	153 ± 16.0 [a]	104 ± 13.7 [b]	−31	84.6 ± 10.3 [b]	−45	57.4 ± 7.7 [c]	−63
iAUC 240–360	148 ± 18.5 [a]	136 ± 16.3 [a]	−8	120 ± 12.4 [a,b]	−19	92.2 ± 13.1 [b]	−38
iAUC 0–360	312 ± 30.8 [a]	240 ± 31.9 [a,b]	−23	245 ± 37.9 [b]	−22	206 ± 33.3 [b]	−34
Insulin							
II 0–120 min	100 [a]	161 ± 19 [b]	61	129 ± 15 [a,b]	29	57 ± 5.5 [c]	−43
iAUC 0–45 min	5.11 ± 0.79 [a]	8.10 ± 1.02 [b]	59	7.15 ± 0.88 [b]	40	4.01 ± 0.63 [a]	−22
iAUC 0–120	11.3 ± 1.79 [a]	15.8 ± 2.45 [b]	40	12.4 ± 1.90 [a,b]	10	5.95 ± 0.97 [c]	−47
iAUC 0–360	26.4 ± 3.74 [a]	32.2 ± 4.86 [a]	22	26.5 ± 3.81 [a]	0.2	20.2 ± 2.75 [b]	−24
ISI$_{composite}$	703 ± 82 [a]	733 ± 98 [a]	4	865 ± 72 [a]	23	1421 ± 135 [b]	102

[1] Values are presented as mean ± SEM; [2] Values within the same row not sharing superscript letters are significantly different, $p < 0.05$. GI, glycemic index; iAUC, incremental area under the curve; II, insulin index; ISI$_{composite}$, insulin sensitivity index; WWB, white wheat bread; CANPBol, canned mixed meal; MWP_CANBol, canned Bolognese sauce served with microwave-cooked spaghetti; MWPBol, microwave-cooked mixed meal.

4.2.2. Insulin Response

No differences were observed in fasting insulin levels. There was no significant time × meal interaction over the 360 min study period (Figure 2). During the first 45 min, the insulin level was significantly higher following the CANPBol meal (59%) and the MWPBol meal (40%) than the MWP_CANBol meal and the WWB meal. The incremental insulin responses during the periods 0–120 and 0–360 min were significantly lower after the MWP_CANBol meal than after all other meals. In addition, the insulin response during 0–120 min was significantly higher following the CANPBol meal than the WWB reference meal.

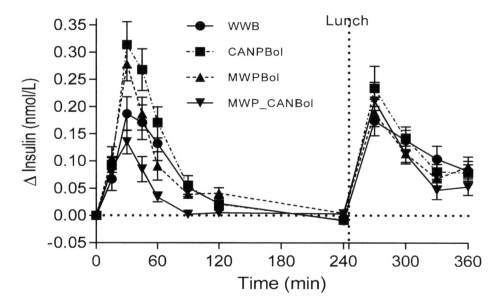

Figure 2. Mean (±SEM) changes in insulin response after the intake of the test meals and reference meal, and subsequent standardized lunch (Study 2).

4.2.3. Blood Lipids

No differences were observed in fasting levels of NEFAs or TGs and no significant time × meal interactions were observed for either of the lipid variables ($p < 0.0001$). Pairwise comparisons of NEFA levels at 240 min showed that they were significantly lower after the MWPBol and MWP_CANBol meals than after the WWB meal ($p = 0.0392$ and 0.0001, respectively, Figure S1). The overall TG response was significantly higher after the CANPBol ($p = 0.0216$) and MWPBol ($p = 0.0008$) meals than after the WWB meal (Figure 3). Furthermore, the level of TGs was significantly higher following the MWPBol meal than after the MWP_CANBol meal ($p = 0.0041$) over the 360 min.

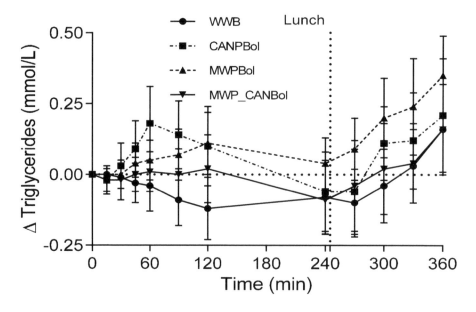

Figure 3. Mean (±SEM) changes in triglyceride response after the intake of the test meals and reference meal, and a subsequent standardized lunch (Study 2).

5. Discussion

The major finding of this study is that canned composite pasta Bolognese meals, processed according to a common procedure for infant meals, elicited substantially higher postprandial metabolic responses in healthy adults than meals intended for adults prepared with conventional cooking conditions. In fact, the infant CANPBol meal elicited an almost two-fold higher postprandial glucose and a 2.6 times higher insulin level during the first 2 h, compared with a meal of canned meat sauce served with gently and separately cooked pasta (MWP_CANBol). When combining the glucose and insulin data in a composite index, $ISI_{composite}$, the insulin sensitivity was improved by 94% after the MWP_CANBol meal, compared with the CANPBol meal. The significantly higher insulin response (+59%) during the first 45 min after the CANPBol meal, compared to the WWB meal, cannot be explained by the corresponding increase in glucose, since this was reduced by 10% (not statistically significant). Instead, we suggest that a fraction of the proteins was rendered highly soluble by the canning process, and may thus exert insulinotrophic effects. Surprisingly, the microwave-cooked composite meal (MWPBol) also led to a significant increase in early insulin response, but no significant differences were found in insulin, compared with WWB, over 120 min. The separately processed meal, MWP_CANBol, resulted in substantially lower glucose (−63%) and insulin (−47%) responses, compared with WWB. Apparently, the canning of Bolognese sauce *per se* did not result in an elevated insulin response, and the reduction in both glucose and insulin is in line with previous findings regarding pasta meals, where a low glucose peak and a late net increment with an accompanying lowering of insulin responses have been reported [18]. Holm *et al.* have previously reported a higher postprandial glycemic response in healthy adults to canned pasta, compared to cooked pasta [9]. They observed glucose responses that were twice as high after canned then after boiled spaghetti, and the insulin response was also significantly increased by canning. A suggested mechanism for the rapid uptake of carbohydrates following the intake of canned pasta was the excessive swelling of the starch, resulting in a very soft and easily digestible texture. The significantly reduced glucose response following the canned Meat&Beans in Study 1 is probably the result of some remaining intact cell structures following homogenization and canning of the composite bean meal [19]. This was also illustrated by the lower *in vitro* rate of starch hydrolysis for the bean component in the canned Meat&Beans meal (HI = 44), than in the canned Meat&Pasta meal (HI = 109) and the WWB reference meal (HI = 100). It should be noted though, that only the intact beans were included in HI-analysis, since they stayed in the strainer after washing. The high HI found for canned pasta is in line with the findings of a previous study indicating that homogenized spaghetti (cooked spaghetti treated for 35 s in a food processor) had a higher GI (73) than intact spaghetti (60), but was still lower than that for bread baked using spaghetti ingredients (100) [18]. Taken together, these findings indicate that canning of pasta disrupts the texture.

The substantial reduction in postprandial glycemic response after the MWP_CANBol meal, compared to the other meals, is further reflected by the improved glucose tolerance following a standardized lunch, manifested by a 38% lower glucose response, than after the WWB breakfast. Another indication of improved insulin sensitivity at the time of lunch (240 min) following the MWP_CANBol breakfast was the reduced NEFA levels. This is in agreement with other reports showing that suppressed NEFA levels between meals improves glucose tolerance following a second meal [20]. The increase in TG levels tended to be higher after the intake of CANPBol than after the other meals over the first postprandial hour. This may be related to a higher availability of lipids from this particular canned composite meal.

It has been suggested that the mechanism behind the increased risk of obesity associated with high protein intakes during infancy may be the protein-associated stimulation of insulin and IGF-1 release [21]. The results of the present study show that insulin stimulation by infant food may be related not only to the quantity of protein, but possibly also to process-induced changes in protein availability. In line with this, hydrolyzed protein appears to stimulate insulin release to a higher extent than intact protein [22].

The CML content in the MWP_CANBol meal was significantly lower than in the MWPBol meal (−34%) and the CANPBol meal (−39%). Gentle processing of the composite meal, as in the case of the MWPBol meal, was, thus, not as effective as expected in terms of reducing CML contents and no significant difference was found between the CML levels in the MWPBol and CANPBol meals. These results indicate that it may be more important to separate the protein- and carbohydrate-rich meal components during processing, than to use gentle heat treatment of a composite meal. The CML comparison in Study 1 indicates that freezing may be an interesting way forward to allow for both gentle and separate heat treatment of the different meal components. It is important to note that the formation of CML renders lysine less available. The fact that lysine is an essential amino acid is one reason to counteract CML formation during processing of all foods, and especially in products intended for infants. Additionally, dietary exposure to CML has repeatedly been linked to impaired metabolism. Consequently, a cross-over study in healthy subjects has shown that exposure to CML-levels of 5.4 mg CML/day (GC-MS analysis) for one month resulted in lower insulin sensitivity, lower plasma levels of omega-3 fatty acids, and higher concentrations of blood lipids than after a low-AGE diet (2.2 mg CML/day) [3]. Similarly, the consumption of a high-AGE diet (24.6 mg CML/day, LC-MS analysis) for one month led to increased fasting insulin and insulin resistance (HOMA-IR), compared to a diet low in AGEs (10.7 mg CML/day), in overweight women [23]. The CML content in one portion of CANPBol was 9.7 mg (LC-MS analysis), and a single meal of canned infant food would thus provide 0.75 mg CML/kg body weight in 12-month-old infants (assuming a body weight of 13 kg). This is more than twice the amount of CML ingested in the case of the high-CML diet previously mentioned where the intake in adults corresponded to 0.35 mg/kg body weight per day [23]. A recent review of randomized controlled trials has shown that high AGE intakes are associated with increased levels of TNF-alpha, which is an established biomarker of inflammation in healthy humans [24]. Furthermore, high postprandial glycemia *per se*, as seen in the current study in the case of CANPBol, has been associated with low-grade inflammation [2,25]. In summary, the intake of canned infant meals appears to result in reduced postprandial insulin sensitivity and high intakes of AGE (measured as CML). The latter is due to favorable conditions for the Maillard reaction, which may result in lower lysine availability and pro-inflammatory responses.

It should be noted that the sample size in Study 1 was lower than that recommended for GI determinations, which may partly explain the larger variation in insulin response after the canned Meat&Pasta meal than after the CANPBol meal. It cannot be excluded that the inclusion of coffee/tea at both test and reference breakfasts in Study 1 may have influenced the postprandial insulin sensitivity and it was therefore removed from the study design in Study 2. Although the metabolic responses to the infant meals were measured in healthy adults, it is reasonable to assume that the differences seen, depending on the type of processing, would be similar in infants.

6. Conclusions

The findings of this study indicate an urgent need for more research on the metabolic effects of food products intended for infants and young children. The importance of considering both the quantity and quality of macronutrients when designing diets for infants was also recently pointed out by Alvisi *et al.* [26]. Gentle and separate processing of meal components seems to have a beneficial impact on human metabolism compared to canning or microwave heated mixed composite meals. With respect to CML contents, conventional cooking and freezing of meal components appears to be more beneficial in comparison with canning.

Acknowledgments: The work in Study 1 was funded by The Swedish Research Council Formas, while the work in Study 2 was funded by the Lund University Antidiabetic Food Centre, a VINNOVA VINN Excellence Centre.

Author Contributions: Elin Östman and Inger Björck conceived and designed the experiments; Inger Björck performed the experiments in Study 1; Elin Östman analyzed the data from Study 1; Anna Forslund performed the experiments and analyzed the data in Study 2; Anna Forslund and Eden Tareke performed the experiments and analyzed the data regarding CML; all authors contributed to writing the manuscript; Elin Östman was primarily responsible for the final content.

References

1. Augustin, L.S.A.; Kendall, C.W.C.; Jenkins, D.J.A.; Willett, W.C.; Astrup, A.; Barclay, A.W.; Björck, I.; Brand-Miller, J.C.; Brighenti, F.; Buyken, A.E.; *et al.* Glycemic index, glycemic load and glycemic response: An international scientific consensus summit from the international carbohydrate quality consortium (ICQC). *Nutr. Metab. Cardiovasc. Dis.* **2015**, *25*, 795–815. [CrossRef] [PubMed]

2. Dickinson, S.; Hancock, D.P.; Petocz, P.; Ceriello, A.; Brand-Miller, J. High-glycemic index carbohydrate increases nuclear factor-kappab activation in mononuclear cells of young, lean healthy subjects. *Am. J. Clin. Nutr.* **2008**, *87*, 1188–1193. [PubMed]

3. Birlouez-Aragon, I.; Saavedra, G.; Tessier, F.J.; Galinier, A.; Ait-Ameur, L.; Lacoste, F.; Niamba, C.N.; Alt, N.; Somoza, V.; Lecerf, J.M. A diet based on high-heat-treated foods promotes risk factors for diabetes mellitus and cardiovascular diseases. *Am. J. Clin. Nutr.* **2010**, *91*, 1220–1226. [CrossRef] [PubMed]

4. Stirban, A.; Tschope, D. Vascular effects of dietary advanced glycation end products. *Int. J. Endocrinol.* **2015**, *2015*, 836498. [CrossRef] [PubMed]

5. Vlassara, H.; Cai, W.; Crandall, J.; Goldberg, T.; Oberstein, R.; Dardaine, V.; Peppa, M.; Rayfield, E.J. Inflammatory mediators are induced by dietary glycotoxins, a major risk factor for diabetic angiopathy. *Proc. Natl. Acad. Sci. USA* **2002**, *99*, 15596–15601. [CrossRef] [PubMed]

6. Tareke, E.; Forslund, A.; Lindh, C.; Fahlgren, C.; Östman, E. Isotope dilution esi-lc-ms/ms for quantification of free and total nε-(1-carboxymethyl)-l-lysine and free nε-(1-carboxyethyl)-l-lysine: Comparison of total nε-(1-carboxymethyl)-l-lysine levels measured with new method to elisa assay in gruel samples. *Food Chem.* **2013**, *141*, 4253–4259. [CrossRef] [PubMed]

7. Plaza, M.; Östman, E.; Tareke, E. Maillard reaction products in powder based food for infants and toddlers. *Eur. J. Food Saf. Nutr.* **2016**, *6*, 65–74. [CrossRef]

8. Canella, D.S.; Levy, R.B.; Martins, A.P.B.; Claro, R.M.; Moubarac, J.C.; Baraldi, L.G.; Cannon, G.; Monteiro, C.A. Ultra-processed food products and obesity in brazilian households (2008–2009). *PLoS ONE* **2014**, *9*. [CrossRef] [PubMed]

9. Holm, J.; Koellreutter, B.; Wursch, P. Influence of sterilization, drying and oat bran enrichment of pasta on glucose and insulin responses in healthy subjects and on the rate and extent of *in vitro* starch digestion. *Eur. J. Clin. Nutr.* **1992**, *46*, 629–640. [PubMed]

10. Järvi, A.E.; Karlström, B.E.; Granfeldt, Y.E.; Björck, I.M.E.; Vessby, B.O.H.; Asp, N.-G.L. The influence of food structure on postprandial metabolism in patients with non-insulin-dependent diabetes mellitus. *Am. J. Clin. Nutr.* **1995**, *61*, 837–842. [PubMed]

11. Liljeberg, H.G.M.; Björck, I.M.E. Bioavailability of starch in bread products. Postprandial glucose and insulin responses in healthy subjects and *in vitro* resistant starch content. *Eur. J. Clin. Nutr.* **1994**, *48*, 151–163. [PubMed]

12. Holm, J.; Bjorck, I.; Drews, A.; Asp, N.G. A rapid method for the analysis of starch. *Starch-Starke* **1986**, *38*, 224–226. [CrossRef]

13. Granfeldt, Y.E.; Björck, I.M.E.; Drews, A.; Tovar, J. An *in vitro* procedure based on chewing to predict metabolic response to starch in cereal and legume product. *Eur. J. Clin. Nutr.* **1992**, *46*, 649–660. [PubMed]

14. Rosen, L.A.; Östman, E.M.; Björck, I.M. Effects of cereal breakfasts on postprandial glucose, appetite regulation and voluntary energy intake at a subsequent standardized lunch; focusing on rye products. *Nutr. J.* **2011**, *10*. [CrossRef] [PubMed]

15. Brouns, F.; Bjorck, I.; Frayn, K.N.; Gibbs, A.L.; Lang, V.; Slama, G.; Wolever, T.M.S. Glycaemic index methodology. *Nutr. Res. Rev.* **2005**, *18*, 145–171. [CrossRef] [PubMed]

16. DeFronzo, R.A.; Matsuda, M. Reduced time points to calculate the composite index. *Diabetes Care* **2010**, *33*. [CrossRef] [PubMed]

17. Matsuda, M.; DeFronzo, R.A. Insulin sensitivity indices obtained from oral glucose tolerance testing: Comparison with the euglycemic insulin clamp. *Diabetes Care* **1999**, *22*, 1462–1470. [CrossRef] [PubMed]

18. Granfeldt, Y.; Bjorck, I. Glycemic response to starch in pasta: A study of mechanisms of limited enzyme availability. *J. Cereal Sci.* **1991**, *14*, 47–61. [CrossRef]

19. Tovar, J.; Granfeldt, Y.; Bjorck, I.M. Effect of processing on blood glucose and insulin responses to starch in legumes. *J. Agric. Food Chem.* **1992**, *40*, 1846–1851. [CrossRef]

20. Gonzalez, J.T. Paradoxical second-meal phenomenon in the acute postexercise period. *Nutrition* **2014**, *30*, 961–967. [CrossRef] [PubMed]

21. Holland-Cachera, M.F. Prediction of adult body composition from infant and child measurements. In *Body Composition Techniques in Health and Disease*; Davies, P.S.W., Cole, T.J., Eds.; Cambridge University Press: Cambridge, UK, 1995; pp. 100–135.

22. Koopman, R.; Crombach, N.; Gijsen, A.P.; Walrand, S.; Fauquant, J.; Kies, A.K.; Lemosquet, S.; Saris, W.H.; Boirie, Y.; van Loon, L.J. Ingestion of a protein hydrolysate is accompanied by an accelerated *in vivo* digestion and absorption rate when compared with its intact protein. *Am. J. Clin. Nut.* **2009**, *90*, 106–115. [CrossRef] [PubMed]

23. Mark, A.B.; Poulsen, M.W.; Andersen, S.; Andersen, J.M.; Bak, M.J.; Ritz, C.; Holst, J.J.; Nielsen, J.; de Courten, B.; Dragsted, L.O.; *et al.* Consumption of a diet low in advanced glycation end products for 4 weeks improves insulin sensitivity in overweight women. *Diabetes Care* **2014**, *37*, 88–95. [CrossRef] [PubMed]

24. Clarke, R.; Dordevic, A.; Tan, S.; Ryan, L.; Coughlan, M. Dietary advanced glycation end products and risk factors for chronic disease: A systematic review of randomised controlled trials. *Nutrition* **2016**, *8*. [CrossRef] [PubMed]

25. Esposito, K.; Nappo, F.; Marfella, R.; Giugliano, G.; Giugliano, F.; Ciotola, M.; Quagliaro, L.; Ceriello, A.; Giugliano, D. Inflammatory cytokine concentrations are acutely increased by hyperglycemia in humans: Role of oxidative stress. *Circulation* **2002**, *106*, 2067–2072. [CrossRef] [PubMed]

26. Alvisi, P.; Brusa, S.; Alboresi, S.; Amarri, S.; Bottau, P.; Cavagni, G.; Corradini, B.; Landi, L.; Loroni, L.; Marani, M.; *et al.* Recommendations on complementary feeding for healthy, full-term infants. *Ital. J. Pediatr.* **2015**, *41*. [CrossRef] [PubMed]

5

The Essentiality of Arachidonic Acid in Infant Development

Kevin B. Hadley [1], Alan S. Ryan [2,*], Stewart Forsyth [3], Sheila Gautier [1] and Norman Salem Jr. [1]

[1] DSM Nutritional Products, 6480 Dobbin Road, Columbia, MD 21045, USA; kevin.hadley@dsm.com (K.B.H.); sheila.gautier@dsm.com (S.G.); norman.salem@dsm.com (N.S.Jr.)
[2] Clinical Research Consulting, 9809 Halston Manor, Boynton Beach, FL 33473, USA
[3] School of Medicine, Dentistry & Nursing, University of Dundee, Ninewells Hospital and Medical School, Dundee, UK; stewartforsyth@btinternet.com
* Correspondence: alan_s_ryan@yahoo.com

Abstract: Arachidonic acid (ARA, 20:4n-6) is an n-6 polyunsaturated 20-carbon fatty acid formed by the biosynthesis from linoleic acid (LA, 18:2n-6). This review considers the essential role that ARA plays in infant development. ARA is always present in human milk at a relatively fixed level and is accumulated in tissues throughout the body where it serves several important functions. Without the provision of preformed ARA in human milk or infant formula the growing infant cannot maintain ARA levels from synthetic pathways alone that are sufficient to meet metabolic demand. During late infancy and early childhood the amount of dietary ARA provided by solid foods is low. ARA serves as a precursor to leukotrienes, prostaglandins, and thromboxanes, collectively known as eicosanoids which are important for immunity and immune response. There is strong evidence based on animal and human studies that ARA is critical for infant growth, brain development, and health. These studies also demonstrate the importance of balancing the amounts of ARA and DHA as too much DHA may suppress the benefits provided by ARA. Both ARA and DHA have been added to infant formulas and follow-on formulas for more than two decades. The amounts and ratios of ARA and DHA needed in infant formula are discussed based on an in depth review of the available scientific evidence.

Keywords: arachidonic acid; docosahexaenoic acid; infant formula; growth; human milk; long-chain polyunsaturated fatty acids

1. Introduction

During the first year of life, infants have special nutritional requirements to maintain a healthy body and support rapid growth and development. Human milk is typically the sole source of nutrition that must supply the infant with appropriate amounts of energy and nutrients. The long-chain polyunsaturated fatty acids (LCPUFA), docosahexaenoic acid (DHA, 22:6n-3) and arachidonic acid (ARA, 20:4n-6) are always present in human milk. These fatty acids play key roles in the structure and function of human tissues, immune function, and brain and retinal development during gestation and infancy [1,2]. Although breastfeeding is considered the ideal way to nourish infants, recent nutrition surveys report that the majority of infants in developed countries receive at least some infant formula during the first year of life [3,4].

Both ARA and DHA have been added to infant formulas in the United States since 2001, although supplementation began in Europe much earlier. Most infant formulas contain 0.2% to 0.4% of total fatty acids as DHA and between 0.35% and 0.7% of total fatty acids as ARA based on worldwide averages of DHA and ARA content in human milk [5] and the recommendations from a number of international expert groups [6–9]. Thus, all commercially available infant formulas contain preformed

ARA at levels equal to or higher than the DHA content in order to maintain adequate DHA and ARA status in non-breastfed infants.

Both α-linolenic acid (ALA, 18:3*n*-3) and linoleic acid (LA, 18:2*n*-6) are regarded as nutritionally essential fatty acids [10]. However, as Lauritzen *et al.* [10] point out, all classic signs of essential fatty acid (EFA) deficiency can be completely reversed by the administration of *n*-6 fatty acids alone, particularly ARA. With respect to infants, the presence of a relatively fixed level of preformed ARA in human milk and the active accumulation of ARA by tissues throughout the body support the concept of the essentiality of ARA. Previously, a description of the essentiality of ARA during infancy has not been considered in detail, although a brief outline of the essentiality of *n*-6 and *n*-3 polyunsaturated fatty acids was presented by Lauritzen *et al.* [10] in 2001.

The purpose of this paper is to review the essentiality of ARA for infant growth and development. We consider both animal models and human studies of ARA. We describe: (1) ARA accumulation and function in brain and tissues; (2) ARA content in human milk and in various tissues, including rates of accretion during gestation and early infancy; (3) the structure and biosynthesis of ARA from LA and its role as a precursor to leukotrienes, prostaglandins, and thromboxanes, collectively known as eicosanoids; (4) dietary intakes of ARA during late infancy and early childhood when non-breast milk food items are introduced into the diet; (5) immune system development and the dual role of PGE_2 and its receptors in modulating the inflammatory response during infancy; (6) bone metabolism and growth; (7) regulation of cardiac function; (8) consequences of ARA deficiency; (9) the importance of ARA for optimal brain and central nervous system development; (10) the history, reasons for, and nutritional effects of adding both DHA and ARA to infant formulas, with an emphasis on the effects of ARA; (11) the importance of ARA in infant health; and (12) the regulatory requirements for ARA and DHA in infant formulas. Based on a detailed review of the scientific literature presented herein, recommendations for dietary intakes ARA during infancy are provided.

2. ARA Accumulation and Function in Brain and Tissue

Over the last decade, there has been increased understanding of the molecular roles that the *n*-3 and *n*-6 PUFA play in brain and cellular function. The variety of functions shown to be related to ARA indicates its importance and essentiality in the metabolic chain of events leading to brain structural lipid development, signaling, and many basic cellular functions.

ARA is indispensable for brain growth where it plays an important role in cell division and signaling [11]. The brain in mammals consists of 60% fat, which requires DHA and ARA for its growth and function [12]. Across different species of mammals there is little variation in DHA and ARA composition of the brain. ARA is one of the most abundant fatty acids in the brain, and compared with DHA, ARA is present in similar quantities [13,14]. The two fatty acids account for approximately ~25% of its total fatty acid content predominately in the form of phospholipids and thus are major structural components of neural cellular membranes.

ARA rapidly accumulates in the brain during development [1,14,15] which takes place from the beginning of the third trimester of gestation up to about 2 years of age [16] (Figure 1). As shown in brain kinetics in fetal baboons, [17] in addition to maternal preformed ARA, LA may be transported across the blood-brain barrier despite its very low content within brain lipids. The brain has an active desaturation/elongation system that converts LA to ARA [17]. ARA activity is higher in brain than in other organs such as the liver. However, the conversion of LA to ARA is low (see below).

The maximum rate of brain growth is primarily associated with myelination [14]. In animal models, approximately 50% of the adult amounts of ARA and DHA accumulate in rat brain during the period before myelination and at 15 days after birth when myelination has just started [14]. Diets low in LCPUFA adversely affect the development of the myelin lipids needed early in brain development [14].

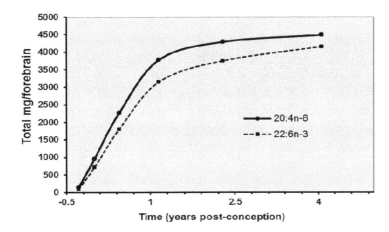

Figure 1. Long-chain polyunsaturated fatty acids (LCPUFA) accretion in the human brain during perinatal development (Data from Martinez [15]).

ARA has several functions in the brain. ARA mediates neuronal firing [18], signaling [19], and long-term potentiation [20]. ARA also helps maintain membrane order and hippocampal plasticity [21], defends the brain against oxidative stress in the hippocampus by activating the peroxisome proliferator-activated receptor gamma (PPARγ), and aids in the synthesis of new protein in tissue [22].

A potentially important aspect of ARA metabolism *in vivo* is its function as an immediate precursor for adrenic acid (22:4*n*-6) [23]. Adrenic acid is the third most abundant PUFA in the brain that is found in large quantities in myelin lipids, particularly in phosphatidylethanolamine (PE) [1]. Rapid accumulation of adrenic acid, like ARA, occurs during the early post-natal period of the brain growth spurt in infants. The conversion of ARA to adrenic acid may represent an important pathway for ARA utilization in infants in order to meet the rapid increase of adrenic acid needed for neural tissue development.

Using a single dose of U-^{13}C-labeled ARA to investigate preformed ARA utilization in baboon neonates, Wijendran *et al.* [23] reported that a major portion of ARA consumed (79%–93%) was accumulated as ARA in tissue lipids, consistent with its primary function as a principal constituent of membrane lipids. Approximately 5% to 16% of ARA was converted to adrenic acid. Based on tracer data, net accretion of ARA and adrenic acid during the first 4 weeks of age in the neonate baboon brain was 17% and 8%, respectively, corresponding to efficiencies (*i.e.*, percentage of dose recovered in brain) of 0.48% and 0.54% of dietary levels, respectively.

To determine the effects that differing DHA to ARA ratios have on tissue fatty acids, twelve-week-old full term baboons were randomized to one of three diets: control (no DHA or ARA), moderate (0.33% DHA, 0.67% ARA) and high LCPUFA (1.00% DHA, 0.67% ARA) [24]. In all groups, DHA levels increased significantly in liver, heart, plasma and in the central nervous system (CNS) regions (precentral gyrus, frontal cortex, inferior and superior colliculi, globus pallidus, and caudate). The formula with the highest level of DHA significantly reduced ARA levels in two areas of the brain (superior colliculus and globus pallidus), indicating its competition with ARA and the importance of a proper balance of DHA to ARA.

Phosphatidylcholine (PC) is a lipid class that is a major component of most intracellular membranes [25]. Some intracellular lipid bilayers include PC containing ARA (ARA-PC). ARA-PC functions as a retrograde messenger in long-term potentiation of synapses in the hippocampus CA1 region [26] and is involved in migration of neurons in the cerebral cortex [27].

Using imaging mass spectrometry, Yang *et al.* [25] characterized the distribution of ARA-PC within cultured neurons of the superior cervical ganglia and found an increasing gradient of ARA-PC along the proximodistal axonal axis that may provide a source for free ARA release [25]. Released free ARA is known to activate protein kinases and ion channels, inhibit neurotransmitter uptake, and enhance synaptic transmission [11]. Free ARA therefore modulates neuronal excitability. As ARA mediates intracellular signaling the concentration of free ARA must be maintained at precise levels within the cells. A higher concentration of ARA-PC near the axon terminal might provide a timely source of ARA when needed during the activated period [25].

ARA also is responsible for the activation of syntaxin-3 (STX-3), a plasma membrane protein involved in the growth and repair of neurites [28]. Growth of neurite processes from the cell body is a critical step in neuronal development. STX-3 serves as a single effector molecule and direct target for ARA [28]. Neurite growth closely correlates with the ability of ARA to activate STX-3 in membrane expansion at growth cones [28].

ARA also enhances the engagement of STX-3 with the fusogenic soluble N-ethylmaleimide-sensitive factor attachment protein receptors (SNARE complex), proteins that form a ternary complex that drives exocytosis [29]. In the brain, at the neuromuscular junction, and in endocrine organs, a set of three SNARE proteins has a primary role in producing fusion of vesicular and plasma membranes. The formation of this SNARE complex drives membrane fusion which leads to the release of vesicular cargo into the extracellular spaces [29]. Darios and colleagues [29] report that α-synuclein, a synaptic modulatory protein implicated in the development of Parkinson disease, can sequester ARA and thereby block the activation of the SNARE complex. This finding underlines the importance of ARA for the regulation of synaptic transmission and transport.

Detergent resistant microdomains, also referred to as lipid rafts, are specialized regions within plasma membranes [30]. These microdomains serve as platforms for biomechanical interactions between the lipid and protein components of signal transduction pathways [30–32]. The outer leaflet of lipid rafts is highly enriched with glycol-sphingolipids and cholesterol [32]. The inner, or cytosol facing leaflet is enriched with alkenyl forms of PE which have been termed plasmenylethanolamine. Electrospray ionization/mass spectrometric analysis has shown that the ARA-containing plasmenylethanolamine represents as much as 50% of the phospholipids of the cytosolic leaflet [31]. This is consistent with a role of PE as an important source of ARA within the cell.

Stearoyl-2-arachidonoyl is a highly abundant species of phosphatidylinositol (PI) found in the phosphorylated forms of PI, the phosphoinositides [33–38]. In addition to serving as a substrate for phospholipase C to produce inositol-triphosphate and diacylglycerol, phosphoinositides serve important biochemical functions including lipid signaling, cell signaling and membrane trafficking. Phosphoinositides perform these roles in part by serving as adaptors for protein-protein and protein-membrane interactions in order to facilitate and/or regulate G-receptor protein activity and signal transduction, and trafficking of various metabolites such as cholesterol or calcium, or other ions, between cellular compartments [39–43]. These biochemical functions of ARA demonstrate its importance for cell signaling, trafficking and regulation of spatial-temporal interactions between cellular structures.

3. Levels of ARA in Human Milk, Brain, and Tissues

Fat is a critical component of human milk that provides energy and nutrients needed for the development of the CNS [10]. DHA and ARA are the principal LCPUFA found in human milk. The synthesis of DHA and ARA is limited in infants [5] and both DHA and ARA must be obtained from dietary sources. Amounts of DHA and ARA in human milk tend to vary by diet, nutritional status, and other factors [5]. Based on data from 65 studies of human milk from 2474 women, the mean concentration of ARA (by weight) was 0.47% ± 0.13% (range 0.24% to 1.0%) whereas the mean concentration of DHA was 0.32% ± 0.22% (range 0.06% to 1.4%) [5]. The DHA concentration in human milk is lower and more variable than ARA. The level of ARA in human milk is much more stable. The relatively stable content of ARA in human milk is biologically important because it provides preformed ARA consistently at a time when brain growth and development is most critical. The majority of ARA in human milk does not derive from dietary LA but rather from maternal stores of ARA [44]. The correlation between DHA and ARA is low, which may reflect a higher degree of variability in the ratio of DHA to ARA in individual human milk samples [5].

The composition of the brain is dominated by ARA and DHA [45]. During pregnancy, both ARA and DHA are preferentially transferred across the placenta [46] and sequestered in the developing brain from the earliest phases of its growth. After birth, human milk provides both DHA and ARA to the breastfed infant [47] with a rapid rise towards adult levels of DHA and ARA in the brain within the first two years of life [48]. ARA is found at a level comparable to that of DHA in neural membranes, particularly those of the brain [49].

Based on estimated total body content of ARA from fetal organ weights during the last trimester of pregnancy and early infancy the relative amount of brain ARA decreases, but because of brain growth the absolute amount of ARA increases [50]. In fact, the absolute amount of ARA increases in all organs with increasing gestational age while the relative contribution (g per 100 g fatty acids; g %) decreases [50]. At 25 weeks gestation, the whole fetal body contains about 1.1 g ARA which increases to 4.2 g ARA at 35 weeks gestation. A full-term infant (3500 g) has about 7.6 g of ARA. The accretion rate of ARA is estimated to be 6.1 mg/day during the first 25 weeks and increases to 95.2 mg/day by 35–40 weeks gestation. The fetal accretion rate for ARA is 2-fold that of DHA [50]. Most of the bodily ARA at 25 and 40 weeks is located in skeletal muscle, adipose tissue and the brain, in that order [50].

In human infant central nervous tissue (cerebral cortex and retina) ARA comprises approximately 10%–12% of total fatty acids [49]. The amount of ARA in central nervous tissue appears to be influenced to a greater extent by postnatal age than by dietary ARA supply [49]. Samples of frontal cerebral cortex obtained from 58 human autopsies (mean age 40 ± 29 years) indicated that the relative levels of PUFA expressed as a percentage of total fatty acids generally decrease with age with the exception of DHA [51].

The distribution of n-6 and n-3 PUFA was determined in various viscera and tissues within the whole body of rats fed a diet containing 10 wt % fat (15% linoleate and 3% α-linolenate) until 7 weeks of age when they were sacrificed [52] (Figure 2).

The rat whole body was comprised of primarily saturated fatty acids (48.4% of total fatty acids) while the monounsaturated fatty acids were present in the second greatest amount (34.8%). The total amount of n-6 PUFA was 12.0% and was more than 5-fold greater than the total n-3 PUFA. The n-6 PUFA with the highest content was LA (10.1%) followed by ARA (1.4%). ARA was the major PUFA in nearly every tissue and was the major PUFA in most internal organs. The tissues with the highest content of ARA were plasma (25.3%) followed by kidney, red blood cells (RBC), and spleen, ranging from 18.7% to 23.5%. Brown adipose, white adipose and the eye contained very low amounts of ARA (<1.0%). For each compartment in the rat body, the total ARA/organ was highest for muscle, then liver, adipose, and carcass. In terms of fatty acid composition expressed as a percentage, ARA was highest in the circulation, kidney, and the spleen.

As shown in rat pups, when tissues are deprived of n-3 PUFA, the accretion of ARA from LA is increased and ARA is further metabolized to produce docosapentaenoic acid (22:5n-6, DPA) which accumulates in tissues [53], particularly in the nervous system. The accumulated DPA in turn reciprocally replaces lost DHA in tissue [53].

Pigs fed varying amounts of ARA and DHA levels after birth and then sacrificed at day 28 showed that dietary ARA had little effect on tissue DHA accretion [54], but heart tissue was particularly sensitive to ARA intake. These observations are particularly notable because the pigs were fed ARA at a level of 0.53% of total fatty acids. This level is slightly above the worldwide ARA mean in human milk and 0.67% of total fatty acids is the level currently added to many infant formulas and is near the high end of human milk ARA levels [5]. Neonatal pigs serve as a practical biomedical model of human infant development due to their similar metabolic responses, genetics of the fatty acid desaturases, and rates of perinatal brain growth [5]. The importance of ARA for the heart is discussed in greater detail in Section 8.

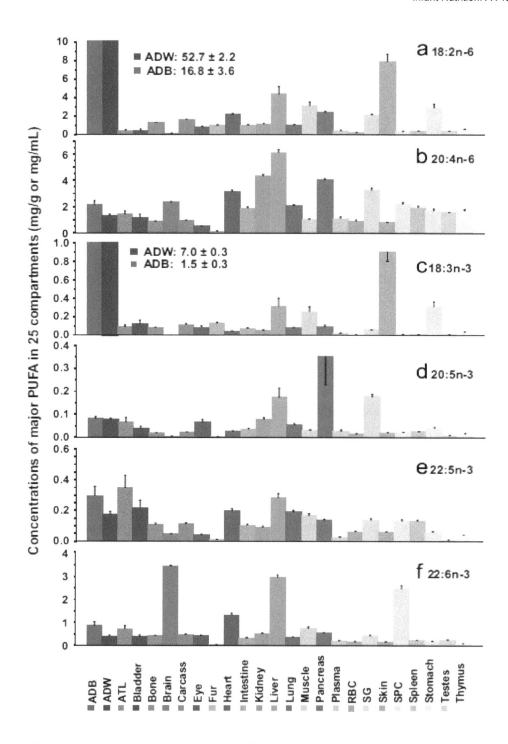

Figure 2. Distribution of fatty acids in 25 different tissue compartments in young male rats. Abbreviations: ATL, adrenal gland, thyroid gland, mandibular gland, and lymph nodes; RBC, red blood cell; SG, salivary gland; ADB, brown adipose tissue; ADW, white adipose tissue (from Salem *et al.* [52]).

4. ARA Biosynthesis and Metabolism

ARA is an *n*-6 polyunsaturated 20-carbon essential fatty acid formed by biosynthesis from LA [10]. ARA is a precursor to leukotrienes, prostaglandins, and thromboxanes, collectively known as eicosanoids [55,56]. ARA is found in membrane phospholipids throughout the body and is particularly abundant in the brain, muscles and liver. The metabolic pathways of the *n*-6 series and *n*-3 series are shown in Figure 3.

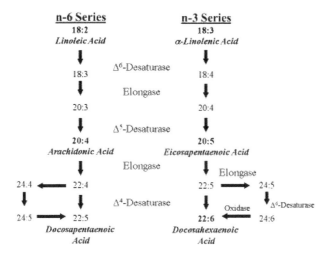

Figure 3. Metabolic pathways of linoleic and α-linolenic acid (Adapted from Lauritzen *et al.* [10]).

The use of stable isotope labelled fatty acids to investigate essential fatty acid metabolism was pioneered in the 1930s with the first identifiable study done by Schoenheimer and Rittenberg [57]. Several decades later, Nichaman *et al.* [58] gave four adult subjects ^{14}C-labeled LA and found a very small but significant incorporation into plasma phospholipid ARA acid based on responses in gas-radiochromatography. Similarly, ^{14}C-labeled LA was shown to be converted to ^{14}C-ARA in human fetal liver microsomes, *in vitro* [59]. El Boustani *et al.* [60] studied the conversion of deuterated dihommo-gamma linoleic acid (20:3*n*-6, DGLA) into ARA in plasma phospholipid and triglyceride fractions *in vivo* in diabetic patients. After a 2 g isotope ingestion, a maximum of 5 mg of labelled ARA/L was observed in plasma. The authors stated that "this was consistent with the very low Δ5 desaturase activity observed *in vitro* in the human liver".

In the 1980s, Emken and colleagues [61] developed stable isotope technology in adult humans. In an early study of deuterated-LA metabolism *in vivo*, when a large dose of over 14 g of isotope was given, the authors concluded that "interconversion products such as deuterium-labeled . . . 20:3 and 20:4 were not detected in any of the lipid classes" [62]. They calculated that a conversion of as little as 0.00012% would have been detectable. The absence of any LA metabolism to ARA was confirmed in a subsequent study even where labelled-ALA was clearly incorporated into EPA and DHA [61].

In 1995, Demmelmair *et al.* [63] used natural abundance ^{13}C measurements in corn oil fed infants to demonstrate LA conversion to ARA. They observed conversion but concluded that "the activity of the enzyme system seems to be limited". Shortly afterwards, the conversion of LA to ARA was conclusively and directly demonstrated in newborn infants using stable isotope technology by Salem *et al.* [64]. The D5-LA was used together with a highly sensitive NCI GC/MS method after PFB derivatization [65]. With this new methodology, the deuterated fatty acid could be chromatographically separated from its corresponding endogenous analogue and so the signal of the stable isotope labeled metabolite would not be obscured by the much larger signal from the endogenous fatty acid. A crude estimate was made of the net accretion of ARA over the six day period of the study which was 53 mg, or about 9 mg ARA/day. Such estimates of "net synthesis" treated the organism as if the synthesis was occurring within the bloodstream and this is clearly not the case. In addition, what was being measured is the synthesis, minus the catabolism, plus the transport/release into a compartment such as the bloodstream where it can be sampled. Carnielli *et al.* [66] used a similar methodology to confirm the conversion of LA to ARA in very low birth-weight infants using ^{13}C-labeled LA.

Pawlosky *et al.* [67] studied stable isotope labeled LA and DGLA metabolism to ARA in 10 newborn human infants within the first week of life *in vivo* and performed compartmental modeling to provide an estimate of the synthetic rates. Formula and breast milk intakes were considered so that ARA and other PUFA intake could be estimated; LA and ARA intake was estimated at 3 g/kg/day and

2.8 mg/kg/day, respectively. They concluded that "the mean daily rate of synthesis and turnover of 20:4n-6 in plasma of infants were estimated to be from 0.06 to 2.1 mg/day ... and from 0 to 51 mg/day (mean 10.2)" [67]. They went on to say that "such rates of synthesis are incapable of sustaining plasma 20:4n-6 concentrations in nearly all of these subjects necessitating an intake of ~4 mg/kg/day from either human milk or a supplement". The fractional rate of conversion (FRC) observed in this study was 2.7% which is even more than that observed by Sauerwald et al. [68] who calculated an FSR of 0.4% to 1.1% depending upon the ALA content of the formula.

Carnielli and colleagues in 2007 [69] studied LA conversion to ARA using natural abundance ^{13}C measurements in preterm infants in vivo in those fed LCPUFA or no LCPUFA-containing formulas at 1, 3 and 7 months of age. These authors show that ARA synthesis is decreasing with age as it fell from 26.7 mg/kg/day to 14.4 mg/kg/day and then to 11.6 mg/kg/day from 1 to 3 to 7 months of age, respectively. It seems that the endogenous synthesis rate in these infants was inadequate as the ARA plasma phospholipid level fell from 5.6 mol% in the ARA fed group to 1.9 mol% in the no ARA group, a 66% drop. This underlines the inadequacy of LA alone as a source of ARA and the requirement for preformed ARA in the infant diet if blood levels of ARA are to be maintained similar to those in breastfed infants.

5. Global Intake of ARA in Early Life

In contrast to n-3 LCPUFA, there are few data relating to dietary intakes of n-6 LCPUFA in early life. In relation to dietary ARA, many regulatory agencies have tended to assume that beyond the age of 6 months, the endogenous synthesis of ARA will meet the needs of infants and young children during this period of rapid growth and development [70,71]. However, studies have shown that the endogenous synthesis of both DHA and ARA may be insufficient with evidence of blood and tissue concentrations decreasing after birth if there is not an exogenous supply [49,72].

The World Health Organization (WHO) [73,74] and the American Academy of Pediatrics [75] recommend that infants should be exclusively breastfed for the first six months of life to achieve optimal growth, development and health. Thereafter, to meet their dietary requirements during growth, infants should receive nutritionally adequate and safe complementary foods while breastfeeding continues for up to two years of age or beyond [73,74]. However, there is widespread variation in compliance with this recommendation in both developed and developing countries. In an evaluation of 33 developing countries, where the health benefits of this policy could have the greatest impact, exclusive breastfeeding occurred in 46% of countries, the median duration of breastfeeding was 18.6 months and over 30% received complementary foods before 6 months of age [76]. The extent to which variation in feeding practices may influence global intakes of ARA and infant growth and development in early life needs to be further evaluated.

5.1. ARA Intake from Human Milk

In exclusively breastfed infants, the mean human milk intake at 6 months has been measured to be 854 g/day [73,74]. Based on those data and an estimation that 4.2% of human milk is composed of fatty acids [77] the average ARA and DHA intakes in exclusively breastfed infants at 6 months of age are about 169 mg/day and 115 mg/day, respectively. Moreover, many infants continue to receive human milk throughout the first year of life and longer. It is estimated that at 12 months of age the intake of human milk is in the range of 600–900 g/day [73,74]. This amount provides infants with an ARA intake from human milk in the range of 118–178 mg/day. The mean estimated ARA intake is approximately 12–18 mg/kg/day when adjusted for body weight using weight-for-age percentiles [78].

5.2. ARA Intake from Infant Formula

Infant formulas typically contain levels of ARA and DHA at 140 mg/day and 100 mg/day, respectfully, based on worldwide averages of ARA and DHA content in human milk [5]. Therefore, intakes of ARA and DHA from infant formula are similar to those provided from human milk.

5.3. ARA Intake from Weaning Foods

In both developed and developing countries weaning foods contain low amounts of fat, which results in a sharp transition from adequate fat intake during breastfeeding to significantly lower fat intake when children are weaned from the breast [79,80]. The main food sources of ARA are beef, poultry, eggs and seafood. Complementary foods in low-income countries are typically cereal-based and therefore LCPUFA dietary intake from these weaning foods may be minimal [79]. Countries with the lowest gross national product (GNP) (e.g., Malawi, Ethiopia, Bangladesh, Burkina Faso, Ghana and India) had a mean percentage of total PUFA from animal source foods of 4.9% *vs.* countries with a higher GNP (Vietnam, Bolivia, Indonesia, Guatemala, China, South Africa, Mexico) where the mean percentage of total PUFA from animal food sources was 18.1% [79].

Intakes of ARA (mean mg/day and estimated mean mg/kg/day) from several developing and developed countries are presented in Table 1. In the village of Keneba, Gambia, estimated mean intake of ARA during the period of 0–6 months when infants are predominantly breastfed was 90 mg/day and as complementary foods were introduced the ARA intake fell steadily to 10 mg/day at 24 months [81]. In Heqing County, Yunnan Province China, the mean intake of ARA was 55 mg/day at 1 to 3 years of age and 50 mg/day at 4 to 5 years of age [82].

Vulnerable infants and young children need energy- and nutrient-dense foods to grow and develop both physically and mentally [83]. For these reasons, dietary diversity is now included as a specific recommendation in the guidance for complementary feeding of the breastfed child aged 6 to 23 months [83]. Many factors contribute to limited dietary diversity including economic limitations, religious beliefs, and a concern that infants under 1 year of age cannot digest animal sourced foods [84,85]. There is also a widely held perception by parents that fish may be associated with allergic reactions [85,86].

Even in developed countries where dietary diversity is higher and meat and eggs contribute more to the complementary diet, the detrimental impact of the introduction of complementary feeding with low amounts of ARA and DHA content is evident. For example, mean ARA intake in German infants/toddlers decreased from 72 mg/day at 6 months of age to 24 mg/day at 9 months of age [87] (Table 1). In a separate study, these authors reported that predominately breastfed German infants had an ARA intake of 103 mg/day at 3 months of age and this amount declined to 24 mg/day at 9 months when human milk represented only 20% of the diet [88].

One hundred-seventy-four Italian breastfed children were followed from birth to 12 months of age [89]. Human milk samples were analyzed. The mean ARA intake from human milk was 95.6 mg/day at 1 month, 109.6 mg/day at 2 months, and 101.1 mg/day at 3 months. However, at 6 months of age, ARA intake sharply declined to 58.7 mg/day.

In Belgium, mean intakes of ARA were very low at 2.5 to 3 years of age and at 4 to 6.5 years of age (17 and 18 mg/day, respectively) [90] (Table 1). In Australia, national intake data indicated that 2 to 3 year-old and 4 to 7 year-old children consumed 16 mg/day and 22 mg/day of ARA, respectively [91]. Much higher mean ARA intakes were reported for Canadian children living in Vancouver where intakes ranged from 133 to 260 mg/day among children 1.5 to 5 years of age [92]. However, in children aged 4 to 7 years of age from Ontario, Canada, mean intake of ARA was lower (57 mg/day) [93].

Based on food records from the National Health and Nutrition Examination Survey (NHANES 2003–2008), the mean intake of ARA in American children at 1 to 4 years of age was 60 mg/day [94]. Most of the ARA was obtained from poultry (32.5%), eggs (27.5%), and meat dishes (20.9%). The latest NHANES data from 2015 indicate that the mean ARA intake of American children at 2 to 5 years of age increased to 80 mg/day [95].

Table 1. ARA intakes in developed and developing countries during the first 2 years of life.

Country	Age	Method	Mean ARA Intake (mg/Day) (mg/kg/Day) [1]
Australia [91]	2–3 years	1-day weighed food record	16 (1.3)
		1-day weighed food record	22 (1.8)
Belgium [90]	2–5 years	3 days food record	17 (1.4)
	4–6.5 years	3 days food record	18 (1.0)
Canada [92,93]	1.5–2 years	1 day food frequency	133 (11.0)
	2.1–3 years	I day food frequency	260 (22.0)
	3.1–5 years	1 day food frequency	226 (15.0)
	4–7 years	3-days food records	57 (2.9)
China [82]	1–3 years	3 days 24 h recall	55 (4.6)
	4–5 years	3 days 24 h recall	50 (2.5)
Gambia [82]	0–6 months	1 day weighed food monthly	90 (15.0)
	7–12 months	1 day weighed food monthly	70 (7.8)
	13–17 months	1 day weighed food monthly	60 (6.7)
	24 months	1 day weighed food monthly	10 (0.8)
Germany [87,88]	6 months	3 days weighed food record	72 (12.0)
	9 months	3 days weighed food record	24 (2.7)
Italy [89]	1 month	Human milk composition	95.6 (29.0)
	2 months	Human milk composition	109.6 (33.0)
	3 months	Human milk composition	101.1 (16.9)
	6 months	Human milk composition	58.7 (9.8)
U.S. 2003–2008 [94]	1–4 years	1 day weighed food record	60 (5.0)
U.S. 2015 [95]	2–5 years	1 day weighed food record	80 (6.7)

Notes: [1] Estimated mean intake for ARA (9 mg/kg/day) for ages 0 month to 3 years was calculated using median weight-for-age percentiles for boys, birth to 36 months, and from median body mass index for ages 4 through 19 years; from the Centers for Disease Control and Prevention-Growth Charts (CDC, [78]).

Based on these dietary intakes from local and national surveys, it is clear that the diets of young children contain low levels of ARA. Reported mean intakes of ARA at 10 to 18 mg/day in developing and developed countries are only about 10% of the amount of ARA available to infants fed human milk or infant formulas containing DHA and ARA.

Birch *et al.* [96] reported that despite the introduction of a variety of solid foods at 17 weeks of age, infants who did not receive an infant formula supplemented with ARA and DHA throughout the first year of life had significantly lower levels of both of these fatty acids in plasma. The clinical consequences of low intake of ARA have not been adequately investigated.

6. ARA and Its Role in Immune System Development and Function

There is growing evidence from preclinical and clinical studies that ARA plays an important role in maintaining infant health through its effects on the immune system and through the modulation of the inflammatory response [97]. The eicosanoids that ARA produces serve as both mediators and regulators of inflammation [98] (Table 2). These immunomodulatory effects have generated much interest in the potential roles that LCPUFA in general and ARA in particular have in common inflammatory conditions in childhood such as asthma, eczema, atopic dermatitis, and food allergies [97].

In cell membranes, ARA contributes to membrane order, has roles in signal transduction, and gene expression, and provides substrate for production of important chemical mediators [99]. Although ARA has been widely viewed as a pro-inflammatory agent, the eicosanoids that ARA produces serve as both mediators and regulators of inflammation [98]. ARA-derived eicosanoids, and other oxidized derivatives [98] are generated by the metabolic processes as shown in Figure 4.

Table 2. Pro- and anti-inflammatory effects of prostaglandin E_2 (PGE$_2$) and leukotriene B_4 (LTB$_4$) [1].

Eicosanoid	Effects
PGE$_2$	**Proinflammatory**
	Induces fever
	Increases vascular permeability
	Increases vasodilatation
	Causes pain
	Enhances pain caused by other agents
	Anti-inflammatory
	Inhibits production of TNF and IL-1
	Inhibits 5-LOX (decreases 4-series LT production
	Induces 15-LOX (increases lipoxin production)
LTB$_4$	**Proinflammatory**
	Increases vascular permeability
	Enhances local blood flow
	Chemotactic agent for leukocytes
	Induces release of lysomal enzymes
	Induces release of oxygen species by granulocytes
	Increases production of TNF, IL-8, and IL-6

Notes: [1] IL, interleukin; LOX, lipoxygenase; TNF, tumor necrosis factor. From Calder [98].

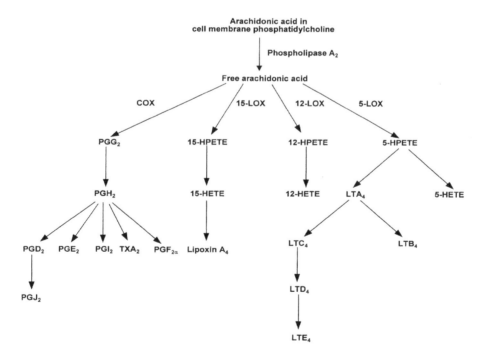

Figure 4. Generalized pathway for the conversion of ARA to eicosanoids. COX, cyclooxygenase; HETE, hydroxyeicosatetraenoic acid; HPETE, hydroperoxyeicosatetraenoic acid; LOX, lipoxygenase; LT, leukotriene; PG, prostaglandin; TX, thromboxane (from Calder [98]).

Another example of the dual role of PGE$_2$ and its receptors in modulating the inflammatory response has been described by Riccioti and FitzGerald [100]. During neuro-inflammation, the LPS-induced PGE$_2$ synthesis causes adverse effects in neurons resulting in lesions and enhanced pain [101]. However, PGE$_2$ also mediates bradykinin-induced neuroprotection by blocking LPS and ATP-induced cytokine synthesis in microglia and in neuron-glia co-cultures [102]. The anti-inflammatory and neuro-protective effects of PGE$_2$ are mediated by microglial EP2- and EP4-receptors [100].

ARA is the substrate for the biosynthesis of prostaglandins. Prostaglandins and thromboxane A_2 are collectively called prostanoids. Prostanoids are formed when ARA is released from the plasma membrane by phospholipase and metabolized by the sequential actions of prostaglandin G/H synthase, or cyclooxygenase (COX), and by respective synthesis [100]. Prostanoids serve a variety of functions. The adhesion-type prostaglandins as well as prostacyclin are important in vasodilation and in anti-thrombus formation [103]. The E series prostaglandins act to dilate arterioles and capillaries to bring about a drop in blood pressure, relax vascular smooth muscle, open the bronchi of the lungs, and enhance blood flow through the kidney [104]. Prostaglandins are also involved in sleep regulation [105], febrile response [106], and in pain perception [107].

As discussed by Calder [98], the overall physiologic (or pathophysiologic) outcome associated with the production of eicosanoids depends on the cells present, the nature of the stimulus, the timing of eicosanoid production, and the sensitivity of the target cells and tissues to the type of eicosanoids that are produced [98,108]. For example, studies have shown that prostaglandin PGE_2, acting as a pro-inflammatory agent, induces cyclooxygenase 2 (COX-2) in fibroblast cells and by doing so up-regulates its own production [109] which in turn stimulates the production of IL-6 by macrophages (see Astudillo *et al.* [108] for a review of ARA metabolism by inflammatory cells). As an anti-inflammatory agent, PGE_2 inhibits 5-lipoxygenase (5-LOX) thereby decreasing production of the 4-series leukotrienes [110].These 4-series leukotrienes induce 15-LOX which in turn promotes the formation of lipoxins that aid the resolution phase of inflammation [110]. Thus, the ARA-derived PGE_2 has both pro- and anti-inflammatory effects (Table 2).

Leukotrienes, eoxins, lipoxins, and hydroperoxyeicosatetranoic acids (HPETEs) are synthesized from ARA by lipoxgenase enzymes and metabolized to LTA_4 [108]. LTA_4 is unstable and can be rapidly converted into LTB_4 or LTC_4. These three leukotrienes constitute the slow-reacting substances involved in anaphylaxis that act in allergic response [111]. They contract smooth muscle and affect vascular permeability. Eoxins are generally proinflammatory and are produced in the same manner as leukotrienes, but by the action of 15-lipoxgenase [108]. Lipoxins are produced by transcellular biosynthesis and have anti-inflammatory properties and are involved in the resolution of inflammation [112].

In vitro and animal studies suggest that ARA has a critical role in immune cell growth in the thymus, and in differentiation, migration, and proliferation of immune cells [98]. During early growth, there is substantial accretion of ARA in the mouse thymus which corresponds to the enrichment of the placental ARA for the fetus [98].

The immune system is composed of an integrated network of organs, tissues, cells and molecules that work together to resist infection, but maintain tolerance to harmless factors such as "self", antigens, and allergens [113]. When a challenge is detected (e.g., an allergen or pathogen), cell signaling between immune cells produces a coordinated immune response involving the release of cytokines and eicosanoids, which under normal circumstances allows cells to communicate with each other to neutralize and eliminate the challenge [114,115].

ARA is highly abundant in platelet membranes and is closely linked to many platelet functions [116]. Due to their high numbers (*i.e.*, normal platelet count of $1.50–4.00 \times 10^{11}$ platelets per liter of blood [117] and their ability to release inflammatory mediators, platelets perform several sentinel tasks and can quickly communicate with the cells of the immune system [118]. For example, in inflammatory skin disorders, platelets recognize bacterial pathogens through interactions with Toll-like receptors leading to the elimination of bacteria by release of antimicrobial peptides or by aggregation of platelets around the bacteria [119]. An array of receptors present on platelet membranes facilitate transduction of signals and coordinate release of chemokines, cytokines, and other inflammatory mediators to regulate inflammation and respond to invading pathogens [118,119].

Inflammation is the immune's systems response to infection and injury [98]. Inflammation disorders are observed in infants, particularly those born prematurely [120]. Inflammation is characterized by the production of inflammatory cytokines, inflammatory agents such as reactive oxygen species, adhesion molecules, and the ARA-derived eicosanoids, and other oxidized derivatives [98]. *N-3* LCPUFA decrease the production of the inflammatory mediators (eicosanoids, cytokines, and reactive oxygen species) and expression of adhesion molecules [98] by replacing ARA as an eicosanoid substrate and inhibiting ARA metabolism [98,121]. Aspirin and nonsteroidal anti-inflammatory drugs (NSAIDs) also inhibit the cyclooxygenase-catalyzed conversion of ARA to prostaglandins [122].

Although inflammation is perceived to be a serious health problem, the inflammation process is in fact an intrinsically beneficial event. Offending factors are removed or destroyed and as a result the affected tissues and physiological functions are restored. During the acute phase of inflammation, there is a rapid influx of blood granulocytes, typically neutrophils, followed by monocytes that mature into inflammatory macrophages [100]. The macrophages proliferate and affect the functions of resident tissue macrophages. This initial acute phase causes the usual signs of inflammation: redness, heat, swelling, and pain [100]. Once the initial adverse stimulus is removed via phagocytosis, the inflammation reaction typically decreases and ultimately resolves. During the resolution phase of inflammation, granulocytes are eliminated and macrophages and lymphocytes return to their normal pre-inflammatory levels [100]. The usual outcome of the acute inflammatory process is successful resolution and repair of tissue damage.

Eicosanoids and Their Effects on Hormones and Bone Formation

The typical definition of a hormone is a chemical substance produced in the body that controls and regulates the activity of certain cells or organs [123]. Many hormones are secreted by special glands, such as thyroid hormone produced by the thyroid gland. Eicosanoids are recognized as different from hormones because they are not synthesized or stored in select tissues or endocrine organs. Eicosanoids are synthesized in almost all tissues and exert their biological effect near the site of their synthesis rather at a distance such as other hormones [124]. Despite these differences, eicosanoids are generally classified as hormones [125]. Eicosanoids directly affect other hormones including glycoprotein hormones. The glycoprotein hormones include luteinizing hormone, somatostatin, and glucagon. Somatostatin is an important growth hormone that controls and regulates growth and cell division [126]. It is the main hormone that stimulates cell proliferation and growth, and this hormone must be regulated so that growth is controlled [126]. Insulin and glucagon release are also affected by the eicosanoid derivatives, epoxy-eicosatrienoic acids [124].

ARA also plays an important role in the hormonal regulation of normal bone formation and whole body mineral metabolism during infant and childhood growth (Table 3). During skeletal development, the eicosanoids relay cellular, organ, and systemic signals to balance the calcium and phosphate needs for bone formation and other metabolic activities [127,128]. During long bone growth, when bone tissue is created, [127–130] ARA mediates vitamin D_3-regulated chondrocyte maturation [131] and proliferation [127,132–134] for the mineralization of skeletal growth plates (Figure 5).

A product of ARA, prostaglandin PGE_2 is a potent regulator of cartilage formation or chondrogenesis and resorption [135–139]. At low levels, PGE_2 stimulates bone formation by increasing the production of insulin-like growth factor, a powerful growth stimulator for bone, cartilage, and muscle [140]. At high levels, PGE_2 has the opposite effect: bone formation is reduced and resorption is increased [140].

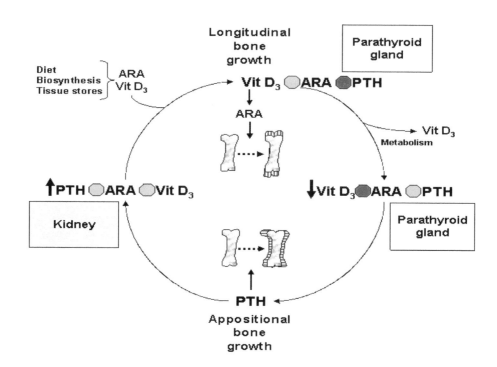

Figure 5. The role of ARA in bone development and homeostatic regulation of vitamin D_3 and parathyroid hormone (PTH) levels along the parathyroid gland-kidney axis during growth. ARA and vitamin D_3 are acquired from the diet and/or from endogenous sources. ARA mediates vitamin D_3 regulation of chondrocyte proliferation and growth plate mineralization during bone elongation. As vitamin D_3 is metabolized and levels subside, ARA-dependent PTH suppression is diminished and PTH production by the parathyroid gland is upregulated. This results in increased periosteal bone mineral content (appositional bone growth). In kidney, PTH induces the ARA-mediated increase in vitamin D_3 activation and secretion, elevating the amount of vitamin D_3 in circulation. The cycle continues as the restoration of vitamin D_3 results in the ARA-dependent suppression of PTH and stimulates longitudinal bone growth.

These differential effects of osteoclast formation and resorption are mediated through multiple subtypes of G-protein coupled PGE_2 cell surface receptors (EP1, EP2, and EP4) [141]. Activation of the EP2 and EP4 receptor subtypes are linked to an elevated level of cyclic adenosine monophosphate (cAMP) and bone formation. EP2 also acts as a selective agonist which has the ability to heal long bone fractures as demonstrated in animal models [141,142].

PGE_2 is also critically important for bone strength [141]. When different doses (3 or 6 mg PGE2/kg/day) of prostaglandin PGE_2 were given to Sprague-Dawley rats for 3 weeks an increase in bone and hard tissue mass, calcified cartilage cores, and a decrease in osteoclasts were observed [143]. PGE_2 increased metaphyseal calcified tissue mass by depressing hard tissue resorption and stimulating the replication and differentiation of osteoblast precursors to form new bone [143].

Other prostaglandins play multiple roles for bone metabolism and remodeling by regulating various signaling pathways [144]. For example, $PGF2\alpha$, through the activation of protein kinase C (PKC), stimulates the Na-dependent inorganic phosphate transport in osteoblasts [144]. $PGF2\alpha$ also up-regulates interleukin (IL-6) to stimulate osteoclast formation and increases vascular endothelial growth factor (VEGF) associated with the growth of blood vessels from pre-existing vasculature [144]. $PKC\alpha$, in particular, appears to play a critical role in the regulation of osteoblastic function under load-bearing conditions [145]. During exposure to mechanical strain, $PKC\alpha$ is activated in osteoblast-like cells [146] while PKC signaling has been implicated in the regulation of various mechanically response genes including the osteoblast differentiation marker osteocalcin [147,148].

Table 3. Roles of ARA in bone formation, metabolism, and mineral balance.

Metabolic Effector	Physiological Roles of ARA
ARA [149]	Maintain normal balance between bone mineral accrual and bone resorption during infant development
ARA, growth hormones [150,151]	Increase insulin-like growth factor gene expression and induction of osteoblast-dependent bone formation
Vitamin D$_3$ [128,133]	Mediate vitamin D$_3$ coordination of chondrocyte proliferation in the epiphyseal growth plates of long bones. Parathyroid hormone secretion
Calcium and phosphorous [152]	Regulation of parathyroid hormone secretion in response to blood mineral concentrations
Parathyroid hormone [149,150]	ARA mediated/activated pathway involved in the activation and secretion of vitamin D$_3$ by kidneys
Physical activity [153]	ARA mediates bone adaptation to changes in physical stress through mechanisms which mediate resorption and remodeling

In studies of piglets fed formulas with differing levels of ARA (0.30%, 0.45%, 0.60% or 0.75% of fat) plus the same level of DHA (0.1% of fat), proportions of ARA in plasma, liver and adipose were dose dependent but bone modeling was not [150]. Whole-body bone mineral content was elevated in the piglets fed the highest levels of ARA (0.60% and 0.75%) and was best predicted by dietary ARA [150,154]. In addition, the 0.60% and 0.75% ARA groups had bone mineral content values closest to that of a reference group of suckled piglets [150,155].

Overall, dietary provision of ARA serves a number of important roles in skeletal metabolism. ARA functions as an important modulator of vitamin D regulation of chondrocyte proliferation and growth plate mineralization. ARA derived metabolites are important inducers of osteoclast [156,157] and osteoblast differentiation [158,159], and in modulating resorption of bone [139,149] by increasing IGF-1 gene expression [104,151] and circulating levels of IGF-1 [150]. ARA also responds to changes in stress and mechanical loading [153,160], and accelerates bone repair and healing [142,161]. Additionally, in term infants, cord blood ARA levels correlate positively with bone mineral density [155]. Thus, ARA represents an important nutrient for infant and childhood bone development and metabolism.

7. ARA in Skeletal and Cardiac Muscle

Several animal studies have shown that the concentration of ARA in the heart is highly sensitive to levels and ratios of ARA and DHA of the diet [24,54,162–164]. The amount of ARA in cardiac tissue muscle is at concentrations 2 to 3 times greater than observed in skeletal muscle [52]. Analysis of the phospholipid composition of skeletal muscle biopsies collected from 56 children <2 years of age indicated that ARA represented 16.5% of the total percentage of LCPUFA in muscle phospholipids [165].

Repetitive force loading and unloading during ATP-dependent contraction of actin filaments are major mechanical functions of heart muscle, and to a lesser extent, skeletal muscle [166]. ARA is critical for muscle contraction [166–168]. In skeletal muscle, excitation–contraction coupling is the process by which muscles contract [166] when a muscle action potential in the muscle fiber causes the myofibrils to contract [169]. Excitation–contraction coupling relies on a direct coupling between key proteins, the sarcoplasmic reticulum calcium release channel (the release of Ca^{2+} ions), and the voltage-gated L-type calcium channels [170]. The release of Ca^{2+} ions from the sarcoplasmic reticulum causes binding between actin and myosin to induce muscle contraction. This cycle is reset as calcium declines back to resting levels [166]. Cardiac and skeletal muscle require tight regulation of voltage-gated calcium channels and calcium homeostasis to coordinate the excitation-contraction coupling process [170].

Phosphatidylinositol (4,5) bisphosphate (PIP_2), a phospholipid component of cell membranes, serves as an important regulator for Ca^{2+} release from the sarcoplasmic reticulum and assists in the maintenance of normal calcium signaling to control contractile forces [167,168,171]. The fatty acids of PIP_2 are variable in different species and tissues, but studies show the most common fatty acids are stearic in position 1 and ARA in position 2 [37].

Calcium homeostasis, regulation and maintenance are critical elements for normal muscle function. Wolf *et al.* [34] have shown that the endoplasmic reticulum is directly responsible for the regulation of intracellular Ca^{2+} concentrations. ARA plays an important cooperative role with myo-inositol 1,4,5-triphosphate (IP_3) in glucose-induced calcium mobilization and insulin secretion by pancreatic islets.

PIP_2 and phosphatidylinositol 3,4,5-triphosphate (PIP_3) are also critical for cardiac function [172]. In the heart, PIP_2, as a key second messenger, controls the activity of ion channels involved with the modulation of heart rhythm. PIP_3, on the other hand, is primarily involved in the control of cardiomyocyte apoptosis, hypertrophy, and contractility [172]. In adults, deregulation of the phosphoinositide metabolism is associated with the onset and progression of several cardiovascular pathologies including atherosclerosis and heart failure [172].

Muscle growth and atrophy depend on the balance between the rates of protein synthesis and degradation [173]. *In vitro* experiments with animal and human skeletal and cardiac muscle tissue indicate that prostaglandins are involved in the regulation of protein synthesis and degradation in various types of striated muscle [173,174]. While PGE_2 increases degradation of muscle in young rats and causes net protein balance to become more negative, $PGF_{2\alpha}$ causes a large stimulation of protein synthesis in muscle tissue [173]. These findings are consistent with the many important roles played by prostaglandins PGE_2 and $PGF_{2\alpha}$ in muscle protein balance and indicate that overall, ARA serves multiple functions in cardiac and skeletal muscle function and physiology.

8. Biomagnification and Accretion of ARA in Infants

Biomagnification is when infants have higher levels of LCPUFA in plasma lipid fractions and erythrocytes as compared with their mothers [45]. Biomagnification can be especially marked for ARA with levels more than 2-fold of that from the maternal side and independent from the amount of its precursor LA available maternally. The stability of LA content implies that any conversion to ARA is not keeping up with the fetal demand for ARA [45]. Biomagnification by the placenta serves to preferentially obtain preformed ARA and DHA from the mother in order to deliver it to and nourish the fetus [45].

As shown by Kuipers *et al.* [175], biomagnification is independent of maternal ARA status at both delivery and at 3 months of age and is found to be similar across different populations with differing diets. These findings indicate that biomagnification as a biological process seeks to achieve a uniform ARA status in infants at the expense of their mothers. The process of biomagnification suggests that a certain level of infant prenatal ARA status must be maintained for optimal infant growth.

Infants with the lowest birthweights have the lowest levels of ARA, and those born earliest have the lowest levels of DHA [45]. The process of biomagnification initially protects vascular growth which is a requirement for brain growth. Vascular growth must precede brain growth to meet the brain's demand for energy, which can be as high as 70% of the total fetal demand for energy in the last trimester of pregnancy [45].

At delivery, as shown by Luxwolda *et al.* [176], the maternal RBC-ARA content is consistently higher than that at 3 months postpartum. At delivery, infant RBC-ARA content is similar or higher than their mother's RBC-ARA contents. From delivery to 3 months postpartum, maternal RBC-ARA increases while infant RBC-ARA decreases. The decrease in RBC-ARA content may be due to a lower conversion of LA to ARA since the infant's capacity to synthesize LCPUFA decreases dramatically after delivery [69] and has been shown to decrease with gestational age at birth [64].

There appears to be a tightly regulated synergism between DHA and ARA at low DHA status and an antagonism at high DHA status [50]. Intrauterine DHA biomagnification in mothers with low fish intakes aims at a synergistic increase of fetal DHA to maintain a balance with ARA. Bioattenuation at higher DHA status may in turn prevent abundant passage of DHA across the placenta that leads to antagonism with ARA. Since ARA is important for fetal growth [177] and is rapidly accreted in the fetal brain [178,179] any competition from gestational DHA must be tightly regulated and balanced for optimal neurodevelopment after birth [50]. Dietary depletion of ARA in early infancy may have adverse consequences for brain development [178,179].

9. Consequences of ARA Deficiency

Essential fatty acid (EFA) deficiency impairs lipid and energy metabolism, cell membrane structures, lipid signaling pathways, and ultimately leads to death [180,181]. Mammals are dependent on a dietary supply of LA and ALA which are converted into n-6 and n-3 PUFA, respectively. Δ6-fatty acid desaturase (FADS2) converts LA to γ-linolenic acid (C18:3n-6) and Δ5-fatty acid desaturase (FADS1) converts dihommo-γ-linolenic acid (C20:3n-6) to ARA [182].

Early studies of EFA deficiency considered the effect that various dose levels of intake of LA, ARA and ALA esters (0% to 10% of total calories for 100 days) had on the fatty acid composition in the liver of rats [183]. Fat deficiency symptoms (necrotic tail and scaly feet) appeared in all animals fed LA at less than 0.6% of calories and ARA at less than 0.25% of calories. ARA was 3-fold more effective than LA in liver incorporation and mitigating deficiency. Fat deficiency symptoms affecting the skin were not surprising. In the skin, as in all organs, EFA are principally found in glycolipids and phospholipids. Most of the epidermal fatty acid PUFA is ARA [184]. EFA deficiency causes skin flaking in humans, dogs, and mice, symptoms that can be restored with LA dietary therapy [184].

Since LA deficiency results in disruption of the skin's water barrier function [185] and heat loss from skin [186] the side effects make it difficult to distinguish the specific effects of ARA deficiency independent from those related to LA deficiency. The fads2$^{-/-}$ mouse allows for the specific investigation of ARA deficiency without the underlying complications of LA deficiency [181]. The mutation eliminates Δ-6 desaturase activity leading to a dramatic decrease in the accumulation of ARA in tissues and subsequently, ARA conversion to PGE, TXB, prostacyclin and leukotrienes. Platelet aggregation and thrombosis are therefore also limited.

When fads2$^{-/-}$ mice were followed for several weeks and fed a diet lacking Δ6-fatty acid desaturase products but containing ample amounts of LA, the lack of PUFA and eicosanoids did not impair lifespan but all the mice were sterile, developed ulcerative dermatitis, splenomegaly, and ulceration in the duodenum and ileocecal junction [182]. Liver levels of ARA and DHA declined by 95% and somewhat smaller decreases were observed in the brain and testes (~50%). The absence of γ-linolenic conversion in the fads2$^{-/-}$ mouse deprived the cyclooxygenase and lipoxygenase pathways of their substrates, including the elimination of PGE synthesis, the failure of synthesis of TXBs by thrombocytes, and the failure to produce leukotrienes [181]. PUFA supplementation completely restored the adverse symptoms observed in fads2$^{-/-}$ mice. The mechanism by which ARA prevented dermatitis may be due, at least in part, to lower levels of prostaglandin D$_2$ (PGD$_2$) when skin ARA is decreased [182].

The ulceration of the small intestine in the fads2$^{-/-}$ mouse may have been associated with the decline of prostaglandin synthesis, similar to the effect often seen with the long-term use of NSAIDs [187]. NSAIDs block prostaglandin synthesis by inhibiting cyclooxygenases, leading to an erosion and then ulceration of the mucosal layer of the stomach and small intestine. However, loss of organized stratification of proliferating cells into defined zones is a common feature of EFA deficiency [188].

The Δ6-fatty acid desaturase gene FADS2 was cloned in 1999 [189]. An adult human case of Δ6-fatty acid desaturase deficiency was identified and described in the literature [190]. The patient exhibited growth retardation accompanied by skin abnormalities, corneal ulceration, and feeding intolerance. Treatment with dietary DHA and ARA restored normal growth and eliminated most of the symptoms [190].

A novel genetic model, the FADS1 (Δ5 desaturase) knockout mouse was used to determine the role that the ARA-derived 2-series eicosanoids had in mucosal physiology and inflammation [191]. Fads1$^{-/-}$ mice have very low levels of ARA in tissues (colon mucosa, liver, spleen, serum and fatty acid profiles). The deficiency in ARA resulted in a massive enhancement of dihomo-γ-linolenic acid, the 1-series prostaglandin substrate in tissues and a decrease in 2-series-derived prostaglandins or PGE$_2$. Fads1$^{-/-}$ mice failed to thrive, gradually dying at 5 to 6 weeks of age with no survivors past 12 weeks of age [191]. The lack of PGE$_2$ was associated with disturbed intestinal crypt proliferation, altered immune cell homeostasis, and a heightened sensitivity to acute inflammatory challenge [191]. Dietary supplementation with ARA extended the longevity of fads1$^{-/-}$ mice to levels comparable with normal wild-type mice (Figure 6).

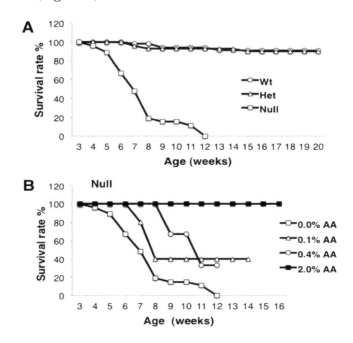

Figure 6. Kaplan-Meier survival curves of *Fads1* mice, AA = ARA. (**A**) *Fads1* null mice exhibited low viability when fed a standard AA-free diet; $n = 37$ for wild-type, $n = 44$ for heterozygous, $n = 11$ for Null; (**B**) Dietary supplementation with AA (0.1% and 0.4%, w/w) partially reversed the *Fads1* null mouse phenotype; $n = 5$ for Null + 0.1% AA, $n = 3$ for Null + 0.4% AA. Supplementation with 2.0% AA completely reverse the Null phenotype; $n = 4$ for Null $\pm$ 2% AA (from Fan *et al.* [191]).

Although fads1$^{-/-}$ and fad2$^{-/-}$ mice are useful to examine the function of ARA *in vivo* PUFA are transferred through the placenta from the heterozygous mother into the homozygous fetus. Additionally, the amount of DHA and ARA in the brain tends to remain tightly controlled even under conditions of PUFA deprivation, but at the expense of other tissues to protect the brain [182]. Lpiat1$^{-/-}$ mice have a mutation that affects the synthesis of ARA-containing PI. PI is unique in its fatty acid composition, *i.e.*, most of the fatty acid that is attached to the sn-2 position of PI is ARA [33]. Other membrane phospholipids such as PC and PE contain other PUFA including DHA.

Lee *et al.* [33] showed that Lpiat1$^{-/-}$ mice had a reduced content of ARA in PI and had deficits in cortical lamination during brain development, delayed neuronal processes in the cortex, and reduced neurite outgrowth *in vitro*. Lpiat1$^{-/-}$ mice died within a month and showed atrophy of the cerebral cortex and hippocampus. These results demonstrate the importance of ARA-containing PI in normal cortical development in mice. By eliminating LPIAT1 in Lpiat1$^{-/-}$ mice, the enzyme responsible for the incorporation of ARA into PI, it was shown that the ARA-containing PI is essential for brain development in mammals [33].

Newborn pups of Δ6-fatty acid desaturase knockout mice were administered artificial milks that contained 3.7% ALA and 16% LA with or without 1.2% ARA and/or 1.2% DHA for 18 days immediately after birth [192]. Compared with wild-type mice, the body weight of the mice fed the control diet was significantly lower, particularly after 6 weeks of age. However, body weights of knockout mice fed milks with DHA and ARA+DHA were similar to that of the wild-type mice. Motor activities of the knockout mice fed ARA were elevated compared with the wild-type mice and those fed the control diet. Better motor performance was also observed in knockout mice fed the ARA + DHA diet. The authors concluded that ARA corrected the decrease in body weight and the combination of ARA and DHA improved the motor dysfunction caused by the deficit of Δ6-fatty acid desaturase.

Taken together, results from these investigations indicate the importance of ARA and its derivatives for the coordination of cellular differentiation, organogenesis, and function during early growth and development.

10. Animal Studies of ARA Supplementation

10.1. Immunomodulatory Effects of ARA and DHA Supplementation

The activation of peroxisomal proliferator-activated receptors (PPARs) has been shown to be protective in brain ischemic and oxidative injury and in many neurological diseases that may affect infants [193] (Figure 7). In addition, transcription of the gene for the Major Facilitator Superfamily of the domain-containing protein 2a (MFSD2A) has been identified as being an important transporter for the uptake of DHA across the blood brain barrier [194] and is under the control of PPAR [195]. Studies indicate that LCPUFA and their metabolites are ligands to PPARs. Diets containing an n-6:n-3 ratio of about 1-2:1 supplied during pregnancy and lactation appear to be optimal for the expression of neuron-specific enolase, glial fibrillary acidic protein and myelin basic protein, markers related to the growth and maturation of neurons, astrocytes and myelin [193].

To investigate the immunomodulatory effects of different PUFA, weanling rats were fed a high-fat diet (178 g/kg) that contained 4.4 g of ALA, γ-linolenic, ARA, EPA, or DHA/100 g total diet [196] for 6 weeks. The proportion of total PUFA content (~35 wt %) was held constant and the n-6 to n-3 ratio was maintained at 5.8 to 7.0. PGE_2 production was enhanced in leukocytes from rats fed the ARA-rich diet and was decreased from leukocytes in rats fed the EPA or DHA diets. ARA did not affect lymphocyte proliferation, NK cell activity, or the cell-mediated immune response. Lack of an effect on T-lymphocyte proliferation and Con A in splenocyte cultures was also observed in mice fed a safflower oil ethyl ester diet +1% ARA for 10 days [197]. The lack of an immunological effect of ARA agrees with findings from a human study that considered 1.5 g of ARA/day for 50 days on the proliferation response of peripheral blood mononuclear cells to Con A, phytohemagglutinin, or poke-weed mitogen [198]. Human peripheral blood NK activity was also unaffected by the consumption of ARA.

Prostaglandins which are involved in inflammatory processes also play a major role in the recovery of intestinal barrier function in ischemia-injured porcine ileum by converting ARA to PGH_2 [199]. The importance of ARA and ARA-derived eicosanoids in the intestinal epithelium was reviewed by Ferrer and Moreno [200]. In a study that considered the effect of supplemental ARA on intestinal barrier repair in ischemia-injured porcine ileum pigs were fed a formula containing no LCPUFA (0% ARA), 0.5% ARA, 5% ARA, or 5% EPA for 10 days. Piglets that were fed 5% ARA exhibited enhanced recovery compared with piglets fed 0% ARA or 0.5% ARA [201]. The EPA-fed piglets had enhanced recovery comparable with piglets fed 0% ARA. The enhanced recovery response observed with 5% ARA was supported by reduction in the mucosal-to-serosal flux of ^{3}H-mannitol and ^{14}C-inulin compared with the other dietary groups. Jacobi et al. [201] concluded that piglets fed a high-ARA diet are less susceptible to ischemia-induced epithelial cell sloughing and that feeding elevated levels of LCPUFA, including ARA, enhances acute recovery of ischemia-injured porcine ileum. For infants affected by necrotizing enterocolitis (NEC) where physiological repair of the intestines is necessary elevated LCPUFA intake including ARA enhances recovery of damaged tissues [201].

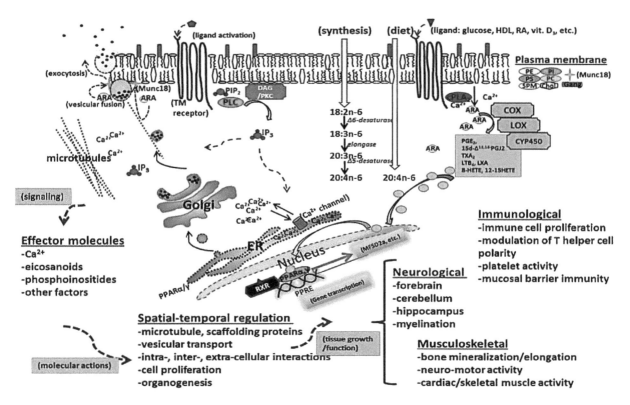

Figure 7. Schematic summary of molecular events and functional outcomes involved in metabolism of ARA. ARA is derived from endogenous synthesis or directly from the diet and is incorporated into cellular membrane complex lipids. Within the lipid bilayer, ARA is enriched in PE and PI in the inner membrane. Coordination of spatial-temporal interactions between molecular and cellular components and activities are mediated by metabolites of, or molecules associated with metabolism of ARA. Metabolism of ARA is triggered by activation of transmembrane receptors as a result of binding a ligand. A few examples of receptor-mediated activation of ARA metabolism include glucose, vitamin D_3, Ca^{2+}, or antigen presentation or detection by immune cells. ARA released from the membrane by the actions of PLA_2 or metabolized by enzymes such as COX, CYP450, and/or LOX can act directly or serve as a substrate for various enzymes to produce second-messengers. ARA-derived eicosanoids, including prostaglandins, leukotrienes, lipoxins, and HETEs regulate numerous activities including passage of ions between subcellular compartments, interactions between various structures or cells, and nuclear regulation of gene transcription by PPARs activators. Within the inner leaflet of cell membranes, ARA is enriched in micro-domains and is involved in regulation of receptor mediated activities. In addition, micro-domains serve as foundations for biophysical interactions between subcellular structures such as microtubules and other cytoskeletal activities including vesicular transport. The consequences of temporal-spatial regulation include coordinated release of hormones, expression of various cell functions, and/or alterations in phenotypes, and cellular motility. Examples of PPAR-regulated gene products involved tissue uptake of LCPUFA and oxidation of stored lipids: MFSD2A, major facilitator of superfamily domain-containing protein 2A. Membrane components: Chol, cholesterol; Gang, gangliosides; PC, phosphatidylcholine; PE, phosphatidylethanolamine; PI, phosphatidylinositol; PS, phosphatidylserine; SPM, Sphingomyelin. Nuclear transcription factors: PPAR, peroxisome-proliferator activator receptors; RXR, retinoid X receptors. TM, transmembrane receptors. Enzymes: COX, cyclooxygenase; CYP450, cytochrome P450; LOX, lipoxygenase; PLA_2, Phospholipase A2; PLC, Phospholipase C. Signaling molecules: PG, prostaglandin (Adapted from Pike [32]).

EFA deficiency also leads to hepatic steatosis. When rats were administered varying amounts of DHA and ARA to determine whether exclusive supplementation with DHA or ARA could prevent

EFA deficiency and inhibit the development of hepatic steatosis mice fed at least 2% of their calories from DHA and 1% of the calories from ARA did not develop clinical or biochemical evidence of EFA deficiency disease or hepatic steatosis [202]. Although hepatic steatosis is an adult disease, the fact that mice fed at least 2% of their calories from DHA and 1% of the calories from ARA prevent the development of EFA deficiency suggests the importance of ARA throughout the lifespan.

To investigate the ability of ARA- and ARA + DHA-enriched formula to modulate immune response in neonatal piglets to an inactivated influenza virus vaccine Bassaganya-Riera *et al.* [203] considered a diet with ARA + DHA in sow milk fed at birth. The diet modulated antigen-specific T-cell responses to an inactivated influenza virus and up-regulated IL-10 expression [203]. Although ARA and DHA have been suggested to elicit opposing immunomodulatory actions, the immunologic outcome in the study was beneficial [203]. The authors concluded that ARA + DHA enriched formulas, with the approximate 2:1 ratio fed during the neonatal period, may prevent or manage autoimmune and allergic reactions in infants by down-modulating T-cell reactions.

10.2. Retinal and Neurodevelopmental Effects of ARA and DHA Supplementation

The retinal DHA content in guinea pigs was considered in relation to diets containing different *n*-6:*n*-3 ratios (from 72.0 to 2.5) [204]. Not surprisingly, diets with the highest *n*-6:*n*-3 PUFA ratios had the highest *n*-6 retinal fatty acid profiles. Weisinger *et al.* [204] reported that retinal function was altered by tissue DHA levels and responded according to an inverted "U-shaped" function. As DHA levels increased past an optimal amount found to be 19%, the result was poorer electroretinographic scores. However, there was no mention that as DHA increased there was a corresponding decrease in ARA levels due to ARA antagonism. The marked decrease in ARA levels may have been the variable of interest that was not fully considered and responsible for the electroretinographic changes at high DHA intakes.

Champoux *et al.* [205] used a neurodevelopmental battery to test the neurological behavior in rhesus macaques neonates fed a control formula without LCPUFA or a LCPUFA-supplemented formula with 1 wt % each of DHA and ARA. Macaque neonates fed the supplemented formula obtained higher scores on motor maturity and orientation than those fed a control formula. Champoux *et al.* [205] concluded that the results supported the view that preformed DHA and ARA in infant formulas are required for optimal neurological development.

Learning behavior in rats fed a diet supplemented with 3% safflower oil (Safflower, *n*-3 fatty acid deficient, high LA acid) was compared to those fed 3% perilla oil (Perilla, high ALA) [206]. Through two generations, the *n*-3 fatty acid deficient group exhibited decreased correct response ratios in a brightness-discrimination behavior test. The altered learning ability in the brightness-discrimination test was restored with supplementation of DHA after weaning, only after levels of ARA in the brain lipids were normalized. The authors concluded that *n*-3 fatty acid is essential for the maintenance of learning performance and that *n*-3 deficiency in the presence of *n*-6 fatty acid during gestation did not lead to irreversible damage to the brain [206]. Thus, both DHA and ARA affected learning performance and a balance of ARA and DHA levels must be maintained.

To investigate the effects that varying dietary levels of LCPUFA have on growth, brain fatty acid composition and behavior in mice, 5 groups of pregnant and lactating mice were fed diets with either very high *n*-6 to *n*-3 ratio of 49 (*n*-3 deficient), a more usual ratio of 4.0, or a low ratio of 0.32 for 15 weeks [207]. There was no effect of diet on birth weights of pups, but on days 15 and 22 the pups in the low *n*-6 to *n*-3 groups weighed less than those in the other treatment groups. Increasing levels of DHA in the diet increased brain DHA and decreased brain ARA. The differing ratios of *n*-6 to *n*-3 had no effect on the ability of mice to learn the place test or perform in the Morris water maze. However, the mice fed the low *n*-6 to *n*-3 ratio swam more slowly, unless ARA was substituted for LA as the source of the *n*-6. The lower body weight in the high *n*-6 to *n*-3 fed mice was not attributed to simply *n*-6 deficiency. The high *n*-3 to *n*-6 ratio led to the inhibition of Δ6-desaturase [207]. Thus, the conversion of LA to ARA was impeded and ARA became unavailable for growth. Mice fed high levels of DHA also had high levels of EPA showing a considerable amount of retroconversion. The findings showed the importance of balancing the amounts of ARA to DHA and that some deficits can be overcome if LA is replaced by ARA as the source of *n*-6 fatty acid [207]. Wainright *et al.* [208] also reported that ARA supplementation increased ARA levels and decreased DHA levels in forebrain membrane phospholipids in Long-Evans rats, whereas DHA supplementation increased DHA levels and decreased ARA levels. Correlational analyses did not show a relationship between DHA and ARA levels in the forebrain and working memory performance [208,209].

Newborn infants of diabetic mothers have lower ARA and DHA levels in cord blood than newborns of normal mothers [210]. The lower levels of the LCPUFA in the newborns of diabetic mothers were associated with impaired and altered sensory-cognitive and psychomotor functions at birth and reduced visual and memory performance at 8 and 12 months [211,212]. Compared with normal controls, most rat models of diabetes are characterized by a lower level of brain ARA only and not a lower level of DHA [213]. Even though both ARA and DHA are important for neurodevelopment, brain accretion of ARA exceeds that of DHA during gestation [214], especially in the first two trimesters during the period of rapid proliferation of neuronal and glial elements [179,215]. When Sprague-Dawley diabetic, pregnant rats were fed either a control diet or an ARA (0.5%) supplemented diet throughout reproduction, the weaned offspring in the ARA group performed significantly better in the water maze and rotarod tests and showed greater exploratory behavior than control-diet offspring [216]. The results indicated that maternal hyperglycemia has long-term consequences during the initial stages of learning and that maternal supplementation with ARA positively influences learning outcomes.

Amusquivar *et al.* [217] reported that rat pups of dams fed diets with *n*-3 fatty acids from fish oil compared with those fed *n*-6 fatty acids from olive oil during pregnancy and lactation had smaller increases in postnatal body weight and length, and delayed body and psychomotor maturation indices. Slower growth and brain development occurred when both dams and fetuses were fed a moderate amount of fish oil (10%) as the only fat source [217]. In the study, the ARA level was lower than the DHA level in brain tissue of the offspring of dams fed high *n*-3 fatty acid diets. The differences in postnatal development disappeared when the fish oil was supplemented with γ-linolenic acid, a precursor of ARA. The growth deficits were also eliminated by the inclusion of ARA in the diet [207]. The studies demonstrate the importance of maintaining adequate levels of ARA during development, and suggest that diets too high in *n*-3 fatty acids during development may have negative effects on development by reducing tissue levels of ARA [218].

To investigate the effects that a DHA-rich maternal diet compared with an ARA-only diet have on brain fatty acid composition of Sprague-Dawley rats, Elsherbiny *et al.* [219] considered a control diet containing ARA (0.4 g/100 g of total fatty acid) *vs.* a DHA + ARA diet (0.9 g/100 of DHA and 0.4 g/100 of ARA of total fatty acid). The results indicated that at three weeks postnatally the DHA-rich diet increased levels of DHA in the brain and decreased ARA by 12.8%. The brain of a three-week-old rat is at a comparable stage as that of a human toddler at 2–3 years of age [219]. At six weeks (comparable to a 12–18 years old human), the DHA-induced decreases in ARA were reversed and disappeared when DHA was continued (*i.e.*, DHA/control group). Thus, elevated dietary levels of DHA decrease the amount of ARA in brain without an adequate supply of dietary ARA.

Prepulse inhibition (PPI) is a normal suppression of a startle response when a low intensity stimulus that elicits little or no behavioral response immediately precedes an unexpected stronger startling response [220]. Deficits in PPI have been reported in individuals that have mental disorders including schizophrenia [220]. Various brain regions including the hippocampus have been associated with PPI problems. To determine whether dietary administration of LCPUFA enhances neurogenesis in the rat hippocampus and improves PPI response in wild-type mice and Pax6[+/−] mice (that exhibit PPI deficits) a control diet or diets supplemented with ARA (4%), DHA (4%) or ARA (4%) + DHA (4%) were administered [220]. Compared with the other diets, the administration of the ARA diet successfully increased neurogenesis not only in the Pax6[+/−] mice but also in the wild-type mice. Treating the

Pax6$^{+/-}$ mice with ARA also resulted in alleviating their PPI deficits. The authors suggested that the ARA diet as compared with the DHA or ARA + DHA diets positively affected postnatal neurogenesis in several regions of the brain including the hippocampus by influencing the fluidity of neuronal membranes and by regulating neuronal transmission [220].

11. Introduction of DHA and ARA in Infant Formulas

Both DHA and ARA have been added to infant formulas in the United States since 2001. In Europe, the addition of DHA and ARA in infant formulas began much earlier in 1994. Most infant formulas contain 0.2% to 0.4% total fatty acids of DHA and between 0.35% and 0.7% total fatty acids of ARA based on worldwide averages of DHA and ARA content in human milk [5]. Several international expert groups [6–9] support the addition of these levels of DHA and ARA in infant formulas to ensure optimal infant growth and development. Thus, all commercially available infant formulas contain preformed ARA at levels equal to or higher than the DHA content in formulas where these LCPUFA are added.

To determine the necessity of adding LCPUFA to infant formula, several studies were performed in the 1990s with preterm and term infants fed formulas containing DHA or EPA with and without ARA (see Fleith and Clandinin [221] for a review). No studies have examined supplementation of infant formula with ARA alone. In most studies, a control group without LCPUFA and/or a breastfed group were included. Studies also investigated the effect of adding ALA to ensure a sufficient endogenous synthesis of DHA [222,223], but not surprisingly, due to the limited conversion of ALA to DHA, the added ALA was not effective in raising DHA plasma status to the same level as that observed in breastfed infants ([223]. Some studies also considered experimental formulas containing added γ-linolenic acid from black current-seed oil, borage oil, or evening primrose oil, DHA and EPA from marine oil, and ARA from egg phospholipids [223–229]. The effects of feeding formula supplemented with soy oil and marine oils containing DHA/EPA showed no abnormalities on growth, tolerance, clotting function, erythrocyte membrane fluidity and vitamin A or E levels in low-birth-weight-term infants [230].

Infant formulas containing DHA and ARA from single cell oils (DHASCO® and ARASCO®, DSM, Columbia, MD, USA), respectively, were evaluated and found to maintain both DHA and ARA status in infants [178,231–233]. After 2001, DHASCO and ARASCO (DSM, Columbia, MD, USA) became predominant as the sources of DHA and ARA added to infant formulas in the United States. Both DHASCO and ARASCO are general recognized as safe (GRAS) for use in infant formulas in the United States and approved as novel foods in Canada [234,235]. DHASCO and ARASCO have an established history of use in Europe, Australia and New Zealand and are not considered novel foods and can be added to infant formulas (see Ryan *et al.* [236] for a review of the safety of single-cell oils).

The clinical studies used to evaluate the effects of DHA and ARA added to infant formulas measured infant growth, body and fatty acid composition, behavioral and sensory functions (retinal function, visual acuity and auditory function). Many of the early studies focused on preterm infants because they provided an opportunity to evaluate the effects of DHA- and ARA-enriched formulas in infants who may be deficient in these LCPUFA. Transfer across the placenta and accretion of ARA and DHA in the developing human brain and retina occurs mainly during the last trimester of pregnancy [179,215] when the rate of brain growth is most rapid [237]. Infants born prematurely thus may have an increased need for dietary ARA due to the interrupted supply during the last trimester [220,238,239].

Four studies with preterm infants considered formulas without added preformed ARA [240–243]. Each was influential in recognizing the importance of ARA for optimal growth. Two of the studies reported an increase in visual acuity at 2 or 4 months postmenstrual age (PMA) in preterm infants fed formulas supplemented with DHA and EPA from fish oil with a low or high ratio of DHA to EPA (2:1, 5:1, respectively) and no ARA [241,244–246].

In one study [240], infants fed formula with a low ratio of DHA to EPA until 79 weeks PMA, compared with controls, had significantly lower z-score values for weight, length and head circumference beginning at 40 weeks PMA. Poorer growth was also associated with lower scores of psychomotor development [244]. The supplemented group also had lower blood levels of ARA [177] suggesting that the effects of growth may have been related to the reduced availability of ARA as a result of the competitive inhibition by the high levels of EPA in marine oil. This finding was supported in a second study [241] in which preterm infants were fed formula with a high DHA to EPA ratio until 48 weeks PMA. Compared with controls, preterm infants fed a high ratio of DHA to EPA and with no ARA consistently had lower mean weight-for-length values at 2, 6, 9, and 12 months PMA, weighed less at 6 and 9 months PMA, and had smaller head circumferences at 9 months PMA [246].

In a third study, three premature infant formulas were compared in a double-blind parallel-group study of the growth of healthy, very-low-birth-weight infants (846–1560 g at birth) [242]. The DHA formula contained 0.34% of fat as DHA and the DHA +ARA formula contained 0.33% as DHA and 0.60% as ARA. The control formula contained no DHA or ARA. A reference group consisted of term infants who were predominately breastfed. Results indicated that infants fed formula with DHA + ARA gained significantly more weight than infants fed formula without DHA+ARA. At 48 and 57 weeks, weight of infants in the DHA + ARA group did not differ from the reference group of term infants. Length of infants in the DHA + ARA group was significantly greater than that of infants fed DHA alone at 40 and 48 weeks, but not at 57 weeks. The authors concluded that supplementation with ARA in addition to DHA supported growth of preterm infants [242].

In a fourth study [243], male but not female preterm infants fed formula with DHA and EPA from fish oil (0.2 wt %, 5:1 ratio) and no ARA, or a control formula to 59 weeks PMA, had significantly smaller gains in weight, length, and head circumference and lower fat-free mass as determined from total body electrical conductivity (TOBEC).

In the Carlson et al. [177,240] studies that reported slower growth in preterm infants a positive association between plasma ARA concentration and measures of growth (weight, length, z-score, weight-to-length, and head circumference) was observed. In the 1990s, when the studies were conducted, it was unknown whether the negative effects of DHA and/or EPA supplementation on growth could be overcome by adding ARA to infant formulas [177]. However, it was known that the bioactive metabolites of ARA mediate the secretion of several hormones associated with growth and basic metabolic functions [247]. These include luteinizing hormone, prolactin, adrenocorticotropic hormone (ATCH), and corticotropin-releasing hormone (CRH) [241] which could influence growth. ARA and its second messengers also appear to be involved in bone formation and resorption [248].

To maintain ARA status in preterm infants, additional studies were performed with infant formulas containing both ARA and DHA [221]. The addition of ARA at levels found in breast milk produced growth comparable to that observed in breastfed infants [221]. Adding both ARA and DHA to preterm infant formulas also resulted in beneficial effects on visual acuity as compared with infants fed a control formula [221].

Concern with a high level of DHA without a concomitant increase of ARA was raised in a randomized, controlled clinical trial of term infants administered formula with no LCPUFA, or differing levels of DHA intakes of 0.32%, 0.64% and 0.96% at the same ARA level of 0.64% [249,250]. There were no formula effects on tests of behavioral and psychophysiological indices of attention at 4, 6, and 9 months of age. However, infants supplemented at the two lower doses of DHA spent proportionately more time engaged in active stimulating processes (increased attention) than infants in the unsupplemented group [249]. Positive results were also observed on vocabulary (Peabody Picture Vocabulary), a card-shorting task, and an intelligence test (Wechler Primary Preschool Scales of Intelligence) at 3 to 6 years of age in the two lower doses of DHA (0.32% and 0.64%) [250]. However, performance of infants and children who were administered the highest dose of DHA (0.96%) but with a reduced ratio of ARA to DHA was attenuated [250]. The results demonstrated that a proper balance of DHA and ARA is needed for optimal cognitive performance as too much DHA may suppress the benefits provided by ARA.

The effects that different ratios of *n*-6 to *n*-3 had on preterm infant neurodevelopment were recently considered by Alshweki *et al.* [251]. Preterm infants (<1500 g and/or <32 weeks gestational age) were given infant formula with an *n*-6 to *n*-3 ratio of 2:1 or 1:1. The infants were followed for up to 2 years. Preterm infants fed formula with a 2:1 ratio of ARA to DHA had higher ARA blood levels during the first year of life and better psychomotor development compared with those fed a 1:1 ratio of ARA to DHA. However, despite the fact that one group received twice the amount of ARA than DHA (66% *vs.* 33%), there was almost no difference between the two groups in plasma *n*-6 to *n*-3 ratio. The balance between *n*-6 and *n*-3 is very complex, but appears to be maintained at a steady level when adequate supplementation of ARA and DHA are available [251].

To date, several systematic reviews of the literature and meta-analyses have been published to evaluate the effects of LCPUFA in preterm and term infants [221,229,252] on various outcomes including growth, cognition and vision. The reviews considered both the earlier and more recent studies on LCPUFA. Fleith and Clandinin [221], in one of the earliest reviews, reported that collectively the body of literature supported the view that LCPUFA are important for growth and development of preterm and term infants. Formula levels of ARA and DHA should be in the same range as those found in human milk and with the same ratio [221]. There needs to be a dietary supply of ARA and DHA to achieve similar accretion levels in plasma and in RBC as compared with breastfed infants [221,253,254].

A Cochrane review of LCPUFA supplementation in term infants reported that there was little evidence that supplementation conferred a benefit on visual or cognitive development [229]. In a recent meta-analysis of four clinical trials including data for preterm and term infants, LCPUFA supplementation was also shown to have no effect on Bailey Developmental scores at 18 months of age [252]. However, as pointed out by Colombo *et al.* [250], the lack of an observed effect at 18 months of age is consistent with the view that the Bailey Scales of Infant Development are not very sensitive to the effects of LCPUFA supplementation. The Bailey Scales of Infant Development yield a composite score obtained from the infant's attainment of normal developmental milestones and may not be able to provide detailed assays of specific cognitive mechanisms that are measured using more sophisticated laboratory tasks [250]. This raises the question of whether the Bailey Scales are appropriate for measuring the effects of LCPUFA on cognitive development in older infants/toddlers.

A systematic review of 20 randomized, controlled trials of term infants who received DHA and ARA supplemented formula or a control formula indicated that infants given formulas containing DHA levels close to the worldwide human milk mean of 0.32% of total fatty acids were more likely to yield positive results on cognitive and visual tests [255]. There was also clinical evidence to suggest than an ARA:DHA ratio greater than 1:1 was associated with improved cognitive outcomes [255].

Since the publication of the Hoffman *et al.* [255] review, several epidemiological and interventional studies of LCPUFA supplementation during infancy have appeared in the literature. These recent publications have been reviewed by Ryan *et al.* [256]. The most recent data indicate that maternal supplementation during pregnancy and/or lactation support the role for LCPUFA in the neurodevelopment of infants [256]. Supplementation with LCPUFA-containing infant formula for more than 6 months increased the likelihood of observing improved cognitive function during infancy [256,257].

The reasons that some studies failed to show a statistically significant association between LCPUFA intake and better neurological performance may have been related to limitations of study design and the use of varying amounts and sources of LCPUFA. For example, in the United States, most of the recent studies that have considered both neurocognitive function and growth have used infant formulas for preterm and term infants that contain DHA and ARA from single cell oils (DHASCO® and ARASCO®). Outside the United States, DHA may be obtained from fish oil [258,259] and ARA may be obtained from eggs [260,261]. As mentioned above, the early studies of the 1990s used a variety of experimental formulas with different sources and amounts of LCPUFA (many of these studies are cited by EFSA in their review, [71]). This is noteworthy because only DHA and ARA from single cell oils have been recently shown to enhance neurodevelopment in both preterm [262–264] and term infants [257,265]. The source of the oil is important because it significantly affects growth. Clandinin *et al.* [264] have shown that body weight at 118 days and length at 79 and 92 weeks of age in preterm infants fed formula containing ARA and DHA from single-cell oils were greater than in those than those fed a formula containing DHA from tuna oil. Additionally, for both weight and length, there were no differences between breastfed infants and those fed ARA and DHA from single-cell oils [264]. The possibility that ARA and DHA derived from single-cell oils or fish oil have differing effects on growth and neurodevelopment may also be due to the EPA at too high a level in fish oil and its propensity to antagonize ARA [257]. An ARA:DHA ratio greater than 1:1 with up to 0.65% of ARA of total fatty acids is associated with improved cognitive performance [255] and balances the potential competition caused by high levels of DHA.

12. The Benefits of ARA for Infant Health

LCPUFA are not only important for growth and neurodevelopment, but recent studies have shown that LCPUFA are also critical for infant health. In an early study, infants fed formula with ARA and DHA developed significantly less stage II and III NEC than those fed a control formula but had similar rates of bronchopulmonary dysplasia, septicemia and retinopathy of prematurity (ROP) [266]. In a recent retrospective cohort study of premature infants (<30 weeks gestation), the relationship between fatty acid profiles during the first postnatal month and infant morbidity due to chronic lung disease, ROP, and late-onset sepsis was analyzed [120]. Results indicated that fatty acid levels of DHA and ARA declined rapidly with a concomitant increase in LA. While the decreased DHA level was associated with increased risk of chronic lung disease, decreased ARA was associated with increased risk of late-onset sepsis. The authors noted that in premature infants, low levels of DHA and ARA contribute to dysregulation of immune and inflammatory responses, predisposing these infants to chronic lung disease and late-onset sepsis [120]. The DHA-derived resolvins decrease neutrophil infiltration and enhance macrophage phagocytosis [267]. DHA also downregulates nuclear factor kB activity in cells either directly or by stimulating the activation of peroxisome proliferator-activated receptors thereby limiting the pro-inflammatory signaling mediated by ARA [267]. Thus, a low level of DHA would predispose these infants to an increased inflammatory response as seen in chronic lung disease. In late-onset sepsis, a decreased ARA level increases the risk of inhibiting the innate immune response through decreased production of eicosanoids, particularly leukotrienes, which enhance chemotaxis of leukocytes, neutrophil activation, and activity of natural killer cells [97,120]. As a consequence, in premature infants, a balance of DHA and ARA levels must be maintained to help reduce the development of morbidity due to prematurity.

Studies have demonstrated that LCPUFA in human milk can modulate immunological responses and affect the T-helper cell (Th) type-1 (Th1)/Th2 balance [268,269]. Th1 cell effectors produce interferon-γ (IFN-γ) and TNF-α which regulate cellular immunity against infection whereas Th2 cells produce interleukin (IL)-4, IL-5, and IL-13 which help mediate immunity against parasitic infections [270,271]. For example, Barakat *et al.* [272] reported that supplementation for 14 days with 10 mg/kg of ARA in *Schistosoma mansoni*-infected schoolchildren induced moderate cure rates (50%) in children with light infection and modest cure rates (21%) in those with high infection. The cure rates associated with ARA were comparable to those produced by 40 mg/kg of praziquantel. The combination of ARA and praziquantel elicited 83% and 78% cure rates in children with light and heavy infections, respectively [272].

The relationship between maternal fatty acid desaturase (FADS) genotype and LCPUFA levels in human milk on infant blood T-cell profiles and cytokine production in 6-month old infants was recently considered [271]. LCPUFA levels in human milk were measured at 4 weeks of age and the FADS genotype was determined in both mothers and infants. Results indicated that ARA levels in human milk were inversely correlated with the production of the cytokines IL-10, IL-17, IL-5 and IL-13 and EPA levels were positively associated with counts of regulatory T-cells and cytotoxic T-cells and decreased T-helper cell counts. The minor FADS alleles were associated with lower ARA and EPA levels in human milk and a higher production of IL-10, Il-17, and IL-5. The major FADS alleles were associated with an increase in the level of ARA in human milk (19%–22%) compared with the minor alleles. There were no association between T-cell distribution and maternal or infant gene variants. Also, there was no relationship between cytokine levels in plasma and levels of LA, EPA, or DHA in human milk.

It has been shown that the FADs gene polymorphism may influence the risk of developing allergies in children [273]. In the study by Muc *et al.* [271] the strongest association between LCPUFA levels and cytokines was observed among those related to the activity of type-2 and type-17 *vs.* those from type-1 responses. The expression of type-2 and type-17 cells have been linked to increased airway inflammation in severe asthma [274]. By reducing type-2 and type-17 activity, LCPUFA including ARA found in human milk may help reduce the risk of childhood asthma and allergies [271].

Notably, Th17 cytokines were initially identified as key factors in the induction of inflammation and tissue destruction associated with a variety of autoimmune response such as multiple sclerosis, arthritis, colitis, celiac disease, and gluten sensitivity [275,276]. However, it is becoming apparent that T17 cells also provide protective immunity against various pathogens at different mucosal sites [270]. Thus, there is a fine balance between protection and pathological manifestation of Th17 responses. As a consequence, a balance of LCPUFA levels similar to that found in human milk is needed to help reduce the risk of developing autoimmune diseases in childhood.

Two studies have compared the frequency of common illnesses in infants fed formula with and without DHA and ARA [277,278]. Both studies used the same LCPUFA-supplemented formula that contained 0.32% DHA and 0.64% ARA of total fatty acids (17 mg of DHA/100 kcal and 34 mg of ARA/100 kcal). In the first study, infants fed the LCPUFA-supplemented formula experienced a lower incidence of bronchiolitis/bronchitis compared with infants fed formula without DHA and ARA [277]. The results from the second study were similar to those of the first. Infants who consumed formula with DHA and ARA had a lower incidence of bronchiolitis/bronchitis, nasal congestion, cough and diarrhea requiring medical attention than infants fed formula without DHA and ARA. The authors indicated that DHA and ARA at present levels in infant formula and follow-on formulas may have a positive effect on moderate to severe common infant illnesses, including diarrhea [277,278].

Two cohorts of children who had previously completed randomized, double-blind trials (one published [72], one unpublished) in which they received a LCPUFA-supplemented formula that contained 0.32%–0.36% DHA and 0.64%–0.72% ARA of total fatty acids or an unsupplemented formula (control) fed during the first year of life were followed up to 3 years of age to determine the incidence of allergies and common respiratory illnesses [279]. The LCPUFA-supplemented group had a significantly lower risk for developing upper respiratory infections, wheezing/asthma, atopic dermatitis, any allergy, and a longer time to first diagnosis than those given an unsupplemented formula.

A subset of children from the Kansas City cohort of the DIAMOND (DHA Intake and Measurement of Neural Development) study [96] were followed to 4 years of age to determine the incidence of childhood allergies [280]. As infants, they were fed either a control unsupplemented formula or one of three formulas with either 0.32%, 0.64% or 0.96% of total fatty acids as DHA with the same amount of ARA (0.64% of total fatty acids). All the different DHA dose and ARA supplemented subjects were pooled into a single supplemented cohort. Results indicated that the incidence of allergic illnesses in the first year of life was lower in the combined LCPUFA group compared with the control. By 4 years of age, LCPUFA supplementation significantly delayed time to first allergic illness and skin allergic illness. LCPUFA supplementation also reduced the risk of any allergic diseases and skin allergic diseases. If the mother had allergies, LCPUFA supplementation reduced the incidence of wheezing/asthma in her offspring. The results of these allergy studies add to the evidence that supplementation of infant formula with both ARA and DHA in the first year of life delays the onset of allergy and may have a protective effect against allergy in early childhood.

Crawford *et al.* [45] reviewed the potential role that ARA and DHA play in protecting against some central nervous system injuries in preterm infants. Deficits of ARA and DHA may contribute to the complications related to prematurity [45]. The mechanism of action responsible for central nervous system injury is reduced vascular or endothelial integrity leading to hemorrhage or ischemia. ARA acts as an endothelial relaxation factor and plays a dominant role in endothelial membrane lipids. The inner cell membrane lipid of the endothelium is especially rich in ARA which provides for membrane properties, signaling and protein kinase C activation [281]. ARA is also a precursor for a range of small molecules that play a key role in cell trafficking, communication and vaso-regulation. As a result, any ARA or DHA deficiency in very preterm infants will be exacerbated after birth during a period of rapid growth. This deficiency may then lead to fragile, leaking vessels and rupture as seen in ROP [45].

The proportion of ARA the placenta delivers to the fetus ranges from 14% to 20% [45]. Infant formula for preterm infants only delivers ~0.4%–0.6% of ARA. For DHA, the placenta delivery to the fetus is ~6% whereas infant formula delivers ~0.3%. That is a 50-fold reduction in ARA and a >10-fold reduction in DHA compared with the infant's apparent physiological need. When plasma levels of ARA and DHA are followed from birth, they continue to decrease to about one third of that of the fetus. Crawford *et al.* [45] argue that higher intakes of ARA and DHA are needed to correct for deficiency during the first year of life.

To explore the impact that deficiency of ARA and DHA may have on immune cell function Moodley *et al.* [282] examined the fatty acid profile and main phosphoglyceride content of cord blood mononuclear cell (CBMC) membranes in healthy preterm infants (30 to 35 weeks) and term infants (37 to 40+ weeks). Results indicated that ARA was the dominant LCPUFA present in both PC and PE membrane fractions of CBMCs in both preterm and term infants. The proportions of ARA, DHA and other LCPUFA were significantly lower in PE and PC of preterm infants compared with those in term infants. The dominance of ARA was consistent with the process of biomagnification that preferentially selects ARA rather than other LCPUFA for transfer to the fetus. Preterm infants also had significantly lower absolute numbers of CD4+ leukocytes and CD4+ and CD8+ naïve T-cells. At birth, there is a period of transition from a sterile environment to one of higher infectious risk. The elevated levels of ARA in CBMCs concomitant with lower levels of other LCPUFA suggest that the acquisition of ARA is needed in preparation for a responsive immune system after birth. These findings indicate that in preterm infants a deficiency in the supply of ARA exists which may compromise their immune system [282].

Infants with mildly abnormal physical movements at 12 weeks of age are reported to have lower ARA content in erythrocyte membranes [283]. This abnormality occurred with maternal supplementation of DHA alone but was not seen when DHA was combined with ARA during pregnancy and lactation [283]. Mildly abnormal movements have been also observed during infancy and linked to increased prevalence of minor neurologic dysfunction and attention deficits at school age [284]. These findings imply that during early brain development of neonates, a supply of ARA is critical.

The effects that feeding preterm infants human milk (HM), infant formula without DHA and ARA (F) or formula with DHA (0.35%) and ARA (0.49%) have on isolated peripheral blood lymphocytes and lipid composition was evaluated by Field *et al.* [285]. Adding DHA and ARA to a preterm infant formula resulted in lymphocyte and cytokine production, phospholipid composition, and antigen maturity similar to those observed in infants fed human milk. These findings suggest that the addition of both DHA and ARA may improve the ability of the infant to respond to immune challenges in a manner similar to breastfed infants [285].

Several epidemiological studies have shown that individuals with learning disorders including attention deficit hyperactivity disorder (ADHD), dyslexia, and autism have signs of EFA deficiency or have lower than normal blood levels of DHA and ARA [286–289]. A meta-analysis of pooled data from RBC and plasma/serum samples indicated that ARA and DHA concentrations were significantly lower than normal in individuals with learning/developmental disorders [290]. In absolute amounts, the level of ARA was as severely depressed as DHA within RBC (both ~0.58 mg/100 mg of fatty acid below normal) but much lower than DHA within plasma/serum (-0.71 $vs.$ -0.34). The reason for lower than normal blood levels of ARA in children with learning disorders is unknown but could be related to a low dietary intake of ARA relative to metabolic requirements or that ARA is not synthesized efficiently from precursor fatty acids, or not delivered or properly incorporated into the brain [290].

The effects of subnormal ARA on brain function seems to be independent of those associated with n-3 deficiency. In Japan where intakes of n-3 fatty acids are relatively high, the incidence of dyslexia in children is similar to that observed in Westernized countries (~6%) [291]. Therefore, although the Japanese population consumes sufficient amounts of n-3 fatty acids, there still may be insufficient intake of ARA to meet the needs for normal brain function during childhood [290]. The important role of ARA in normal growth and development requires as much research emphasis as DHA has received. ARA should be the focus of preclinical and clinical research for a detailed assessment of dietary requirements.

13. The Regulatory Requirements for ARA and DHA in Infant Formulas

A joint International Expert Consultation of the Food and Agricultural Organization of the United Nations (FAO) and the WHO was assembled in 1976 to review the literature on "The Role of Dietary Fats and Oils in Human Nutrition" [292]. The section dealing with infant growth and development indicated that the ideal recommendation for infant formulas would be to match the essential fatty acids found in human milk with respect to LCPUFA content [292]. The FAO further stated that LCPUFA were particularly important during fetal and infant growth when there is a high demand for the synthesis of cell structured lipid [292]. FAO issued a follow-up report in 1994 which provided additional supportive recommendations for adding both ARA and DHA to infant formulas. The FAO stated that "the n-6 and n-3 fatty acids have critical roles in the membrane structure and as precursors of eicosanoids, which are potent and highly reactive compounds. Various eicosanoids have widely divergent, and often opposing effects on, for example, smooth muscle cells, platelet aggregation, vascular parameters (permeability, contractility), and on the inflammatory processes and the immune system. Since they compete for the same enzymes and have different biological roles, the balance between the n-6 and the n-3 fatty acids in the diet can be of considerable importance" [293]. In a follow-up report in 2008–2010, the FAO/WHO Expert Consultancy on Fats and Fatty Acids further concluded that "There can be little doubt about the essentiality of DHA and ARA for the brain" [294].

A global standard for infant formula was established by the Codex Alimentarius Commission in 1981, and revised over the years [295]. The latest revision was issued in 2007 and the latest amendment was added in 2015 [296]. The standard includes details on essential composition of nutrients and a list of food additives that are allowed to be added. Quality control measures such as labeling, packaging, contaminants and hygiene are also specified. In the United States, standards for infant formula are the responsibility of the U.S. Food and Drug Administration (FDA). The U.S. Code of Federal Regulations Title 21, Part 106 specifies infant formula quality control procedures and Part 107 lists the nutrient requirements and other rules concerning labeling for infant formulas. Not surprisingly, the quality and safety standards for infant formulas are extremely high, exceeding most requirements for other food products [297].

In the European Union (EU), the legislation on infant formula and follow-on formulas was adopted in 2006 [298] and at the time of this writing is being revised. Before revising the legislation the European Commission requested the European Food Safety Authority (EFSA) Panel on Dietetic Products, Nutrition and Allergies to provide their scientific advice on the essential nutrient composition of infant and follow-on formulas [70,71]. In the first report of 2013, dedicated to nutrient requirements and dietary intakes of infants and young children in the EU, the EFSA Panel reviewed a variety of nutrients, including the levels of DHA and ARA. In the 2013 EFSA report, adequate intakes were defined as 100 mg/day of DHA and 140 mg/day of ARA from birth to six months of age. From 6 to 24 months of age, 100 mg/day of DHA were considered adequate. These recommendations were also supported by a global expert panel, based on a systematic review of the available scientific literature [299]. However, in the subsequent report of 2014, dedicated to essential composition of infant and follow-on formulae, the EFSA Panel advised that infant and follow-on formulas should contain relatively higher amounts of DHA (20–50 mg/100 kcal). Mandatory addition of ARA was not supported in this EFSA report. Still, the Panel noted that feeding an infant formula containing DHA alone resulted in lower concentration of ARA in erythrocytes compared with a control formula without DHA.

At an assumed mean fat content of 5.2 g 100 kcal in a typical infant formula, this means that the recommendation of higher levels of DHA would result in a DHA content of 0.38% to 0.96% of fatty acids, higher than the 0.2% to 0.3% of DHA currently found in most infant formulas available in the marketplace [2]. Notably, PUFA-supplemented commercially available infant formulas contain preformed ARA at levels equal to or higher than the DHA content. The ESFA Panel's advice of providing up to 1% DHA and no ARA is a unique approach and directly opposite to a consensus reached by international expert groups who have recommended that infant formulas for term infants should contain ARA at levels that range from 0.4% to 0.7% fatty acids (at a 1:1–2:1 ratio to DHA) based on the median worldwide range of ARA and DHA concentrations in breast milk [6–9].

14. Discussion

ARA is the principle LCPUFA in the inner cell membrane lipid of muscle, heart, vascular endothelium, adrenals, kidneys, liver, the placenta, and in almost all other organs [300]. ARA is essential for cell integrity. The cell membrane separates the interior structures of cells from the outside environment. It also controls the movement of substances in and out of the cell [300]. These membranes contain signalers, receptors, ion channels, antioxidant defense enzymes, and rafts. Changing any aspect of the composition of the cell membrane may alter its function [300]).

ARA has very different biological functions than DHA [300]. While DHA controls signaling membranes in the photoreceptor, brain and nervous system, ARA is indispensable in the vasculature and in specific aspects of immunity. ARA is important for brain growth during gestation and early infancy where it plays a critical role in cell division and signaling [11]. A potentially important aspect of ARA metabolism is its function as a precursor for leukotrienes, prostaglandins, and thromboxanes, collectively known as eicosanoids. Eicosanoids have numerous critical and specific functions occurring in almost every tissue of the body. Eicosanoids function to modulate the release of somatostatin, the principal hormone that stimulates cell proliferation and growth. Eicosanoids also have important roles in immunity and inflammation.

This review focused on the essentiality of ARA for infant growth and development. Animal studies demonstrated the importance of ARA for growth and maturation of neurons and myelin and the resolution of inflammation in models of NEC, influenza and EFA deficiency. These studies also provided compelling evidence that both preformed DHA and ARA are required for optimal cognitive and neurological development. The ratio of ARA and DHA added as supplements really matters. Brain tissue analysis of neonatal baboons fed formula with a high level of 0.96% DHA significantly reduced ARA levels in two regions of the brain indicating the importance of a proper balance of DHA and ARA [24].

For over 10 years, both DHA and ARA have been added to infant formulas worldwide in an attempt to match the nutrient supply and functional benefits achieved with human milk. The combination of ARA and DHA in infant formulas has been shown to be safe in many millions of infants globally. The DHA concentration in human milk is lower and more variable than for ARA and the level of ARA in human milk is more stable [5]. The relatively stability of the ARA level in human milk is biologically important because it provides preformed ARA consistently at a time when brain growth and development is most critical [300]. Although DHA is more variable than ARA it is always present in human milk and the balance between ARA and DHA can be as much as 2 to 1.

The biosynthetic capability for providing ARA and DHA for brain growth is low and preformed ARA and DHA are preferentially incorporated into the brain during gestation and early infancy [2,46]. Infant formulas devoid of ARA results in a dramatic decrease of up to 40% of ARA in plasma shortly after birth [223,230,238,239,300,301], especially in preterm infants who do not receive the third trimester's maternal supply of ARA and DHA. The finding that there is a decrease in ARA shortly after birth shows that biosynthetic capability is insufficient to meet the infant's demand [300]. The process of biomagnification and its resulting fatty acid profile further highlights the importance of ARA in infant growth [45]. In several clinical studies, the provision of high amounts of DHA/EPA without a concomitant supply of ARA has been associated with adverse effects on growth in premature infants [240–243].

EFSA [71] recently concluded that "there is no necessity to add ARA to infant formula even in the presence of DHA". This recommendation needs further explanation. One of the possible reasons for this recommendation is that it is generally believed that LA is converted into ARA in sufficient quantities, even though EFSA noted that feeding an infant formula containing DHA alone resulted in lower concentration of ARA in erythrocytes compared with a control formula without DHA. From the limited dietary intake data presented here for non-breastfed infants and young children (Table 1) living in developing and developed countries there is evidence that intakes of ARA from dietary sources are very low, much lower than the average amount of ARA available in human milk or infant formulas containing ARA and DHA. The composition of infant formulas and follow-on formulas should therefore not only be based on human milk composition but also on food/nutrient intake data to address the assumption that complementary foods fill nutrient gaps.

The EFSA Panel's advice of providing higher amounts of DHA (20–50 mg/100 kcal, 0.38% to 0.96% of fatty acids) without a concomitant supply of ARA is also questionable. As discussed here, DHA suppresses ARA concentration in membranes and its function. As a result, an infant formula with DHA and no ARA may result in a potential higher risk of morbidity due to the suppression of favorable eicosanoids that play a key role in cell trafficking, communication and vaso-regulation [45].

EFSA did not take into account the original FAO/WHO publications as well as the earlier 2008–2010 publication which strongly concluded "There can be little doubt about the essentiality of DHA and ARA for the brain" [294]. When infants are exclusively breastfed during the first 6 months of life, "there is evidence of a requirement for preformed ARA and DHA after 6 months of life" [294]. According to the 2010 FAO/WHO statement, DHA and ARA should be included in infant formula with DHA (from 0.2% to 0.5% of total fatty acids) and added ARA should be at least equal to the amount of DHA [294].

The clinical trials considered by EFSA were not designed to consider the specific physiological outcomes related to ARA. Most studies included both ARA and DHA. There were no clinical trials that evaluated the effects of ARA in the absence of DHA. The benefits of ARA + DHA supplementation cannot be ascribed to DHA alone but logically must be ascribed to the variables used in most of these studies, the combination of the two. The combination of ARA and DHA has shown benefits for cognitive development, visual function, and blood pressure well beyond the period of supplementation and into early childhood [249,302].

EFSA's lack of support of ARA in DHA-containing formulas relied almost exclusively on the meta-analysis of infant growth conducted by Makrides *et al.* [303]. However, the meta-analysis of Makrides *et al.* [303] was not comprehensive. The majority of subjects (n = 1050) included in the meta-analysis participated in 8 clinical trials using formula containing both DHA and ARA. Only 341 subjects in the 8 trials were provided infant formula with DHA/EPA without ARA. At 12 months of age, only 99 subjects were supplemented with DHA in the absence of ARA. Additionally, the analysis excluded studies that included preterm infants who are most vulnerable to growth faltering due to nutrition, and excluded studies in which DHA plus ARA supplementation was less than 3 months during which growth velocity is particularly sensitive to nutritional inadequacy. The reason for excluding these studies was not reported.

In the meta-analysis, Makrides *et al.* [303] noted that the results were inconclusive, *i.e.*, LCPUFA supplementation had no detrimental effect on growth. The importance of ARA as a structural and metabolically active lipid, was not addressed. Better visual and mental performance was attributed to the contribution of DHA. However, in one of the studies considered, DHA plus ARA improved mental function [265] compared with an unsupplemented control. In fact, in one study, DHA alone did not perform better than did the unsupplemented controls [72].

Clinical evidence to support the safe removal of ARA from infant formula and follow-on formula containing DHA is lacking. The human and nonhuman primate studies described herein question the EFSA recommendation to provide infant formula from birth with up to 1% of DHA without a proportional amount of ARA [2]. Any major change in infant formula composition should be subjected to a full preclinical and clinical evaluation of safety and nutritional adequacy before its introduction into the marketplace [2]. Without such an assessment, and in light of the universal presence of ARA in human milk and the numerous essential ARA functions for cell structure and function, the most judicious approach is to include ARA in DHA-containing infant formulas to promote optimal infant growth and development.

Acknowledgments: The corresponding author, Alan S. Ryan, has received funds from DSM Nutritional Products to cover the costs to publish this article.

Author Contributions: Kevin B. Hadley, Sheila Gautier and Norman Salem, Jr. conceived the structure of the review. Alan S. Ryan, Kevin B. Hadley, Stewart Forsyth, Sheila Gautier, and Norman Salem, Jr. were involved in drafting and writing of the manuscript, reviewing of scientific literature, and manuscript revision. All authors agreed on the final form of the manuscript.

References

1. Martinez, M. Tissue levels of polyunsaturated fatty acids during early human development. *J. Pediatr.* **1992**, *120*, S129–S138. [CrossRef]
2. Koletzko, B.; Carlson, S.E.; van Goudoever, J.B. Should infant formula provide both omega-3 DHA and omega-6 arachidonic acid? *Ann. Nutr. Metab.* **2015**, *66*, 137–138. [CrossRef] [PubMed]
3. Bolling, K. Infant Feeding Survey, 2005. Available online: http://www.hscic.gov.uk/pubs/ifs2005 (accessed on 17 August 2015).
4. Centers for Disease Control and Prevention, Division of Nutrition, Physical Activity, and Obesity. Breastfeeding Report Card, 2014. Available online: http://www.cdc.gov/breastfeeding/data/reportcard.htm (accessed on 18 August 2015).
5. Brenna, J.T.; Varamini, B.; Jensen, R.G.; Diersen-Schade, D.A.; Boettcher, J.A.; Arterburn, L.M. Docosahexaenoic and arachidonic acid concentrations in human milk worldwide. *Am. J. Clin. Nutr.* **2007**, *85*, 1457–1464. [PubMed]
6. British Nutrition Foundation. *Unsaturated Fatty Acids: Nutritional and Physiological Significance*; Chapman & Hall: London, UK, 1992; pp. 152–163.
7. Food and Agricultural Organization of the United Nations/World Health Organization Joint Expert Consultation. Lipids in early development. In *Fats and Oils in Human Nutrition*; FAO Food and Nutrition Papers; FAO: Rome, Italy, 1994; Volume 57, pp. 49–55.
8. Simopoulos, A.P.; Leaf, A.; Salem, N., Jr. Workshop on the essentiality of and recommended dietary intakes for omega-6 and omega-3 fatty acids. *J. Am. Coll. Nutr.* **1999**, *18*, 487–489. [CrossRef] [PubMed]
9. Koletzko, B.; Baker, S.; Cleghorn, G.; Neto, U.F.; Gropalan, S.; Hernell, O.; Hock, Q.S.; Jirapinyo, P.; Lonnerdal, B.; Pencharz, P.; *et al.* Global standard for the composition of infant formula: Recommendations of an ESPAGHAN coordinated international expert group. *J. Pediatr. Gastroenterol. Nutr.* **2005**, *41*, 584–599. [CrossRef] [PubMed]

10. Lauritzen, L.; Hensen, H.S.; Jorgensen, M.H.; Michaelsen, K.F. The essentiality of long chain *n*-3 fatty acids in relation to development and function of the brain and retina. *Prog. Lipid Res.* **2001**, *40*, 1–94. [CrossRef]

11. Katsuki, H.; Okuda, S. Arachidonic acid as a neurotoxic and neurotrophic substance. *Prog. Neurobiol.* **1995**, *46*, 607–636. [CrossRef]

12. Crawford, M.A.; Broadhurst, C.L. The role of docosahexaenoic and the marine food web as determinants of evolution and hominid brain development: The challenges for human sustainability. *Nutr. Health* **2012**, *21*, 17–39. [CrossRef] [PubMed]

13. Bazan, N.G.; Reddy, T.S.; Bazan, H.E.P.; Birkle, D.L. Metabolism of arachidonic acid and docosahexaenoic acid in the retina. *Prog. Lipid Res.* **1886**, *25*, 595–606. [CrossRef]

14. Crawford, M.A.; Sinclair, A.J. Nutritional influences in the evolution of mammalian brain. In *Lipids, Malnutrition & the Developing Brain*; A Ciba Foundation Symposium: Amsterdam, The Netherlands, 1971; pp. 267–292.

15. Martinez, M. Polyunsaturated fatty acids in the developing human brain, red cells and plasma: Influence of nutrition and peroxisomal disease. In *Fatty Acids and Lipids: Biological Aspects*; Galli, C., Simopoulos, A.P., Tremoli, E., Eds.; Karger: Basel, Switzerland, 1994; Volume 75, pp. 70–78.

16. Dobbing, J.; Sands, J. Comparative aspects of the brain growth spurt. *Early Hum. Dev.* **1979**, *3*, 79–83. [CrossRef]

17. Su, H.-M.; Corso, T.N.; Nathanielsz, P.W.; Brenna, J.T. Linoleic acid kinetics and conversion to arachidonic acid in the pregnant and fetal baboon. *J. Lipid Res.* **1999**, *40*, 1304–1311. [PubMed]

18. Sanchez-Mejia, R.O.; Newman, J.W.; Toh, S.; Yu, G.; Zhou, G.Q.; Halabisky, B.; Cissé, M.; Scearce-Levie, K.; Cheng, I.H.; Gan, L.; *et al.* Phospholipase A2 reduction ameliorates cognitive deficits in a mouse model of Alzheimer's disease. *Nat. Neurosci.* **2008**, *11*, 1311–1318. [CrossRef] [PubMed]

19. Vijayaraghaven, S.; Huang, B.; Blumenthal, E.M.; Berg, D.L. Arachidonic acid as a possible negative feedback inhibitor of nicotinic acetylcholine receptors on neurons. *J. Neurosci.* **1995**, *15*, 3679–3687.

20. Williams, J.H.; Errington, M.L.; Lynch, M.A.; Bliss, T.V. Arachidonic acid induces a long term activity-dependent enhancement of synaptic transmission in the hippocampus. *Nature* **1989**, *341*, 739–742. [CrossRef] [PubMed]

21. Fukaya, T.; Gondaira, T.; Kashiyae, Y.; Kotani, S.; Ishikura, Y.; Fujikawa, S.; Kiso, Y.; Sakakibara, M. Arachidonic acid preserves hippocampal neuron membrane fluidity in senescent rats. *Neurobiol. Aging* **2007**, *28*, 1179–1186. [CrossRef] [PubMed]

22. Wang, Z.-J.; Liang, C.-L.; Li, G.-M.; Yu, C.-Y.; Yin, M. Neuroprotective effects of arachidonic acid against oxidative stress on rat hippocampal slices. *Chem. Biol. Interact.* **2006**, *163*, 207–217. [CrossRef] [PubMed]

23. Wijendran, V.; Lawrence, P.; Diau, G.-Y.; Boehm, G.; Nathanielsz, P.W.; Brenna, J.T. Significant utilization of dietary arachidonic acid is for brain adrenic acid in baboon neonates. *J. Lipid Res.* **2002**, *43*, 762–767. [PubMed]

24. Hsieh, A.T.; Anthony, J.C.; Diersen-Schade, D.A.; Rumsey, S.C.; Lawrence, P.; Li, C.; Nathanielsz, P.W.; Brenna, J.T. The influence of moderate and high dietary long chain polyunsaturated fatty acids (LCPUFA) on baboon neonate tissue fatty acids. *Pediatr. Res.* **2007**, *61*, 537–545. [CrossRef] [PubMed]

25. Yang, H.-J.; Sugiura, Y.; Ikegami, K.; Konishi, Y.; Setou, M. Axonal gradient of arachidonic acid-containing phosphatidylcholine and its dependence on actin dynamics. *J. Biol. Chem.* **2012**, *287*, 5290–5300. [CrossRef] [PubMed]

26. Bazan, N.G. The neuromessenger platelet-activation factor in plasticity and neurodegeneration. *Prog. Brain Res.* **1998**, *118*, 281–291. [PubMed]

27. Hattori, M.H.; Adachi, H.; Tsujimoto, M.; Arai, H.; Inoue, K. Miller-Dieker lissencephaly gene encodes a subunit of brain platelet-activation factor acetylhydrolase. *Nature* **1994**, *370*, 216–218. [CrossRef] [PubMed]

28. Darios, F.; Davletov, B. Omega-3 and omega-6 fatty acids stimulate cell membrane expansion by acting on syntaxin 3. *Nature* **2006**, *440*, 813–817. [CrossRef] [PubMed]

29. Darios, F.; Ruiperez, V.; Lopez, I.; Villanueva, J.; Gutierrez, L.M.; Davletov, B. α-synuclein sequesters arachidonic acid to modulate SNARE-mediated exocytosis. *EMBO Rep.* **2010**, *11*, 528–533. [CrossRef] [PubMed]

30. Smart, E.J.; Graf, G.A.; McNiven, M.A.; Sessa, W.C.; Engelman, J.A.; Scherer, P.E.; Okamoto, T.; Lisanti, M.P. Caveolins, liquid-ordered domains, and signal transduction. *Mol. Cell. Biol.* **1999**, *19*, 7289–7304. [CrossRef] [PubMed]

31. Pike, L.J.; Han, X.; Chung, K.-N.; Gross, R.W. Lipid rafts are enriched in arachidonic acid and plasmmenylethanolamine and their composition is independent of caveolin-1 expression: A quantitative electrospray ionization/mass spectrometric analysis. *Biochemistry* **2002**, *41*, 2075–2088. [CrossRef] [PubMed]

32. Pike, L. Lipid rafts: Bringing order to chaos. *J. Lipid Res.* **2003**, *44*, 655–667. [CrossRef] [PubMed]

33. Lee, H.-C.; Sasaki, J.; Kubo, T.; Matsuda, S.; Nakasaki, Y.; Hattori, M.; Tanaka, F.; Udagawa, O.; Kono, N.; Itoh, T.; *et al.* LPIAT1 regulates arachidonic acid content in phosphatidylinositol and is required for cortical lamination in mice. *Mol. Biol. Cell* **2012**, *23*, 4689–4697. [CrossRef] [PubMed]

34. Wolf, B.A.; Turk, J.; Sherman, W.R.; McDaniel, M.L. Intracellular Ca^{2+} mobilization of arachidonic acid. *J. Biol. Chem.* **1986**, *261*, 3501–3511. [PubMed]

35. Cao, Y.; Pearman, A.T.; Zimmermann, G.A.; McIntyre, T.M.; Prescott, S.M. Intracellular unesterified arachidonic acid signals apoptosis. *PNAS* **2000**, *97*, 11280–11285. [CrossRef] [PubMed]

36. Hicks, A.M.; DeLong, C.J.; Thomas, M.J.; Samuel, M.; Cui, Z. Unique molecular signatures of glycerophospholipid species in different rat tissues analyzed by tandem mass spectrometry. *Biochim. Biophys. Acta* **2006**, *71*, 1022–1029. [CrossRef] [PubMed]

37. Tanaka, T.; Iwawaki, D.; Sakamoto, M.; Takai, Y.; Morishige, J.-I.; Murakami, K.; Satouchi, K. Mechanisms of accumulation of aracidonate in phoshatidylinositol in yellowtail. *Eur. J. Biochem.* **2003**, *270*, 1466–1473. [CrossRef] [PubMed]

38. Jungalwala, F.B.; Evans, J.E.; McCluer, R.H. Compositional and molecular species analysis of phospholipids by high performance liquid chromatography couples with chemical ionization mass spectrometry. *J. Lipid Res.* **1984**, *25*, 738–749. [PubMed]

39. Szentpetery, Z.; Varnai, P.; Balla, T. Acute manipulation of Golgi phosphoinositides to assess their importance in cellular trafficking and signaling. *PNAS* **2010**, *107*, 8225–8230. [CrossRef] [PubMed]

40. Di Paolo, G.; De Camilli, P. Phosphoinositides in cell regulation and membrane dynamics. *Nature* **2006**, *44*, 12. [CrossRef] [PubMed]

41. Malaiyandi, L.M.; Honick, A.S.; Rintoul, G.L.; Wang, Q.L.; Reynolds, I.J. Zn^{2+} inhibits mitochondrial movement in neurons by phosphatidylinositol 3-kinase activation. *J. Neurosci.* **2005**, *25*, 9507–9514. [CrossRef] [PubMed]

42. De Vos, K.J.; Sable, J.; Miller, K.E.; Sheetz, M.P. Expression of phosphatidylinositol (4,5) bisphosphate-specific pleckstrin homology domains alters direction but not the level of axonal transport of mitochondria. *Mol. Biol. Cell* **2002**, *14*, 3636–3649. [CrossRef] [PubMed]

43. Caroni, P. New EMBO members' review: Actin cytoskeleton regulation through modulation of PI(4,5)P(2) rafts. *EMBO J.* **2001**, *20*, 4332–4336. [CrossRef] [PubMed]

44. Del Prado, M.; Villalpando, S.; Elizondo, A.; Rodriguez, M.; Demmelmair, H.; Koletzko, B. Contribution of dietary and newly formed arachidonic acid to human milk lipids in women eating a low-fat diet. *Am. J. Clin. Nutr.* **2001**, *74*, 242–247. [PubMed]

45. Crawford, M.A.; Golfetto, I.; Ghebremeskel, K.; Min, Y.; Moodley, T.; Poston, L.; Phylactos, A.; Cunnane, S.; Schmidt, W. The potential role for arachidonic and docosahexaenoic acids in protection against some central nervous system injuries in preterm infants. *Lipids* **2003**, *38*, 303–315. [CrossRef] [PubMed]

46. Larque, E.; Ruiz-Palacios, M.; Koletzko, B. Placental regulation of fetal nutrient supply. *Curr. Opin. Clin. Nutr. Metab. Care* **2013**, *16*, 292–297. [CrossRef] [PubMed]

47. Koletzko, B.; Agostini, C.; Bergmann, R.; Ritzenthaler, K.; Shamir, R. Physiological aspects of human milk lipids and implications for infant feeding: A workshop report. *Acta Paediatr.* **2011**, *100*, 1405–1415. [CrossRef] [PubMed]

48. Sinclair, A.J.; Crawford, M.A. The accumulation of arachidonate and docosahexaenoate in the developing rat brain. *J. Neurochem.* **1972**, *19*, 1753–1758. [CrossRef] [PubMed]

49. Makrides, M.; Neumann, M.; Byard, R.W.; Simmer, K.; Gibson, R.A. Fatty acid composition of brain, retina, and erythrocytes in breast- and formula-fed infants. *Am. J. Clin. Nutr.* **1994**, *60*, 189–194. [PubMed]

50. Kuipers, R.S.; Luxwolda, M.F.; Offringa, P.J.; Boersma, E.R.; Dijck-Brouwer, D.A.; Muskiet, F.A.J. Fetal intrauterine whole body linoleic, arachidonic, and docosahexaenoic acid contents and accretion rates. *Prostaglandins Leukot. Essent. Fat. Acids* **2011**, *86*, 13–20. [CrossRef] [PubMed]

51. Carver, J.D.; Benford, V.J.; Han, B.; Cantor, A.B. The relationship between age and the fatty acid composition of cerebral cortex and erythrocytes in human subjects. *Brain Res. Bull.* **2001**, *56*, 79–85. [CrossRef]

52. Salem, N.M.; Lin, Y.H.; Moriguchi, T.; Lim, S.Y.; Salem, N., Jr.; Hibbelin, J.R. Distribution of omega-6 and omega-3 polyunsaturated fatty acids in the whole rat body and 25 compartments. *Prostaglandins Leukot. Essent. Fat. Acids* **2015**, *100*, 13–20. [CrossRef] [PubMed]

53. DeMar, J.C., Jr.; DiMartino, C.; Baca, A.W.; Lefkowitz, W.; Salem, N., Jr. Effect of dietary docosahexaenoic acid on biosynthesis of docosahexaenoic acid from alpha-linolenic acid in young rats. *J. Lipid Res.* **2008**, *49*, 1963–1980. [CrossRef] [PubMed]

54. Tyburczy, C.; Kothapalli, K.S.D.; Park, W.J.; Blank, B.S.; Bradford, K.L.; Zimmer, J.P.; Butt, C.M.; Salem, N., Jr.; Brenna, J.T. Heart arachidonic acid is uniquely sensitive to dietary arachidonic acid and docosahexaenoic acid content in domestic piglets. *Prostaglandins Leukot. Essent. Fat. Acids* **2011**, *85*, 335–343. [CrossRef] [PubMed]

55. Axelrod, J. Receptor-mediated activation of phospholipase A2 and arachidonic acid release in signal transduction. *Biochem. Soc. Trans.* **1990**, *18*, 503–507. [CrossRef] [PubMed]

56. Piomelli, D. Eicosanoids in synaptic transmissions. *Crit. Rev. Neurobiol.* **1994**, *11*, 367–373.

57. Schoenheimer, R.; Rittenberg, D. Deuterium as an indicator in the study of intermediary metabolism V. The desaturation of fatty acids in the organism. *J. Biol. Chem.* **1936**, *113*, 505–510.

58. Nichaman, M.Z.; Olson, R.E.; Sweeley, C.C. Metabolism of linoleic acid-1-^{14}C in normolipidemic and hyperlipidemic humans fed linoleate diets. *Am. J. Clin. Nutr.* **1967**, *20*, 1070–1083. [PubMed]

59. Chambaz, J.; Ravel, D.; Manier, M.-C.; Pepin, D.; Mulliez, N.; Bereziat, G. Essential fatty acids interconversion in the human fetal liver. *Neonatology* **1985**, *47*, 136–140. [CrossRef]

60. El Boustani, S.; Descomps, B.; Monnier, L.; Warnant, J. *In vivo* conversion of dihommogamma linolenic acid into arachidonic acid in man. *Prog. Lipid Res.* **1986**, *25*, 67–71. [CrossRef]

61. Emken, E.A.; Adlof, R.O.; Rakoff, H.; Rohwedder, W.K. Metabolism of deuterium-labeled linolenic, linoleic, oleic, stearic and palmitic acid in human subjects. In Synthesis and Applications of Isotopically Labelled Compounds, Proceedings of the Third International Symposium, Innsbruck, Austria, 17–21 July 1988; Baillie, T.A., Jones, J.R., Eds.; Elsevier Science Publishers: Amsterdam, The Netherlands, 1988; pp. 713–716.

62. Emken, E.A.; Rohwedder, W.K.; Adlof, R.O.; Gulley, R.M. Metabolism in humans of cis-12, trans-15-octadecadienoic acid relative to palmitic, stearic, oleic and linoleic acids. *Lipids* **1987**, *22*, 495–504. [CrossRef] [PubMed]

63. Demmelmair, H.; von Schenck, U.; Behrendt, E.; Sauerwald, T.; Koletzko, B. Estimation of arachidonic acid synthesis in full-term neonates using natural variation of 13C content. *J. Pediatr. Gastroenterol. Nutr.* **1995**, *21*, 31–36. [CrossRef] [PubMed]

64. Salem, N., Jr.; Wegher, B.; Mena, P.; Uauy, R. Arachidonic and docosahexaenoic acids are biosynthesized from their 18-carbon precursors in human infants. *Proc. Natl. Acad. Sci. USA* **1996**, *93*, 49–54. [CrossRef] [PubMed]

65. Pawlosky, R.J.; Sprecher, H.W.; Salem, N., Jr. High sensitivity negative ion GC/MS method for detection of desaturated and chain-elongated products of deuterated linoleic and linolenic acids. *J. Lipid Res.* **1992**, *33*, 1711–1717. [PubMed]

66. Carnielli, V.P.; Wattimea, D.J.L.; Luijendijk, I.H.T.; Boerlage, A.; Degenhart, H.J.; Sauer, P.J.J. The very low weight premature infant is capable of synthesizing arachidonic and docosahexaenoic acids from linoleic and linolenic acids. *Pediatr. Res.* **1996**, *40*, 169–174. [CrossRef] [PubMed]

67. Pawlosky, R.J.; Lin, Y.H.; Llanos, A.; Mena, P.; Uauy, R.; Salem, N., Jr. Compartmental analysis of plasma ^{13}C- and ^{2}H-labelled *n*-6 fatty acids arising from oral administrations of ^{13}C-U-18:2*n*-6 and ^{2}H$_5$-20:3*n*-6 in newborn infants. *Pediatr. Res.* **2006**, *60*, 327–333. [CrossRef] [PubMed]

68. Sauerwald, T.U.; Hachey, D.L.; Jensen, C.L.; Chen, H.; Andersen, R.E.; Heird, W.C. Effect of dietary α-linolenic intake on incorporation of docosahexaenoic and arachidonic acids into plasma phospholipids of term infants. *Lipids* **1996**, *31*, S131–S135. [CrossRef] [PubMed]

69. Carnielli, V.P.; Simonato, M.; Verlato, G.; Luijendijk, I.; De Curtis, M.; Sauer, P.J.J.; Cogo, P.E. Synthesis of long-chain polyunsaturated fatty acids in preterm newborns fed formula with long-chain polyunsaturated fatty acids. *Am. J. Clin. Nutr.* **2007**, *86*, 1323–1330. [PubMed]

70. EFSA Panel on Dietetic Products. Scientific opinion on nutrient requirements and dietary intakes on infants and young children in the European Union. *EFSA J.* **2013**, *11*, 3408.

71. EFSA Panel on Dietetic Products, Nutrition and Allergies (NDA). Scientific opinion on the essential composition of infant and follow-on formulae. *EFSA J.* **2014**, *12*, 3760.

72. Birch, E.E.; Castañeda, Y.S.; Wheaton, D.H.; Birch, D.G.; Uauy, R.D.; Hoffman, D.R. Visual maturation of term infants fed long-chain polyunsaturated fatty acid-supplemented or control formula for 12 mo. *Am. J. Clin. Nutr.* **2005**, *81*, 871–879. [PubMed]

73. World Health Organization (WHO). Global Strategy on Infant and Young Child Feeding, 2002. Available online: http://www.who.int/nutrition/topics/infantfeeding_recommendation/en/ (accessed on 15 October 2015).

74. World Health Organization (WHO). Nutrient Adequacy of Exclusive Breastfeeding for the Term Infant during the First Six Months of Life, 2002. Available online: http://www.who.int/nutrition/publications/infantfeeding/9241562110/en/ (accessed on 15 October 2015).

75. American Academy of Pediatrics. Breastfeeding and the use of human milk. *Pediatrics* **2012**, *129*, e827. [CrossRef]

76. International Baby Food Action (IBFAN). The State of Breastfeeding in 33 Countries, 2010. Available online: https://www.google.co.uk/?gws_rd=ssl#q=IBFAN+33+countries (accessed on 15 October 2015).

77. U.S. Department of Agriculture, Agricultural Research Service. USDA National Nutrient Database for Standard Reference, Release 27. Nutrient Data Laboratory Home Page. 2014. Available online: http://www.ars.usda.gov/nutrientdata (accessed on 15 October 2015).

78. Centers for Disease Control and Prevention. Clinical Growth Charts, 2015. Available online: http://www.cdc.gov/growthcharts/cdccharts.htm (accessed on 19 November 2015).

79. Michaelsen, K.F.; Dewey, K.G.; Perez-Exposito, A.B. Food sources and intake of *n*-6 and *n*-3 fatty acids in low-income countries with emphasis on infants, young children (6–24 months), and pregnant and lactating women. *Mater. Child Nutr.* **2011**, *7* (Suppl. S2), 124–140. [CrossRef] [PubMed]

80. Agostoni, C. Docosahexaenoic acid (DHA): From the maternal-foetal dyad to the complementary feeding period. *Early Hum. Dev.* **2010**, *86* (Suppl. S1), 3–6. [CrossRef] [PubMed]

81. Prentice, A.M.; Paul, A.A. Fat and energy needs of children in developing countries. *Am. J. Clin. Nutr.* **2000**, *72*, 1253S–1265S. [PubMed]

82. Barbarich, B.N.; Willows, N.D.; Wang, L.; Clandinin, M.T. Polyunsaturated fatty acids and anthropometric indices of children in rural China. *Eur. J. Clin. Nutr.* **2006**, *60*, 1100–1107. [CrossRef] [PubMed]

83. PAHO/WHO. *Guiding Principles for Complementary Feeding of the Breastfed Child*; PAHO/WHO: Washington, DC, USA, 2003.

84. Joshi, N.; Agho, K.E.; Dibley, M.J.; Senarath, U.; Tiwari, K. Determinants of inappropriate complementary feeding practices in young children in Nepal: Secondary data analysis of Demographic and Health Survey 2006. *Mater. Child Nutr.* **2012**, *1*, 45–59. [CrossRef] [PubMed]

85. Dutta, T.; Sywulka, S.M.; Frongillo, E.A.; Lutter, C.K. Characteristics attributed to complementary foods by caregivers in four countries of Latin America and the Caribbean. *Food Nutr. Bull.* **2006**, *27*, 316–326. [CrossRef] [PubMed]

86. Agostoni, C.; Decsi, T.; Fewtrell, M.; Goulet, O.; Kolacek, S.; Koletzko, B.; Michaelsen, K.F.; Moreno, L.; Puntis, J.; Rigo, J.; *et al.* Complementary feeding: A commentary by the ESPGHAN Committee on Nutrition. *J. Pediatr. Gastroenterol. Nutr.* **2008**, *46*, 99–110. [CrossRef] [PubMed]

87. Schwartz, J.; Dube, K.; Alexy, U.; Kalhoff, H.; Kersting, M. PUFA and LC-PUFA intake during the first year of life: Can dietary practice achieve a guideline diet? *Eur. J. Clin. Nutr.* **2010**, *64*, 124–130. [CrossRef] [PubMed]

88. Schwartz, J.; Dube, K.; Sichert-Hellert, W.; Kannenberg, F.; Kunz, C.; Kalhoff, H.; Kersting, M. Modification of dietary polyunsaturated fatty acids via complementary food enhances *n*-3 long-chain polyunsaturated fatty acid synthesis in healthy infants: A double blinded randomised controlled trial. *Arch. Dis. Child.* **2009**, *94*, 876–882. [CrossRef] [PubMed]

89. Grote, V.; Verduci, E.; Scalioni, S.; Vecchi, F.; Contarini, G.; Giovannini, M.; Koletzko, B.; Agostoni, C. Breast milk composition and infant nutrient intakes during the first 12 months of life. *Eur. J. Clin. Nutr.* **2015**, *70*, 250–256. [CrossRef] [PubMed]

90. Sioen, I.; Matthys, C.; De Backer, G.; Van Camp, J.; De Henauw, S. Importance of seafood as nutrient source in the diet of Belgian adolescents. *J. Hum. Nutr. Diet.* **2007**, *20*, 580–589. [CrossRef] [PubMed]

91. Meyer, B.J.; Mann, N.J.; Lewis, J.L.; Milligan, G.C.; Sinclair, A.J.; Howe, P.R. Dietary intakes and food sources of omega-6 and omega-3 polyunsaturated fatty acids. *Lipids* **2003**, *38*, 391–398. [CrossRef] [PubMed]

92. Innis, S.M.; Vaghri, Z.; King, D.J. *n*-6 docosapentaenoic acid is not a predictor of low docosahexaenoic acid status in Canadian preschool children. *Am. J. Clin. Nutr.* **2004**, *80*, 768–773. [PubMed]

93. Lien, V.W.; Clamdinin, M.T. Dietary assessment of arachidonic acid and docosahexaenoic acid intake in 4–7 year-old children. *J. Am. Coll. Nutr.* **2009**, *28*, 7–15. [CrossRef] [PubMed]

94. Keim, S.A.; Branum, A.M. Dietary intake of polyunsaturated fatty acids and fish among US children 12–60 months of age. *Mater. Child Health Nutr.* **2015**, *11*, 987–998. [CrossRef] [PubMed]

95. U.S. Department of Agriculture, Agricultural Research Service. What We Eat in America. 2015. Available online: http://www.ars.usda.gov/Services/docs.htm?docid=13793# (accessed on 15 October 2015).

96. Birch, E.E.; Khoury, J.C.; Berseth, C.L.; Castaneda, Y.S.; Couch, J.M.; Bean, J.; Tamer, R.; Harris, C.L.; Mitmesser, S.H.; Scalabrin, D.M. The impact of early nutrition on incidence of allergic manifestations and common respiratory illnesses in children. *J. Pediatr.* **2010**, *156*, 902–906. [CrossRef] [PubMed]

97. Calder, P.C. Polyunsaturated fatty acids and inflammation: From molecular biology to the clinic. *Lipids* **2003**, *38*, 343–352. [CrossRef] [PubMed]

98. Calder, P.C. *n*-3 polyunsaturated fatty acids, inflammation, and inflammatory diseases. *Am. J. Clin. Nutr.* **2006**, *83*, 1505S–1519S. [PubMed]

99. Jones, P.J.H.; Kubow, S. Lipids, sterols, and their metabolites. In *Modern Nutrition in Health and Disease*; Shils, M.E., Shike, M., Ross, A.C., Caballero, B., Cousins, B., Eds.; Lippincott Williams & Wilkins: Philadelphia, PA, USA, 2006; pp. 92–122.

100. Ricciotti, E.; FitzGerald, G.A. Prostaglandins and inflammation. *Arterioscler. Thromb. Vasc. Biol.* **2011**, *31*, 986–1000. [CrossRef] [PubMed]

101. Reinhold, H.; Ahmadi, S.; Depner, U.B.; Layh, B.; Heindl, C.; Hamza, M.; Pahl, A.; Brune, K.; Narumiya, S.; Müller, U.; et al. Spinal inflammatory hyperalgesia is mediated by prostaglandin E receptors of the EP2 subtype. *J. Clin. Investig.* **2005**, *115*, 673–679. [CrossRef] [PubMed]

102. Noda, M.; Kariura, Y.; Pannasch, U.; Nishikawa, K.; Wang, L.; Seike, T.; Ifuku, M.; Kosai, Y.; Wang, B.; Nolte, C.; et al. Neuroprotective role of bradykinin because of the attenuation of pro-inflammatory cytokine release from activated microglia. *J. Neurochem.* **2007**, *101*, 397–410. [CrossRef] [PubMed]

103. Min, Y.; Crawford, M.A. Essential fatty acids. In *The Eicosanoids*; Curtis, P., Ed.; John Wiley & Sons, Ltd.: West Sussex, UK, 2004; pp. 257–276.

104. McCarthy, T.L.; Casinghino, S.; Mittanck, D.W.; Ji, C.H.; Centrella, M.; Rotwein, P. Promoter-dependent and -independent activation of insulin-like growth factor binding protein-5 gene expression by prostaglandin E_2 in primary rat osteoblasts. *J. Biol. Chem.* **1996**, *271*, 6666–6671. [PubMed]

105. Urade, Y.; Hayaishi, O. Prostaglandin D2 and sleep regulation. *Biochem. Biophys. Acta* **1999**, *1436*, 606–615. [CrossRef]

106. Ushikubi, F.; Sergi, E.; Sugimoto, Y.; Murata, T.; Matsuoka, T.; Kobayashi, T.; Hizaki, H.; Tuboi, K.; Katsuyama, M.; Ichikawa, A.; et al. Impaired febrile response in mice lacking the prostaglandin E receptor subtype EP3. *Nature* **1998**, *395*, 281–284. [PubMed]

107. Murata, T.; Ushikubi, F.; Matsuoka, T.; Hirata, M.; Yamasaki, A.; Sugimoto, Y.; Ichikawa, A.; Aze, Y.; Tanaka, T.; Yoshida, N.; et al. Altered pain perception and inflammatory response in mice lacking prostacyclin receptor. *Nature* **1997**, *388*, 678–682. [PubMed]

108. Astudillo, A.M.; Balgoma, D.; Balboa, M.A.; Balsinde, J. Dynamics of arachidonic acid mobilization by inflammatory cells. *Biochim. Biophys. Acta* **2012**, *1821*, 249–256. [CrossRef] [PubMed]

109. Bagga, D.; Wang, L.; Faris-Eisner, R.; Glaspy, J.A.; Reddy, S.T. Differential effects of prostaglandin derived from ω-6 and ω-3 polyunsaturated fatty acids on COX-2 expression and IL-6 secretion. *Proc. Natl. Acad. Sci. USA* **2003**, *100*, 1751–1756. [CrossRef] [PubMed]

110. Levy, B.D.; Clish, C.B.; Schmidt, B.; Gronert, K.; Serhan, C.N. Lipid mediator class switching during acute inflammation signals in resolution. *Nat. Immunol.* **2001**, *2*, 612–619. [CrossRef] [PubMed]

111. Samuelsson, B.; Dahlen, S.E.; Lindgren, J.A.; Rouzer, C.A.; Serhan, C.N. Leukotrienes and lipoxins—Structures, biosynthesis, and biological effects. *Science* **1987**, *237*, 1171–1176. [CrossRef] [PubMed]

112. Fredman, G.; Serhan, C.N. Specialized proresolving mediator targets for RvE1 and RvD1 in peripheral blood and mechanisms of resolution. *Biochem. J.* **2011**, *437*, 185–197. [CrossRef] [PubMed]

113. Kelley, D.S. Modulation of human and inflammatory responses by dietary fatty acids. *Nutrition* **2001**, *17*, 669–673. [CrossRef]

114. Calder, P.C.; Kew, S. The immune system: A target for functional foods? *Br. J. Nutr.* **2002**, *88* (Suppl. S2), S165–S176. [CrossRef] [PubMed]

115. Lentz, A.K.; Feezor, R.J. Principles of immunology. *Nutr. Clin. Pract.* **2003**, *18*, 451–460. [CrossRef] [PubMed]

116. Mahadevappa, V.G.; Holub, B.J. The molecular species composition of individual diacyl phospholipids in human platelets. *Biochim. Biophys. Acta* **1982**, *713*, 73–79. [CrossRef]

117. Kaushansky, K. Lineage-specific hematopoietic growth factors. *N. Engl. J. Med.* **2006**, *354*, 2034–2045. [CrossRef] [PubMed]

118. Semple, J.W.; Italiano, J.E., Jr.; Freedman, J. Platelets and the immune system. *Nature* **2011**, *11*, 264–274.

119. Tamagawa-Mineoka, R. Important roles of platelets as immune cells in the skin. *J. Dermatol. Sci.* **2015**, *77*, 93–101. [CrossRef] [PubMed]

120. Martin, C.R.; DaSilva, D.A.; Cluette-Brown, J.E.; DiMonda, C.; Hamill, A.; Bhutta, A.Q.; Coronel, E.; Wilschanski, M.; Stephens, A.J.; Driscoll, D.F.; *et al.* Decreased postnatal docosahexaenoic and arachidonic acid blood levels in premature infants are associated with neonatal morbidities. *J. Pediatr.* **2011**, *159*, 743–749. [CrossRef] [PubMed]

121. Lands, W.F.; LeTellier, P.R.; Rome, L.H.; Vanderhoek, J.Y. Inhibition of prostaglandin biosynthesis. *Adv. Biosci.* **1973**, *9*, 15–227.

122. Vane, J.R. Inhibition of prostaglandin synthesis as a mechanism of action for aspirin-like drugs. *Nature* **1971**, *231*, 232–235. [CrossRef]

123. Hormones. Available online: http://www.medicinenet.com/script/main/art.asp?articlekey=3783 (accessed on 6 February 2016).

124. McMurray, W.C. *A Synopsis of Human Biochemistry*; Harper and Row Publishers: New York, NY, USA, 1982; pp. 193–199.

125. Bowen, R.A. Hormone Chemistry, Synthesis and Elimination. Available online: http://www.vivo.colostate.edu/hbooks/pathphys/endocrine/basics/chem.html (accessed on 15 October 2015).

126. Thorner, M.O.; Vance, M.L.; Hartman, M.L.; Holl, R.W.; Evans, W.S.; Veldhuis, J.D.; Van Cauter, E.; Copinschi, G.; Bowers, C.Y. Physiological role of somatostatin on growth hormone regulation in humans. *Metabolism* **1990**, *39*, 40–42. [CrossRef]

127. Brochhausen, C.; Neuland, P.; Kirkpatrick, C.J.; Nusing, R.M.; Klaus, G. Cyclooxygenases and prostaglandin E_2 receptors in growth plate chondrocytes *in vitro* and *in situ*-prostaglandin E_2 dependent proliferation of growth plate chondrocytes. *Arthritis Res. Ther.* **2006**, *8*, R78. [CrossRef] [PubMed]

128. Boyan, B.D.; Sylvia, V.L.; Dean, D.D.; Del Toro, F.; Schwartz, Z. Differential regulation of growth plate chondrocytes by 1alpha,25-(OH)2D3 and 24R,25-(OH)2D3 involves cell-maturation-specific membrane-receptor-activated phospholipid metabolism. *Crit. Rev. Oral Biol. Med.* **2002**, *13*, 143–154. [CrossRef] [PubMed]

129. Specker, B.; Binkley, T. Randomized trial of physical activity and calcium supplementation on bone mineral content in 3- to 5-year-old children. *J. Bone Miner. Res.* **2003**, *418*, 885–892. [CrossRef] [PubMed]

130. Specker, B.L.; Mulligan, L.; Ho, M. Longitudinal study of calcium intake, physical activity, and bone mineral content in infants 6–18 months of age. *J. Bone Miner. Res.* **1999**, *14*, 569–576. [CrossRef] [PubMed]

131. Del Toro, F., Jr.; Sylvia, V.L.; Schubkegel, S.R.; Campos, R.; Dean, D.D.; Boyan, B.D.; Schwartz, Z. Characterization of prostaglandin E(2) receptors and their role in 24,25-(OH)(2)D(3)-mediated effects on resting zone chondrocytes. *J. Cell Physiol.* **2000**, *182*, 196–208. [CrossRef]

132. Boyan, B.D.; Sylvia, V.L.; Dean, D.D.; Pedrozo, H.; Del Toro, F.; Nemere, I.; Posner, G.H.; Schwartz, Z. 1,25-(OH)2D3 modulates growth plate chondrocytes via membrane receptor-mediated protein kinase C by a mechanism that involves changes in phospholipid metabolism and the action of arachidonic acid and PGE_2. *Steroids* **1999**, *64*, 129–136. [PubMed]

133. Schwartz, Z.; Sylvia, V.L.; Curry, D.; Luna, M.H.; Dean, D.D.; Boyan, B.D. Arachidonic acid directly mediates the rapid effects of 24,25-dihydroxyvitamin D3 via protein kinase C and indirectly through prostaglandin production in resting zone chondrocytes. *Endocrinology* **1999**, *140*, 2991–3002. [CrossRef] [PubMed]

134. Sylvia, V.L.; Schwartz, Z.; Curry, D.B.; Chang, Z.; Dean, D.D.; Boyan, B.D. 1,25(OH)2D3 regulates protein kinase C activity through two phospholipid-dependent pathways involving phospholipase A2 and phospholipase C in growth zone chondrocytes. *J. Bone Miner. Res.* **1998**, *13*, 559–569. [CrossRef] [PubMed]

135. Kosher, R.A.; Walker, K.H. The effect of prostaglandins on *in vitro* limb cartilage differentiation. *Exp. Cell Res.* **1983**, *145*, 145–153. [CrossRef]

136. Copray, J.C.; Jansen, H.W. Cyclic nucleotides and growth regulation of the mandibular condylar cartilage of the rat *in vitro*. *Arch. Oral Biol.* **1985**, *30*, 749–752. [CrossRef]

137. Li, T.F.; Zuscik, M.J.; Ionescu, A.M.; Zhang, X.; Rosier, R.N.; Schwarz, E.M.; Drissi, H.; O'Keefe, R.J. PGE$_2$ inhibits chondrocyte differentiation through PKA and PKC signaling. *Exp. Cell Res.* **2004**, *300*, 159–169. [CrossRef] [PubMed]

138. Raisz, L.G. Prostaglandins and bone: Physiology and pathophysiology. *Osteoarthr. Cartil.* **1999**, *7*, 419–421. [CrossRef] [PubMed]

139. Suzawa, T.; Miyaura, C.; Inada, M.; Maruyama, T.; Sugimoto, Y.; Ushikubi, F.; Ichikawa, A.; Narumiya, S.; Suda, T. The role of prostaglandin E receptor subtypes (EP1, EP2, EP3, and EP4) in bone resorption: An analysis using specific agonists for the respective EPs. *Endocrinology* **2000**, *141*, 1554–1559. [CrossRef] [PubMed]

140. Baylink, D.J.; Finkelman, R.D.; Mohan, S. Growth factors to stimulate bone formation. *J. Bone Min. Res.* **1993**, *8*, S565–S572. [CrossRef] [PubMed]

141. Paralkar, V.M.; Borovecki, F.; Ke, H.Z.; Cameron, K.O.; Lefker, B.; Grasser, W.A.; Owen, T.A.; Li, M.; DaSilva-Jardine, P.; Zhou, M.; *et al.* An EP2 receptor-selective prostaglandin E$_2$ agonist induces bone healing. *PNAS* **2003**, *100*, 6736–6740. [CrossRef] [PubMed]

142. Tanaka, M.; Sakai, A.; Uchida, S.; Tanaka, S.; Nagashima, M.; Katayama, T.; Yamaguchi, K.; Nakamura, T. Prostaglandin E$_2$ receptor (EP4) selective agonist (ONO-4819.CD) accelerates bone repair of femoral cortex after drill-hole injury associated with local upregulation of bone turnover in mature rats. *Bone* **2004**, *34*, 940–943. [CrossRef] [PubMed]

143. Jee, W.S.; Ueno, K.; Kimmel, D.B.; Woodbury, D.M.; Price, P.; Woodbury, L.A. The role of bone cells in increasing metaphyseal hard tissue in rapidly growing rats treated with prostaglandin E$_2$. *Bone* **1987**, *8*, 171–178. [CrossRef]

144. Agas, D.; Marchetti, L.; Hurley, M.M.; Sabbieti, D. Prostaglandin F2α: A bone remodeling mediator. *J. Cell. Physiol.* **2013**, *228*, 25–29. [CrossRef] [PubMed]

145. Galea, G.L.; Meakin, L.B.; Williams, C.M.; Hulin-Curtis, S.L.; Lanyon, L.E.; Poole, A.W.; Price, J.S. Protein kinase Cα (PKCα) regulates bone architecture and osteoblast activity. *J. Biol. Chem.* **2014**, *289*, 25509–25522. [CrossRef] [PubMed]

146. Zaman, G.; Sunters, A.; Galea, G.L.; Javaheri, B.; Saxon, L.K.; Moustafa, A.; Armstrong, V.J.; Price, J.S.; Lanyon, L.E. Loading-related regulation of transcription factor EGR2/Krox-20 in bone cells is ERK1/2 protein-mediated and prostaglandin, Wnt-signaling pathway-, and insulin-like growth factor-I axis-dependent. *J. Biol. Chem.* **2012**, *287*, 3946–3962. [CrossRef] [PubMed]

147. Kido, S.; Kuriwaka-Kido, R.; Umino-Miyatani, Y.; Endo, I.; Inoue, D.; Taniguchi, H.; Inoue, Y.; Imamura, T.; Matsumoto, T. Mechanical stress activates Smad pathway through PKCδ to enhance interleukin-11 gene transcription in osteoblasts. *PLoS ONE* **2010**, *5*, e13090. [CrossRef] [PubMed]

148. Nakura, A.; Higuchi, C.; Yoshida, K.; Yoshikawa, H. PkCα suppresses osteoblastic differentiation. *Bone* **2011**, *48*, 476–484. [CrossRef] [PubMed]

149. Weiler, H.A.; Fitzpatrick-Wong, S. Dietary long-chain polyunsaturated fatty acids minimize dexamethasone-induced reductions in arachidonic acid status but not bone mineral content in piglets. *Pediatr. Res.* **2002**, *51*, 282–289. [CrossRef] [PubMed]

150. Blanaru, J.L.; Kohut, J.R.; Fitzpatrick-Wong, S.C.; Weiler, H.A. Dose response of bone mass to dietary arachidonic acid in piglets fed cow milk-based formula. *Am. J. Clin. Nutr.* **2004**, *79*, 139–147. [PubMed]

151. Pash, J.M.; Canalis, E. Transcriptional regulation of insulin-like growth factor-binding protein-5 by prostaglandin E$_2$ in osteoblast cells. *Endocrinology* **1996**, *137*, 2375–2382. [PubMed]

152. Almaden, Y.; Canalejo, A.; Ballesteros, E.; Anon, G.; Rodriguez, M. Effect of high extracellular phosphate concentration on arachidonic acid production by parathyroid tissue *in vitro*. *J. Am. Soc. Nephrol.* **2000**, *11*, 1712–1718. [PubMed]

153. Klein-Nulend, J.; Burger, E.H.; Semeins, C.M.; Raisz, L.G.; Pilbeam, C.C. Pulsating fluid flow stimulates prostaglandin release and inducible prostaglandin G/H synthase mRNA expression in primary mouse bone cells. *J. Bone Miner. Res.* **1997**, *12*, 45–51. [CrossRef] [PubMed]

154. Weiler, H.A. Dietary supplementation of arachidonic acid is associated with higher whole body weight and bone mineral density in growing pigs. *Pediatr. Res.* **2000**, *47*, 692–697. [CrossRef] [PubMed]

155. Weiler, H.; Fitzpatrick-Wong, S.; Schellenberg, J.; McCloy, U.; Veitch, R.; Kovacs, H.; Kohut, J.; Kin Yuen, C. Maternal and cord blood long-chain polyunsaturated fatty acids are predictive of bone mass at birth in healthy term-born infants. *Pediatr. Res.* **2005**, *58*, 1254–1258. [CrossRef] [PubMed]

156. Akatsu, T.; Takahashi, N.; Udagawa, N.; Imamura, K.; Yamaguchi, A.; Sato, K.; Nagata, N.; Suda, T. Role of prostaglandins in interleukin-1-induced bone resorption in mice *in vitro. J. Bone Miner. Res.* **1991**, *6*, 183–189. [CrossRef] [PubMed]

157. Liu, X.H.; Kirschenbaum, A.; Yao, S.; Levine, A.C. Interactive effect of interleukin-6 and prostaglandin E_2 on osteoclastogenesis via the OPG/RANKL/RANK system. *Ann. N. Y. Acad. Sci.* **2006**, *1068*, 225–233. [CrossRef] [PubMed]

158. Zhang, X.; Schwarz, E.M.; Young, D.A.; Puzas, J.E.; Rosier, R.N.; O'Keefe, R.J. Cyclooxygenase-2 regulates mesenchymal cell differentiation into the osteoblast lineage and is critically involved in bone repair. *J. Clin. Investig.* **2002**, *109*, 1405–1415. [CrossRef] [PubMed]

159. Samoto, H.; Shimizu, E.; Matsuda-Honjyo, Y.; Saito, R.; Nakao, S.; Yamazaki, M.; Furuyama, S.; Sugiya, H.; Sodek, J.; Ogata, Y. Prostaglandin E_2 stimulates bone sialoprotein (BSP) expression through cAMP and fibroblast growth factor 2 response elements in the proximal promoter of the rat BSP gene. *J. Biol. Chem.* **2003**, *278*, 28659–28667. [CrossRef] [PubMed]

160. Cherian, P.P.; Cheng, B.; Gu, S.; Sprague, E.; Bonewald, L.F.; Jiang, J.X. Effects of mechanical strain on the function of Gap junctions in osteocytes are mediated through the prostaglandin EP2 receptor. *J. Biol. Chem.* **2003**, *278*, 43146–43156. [CrossRef] [PubMed]

161. Miyaura, C.; Inada, M.; Matsumoto, C.; Ohshiba, T.; Uozumi, N.; Shimizu, T.; Ito, A. An essential role of cytosolic phospholipase A2alpha in prostaglandin E_2-mediated bone resorption associated with inflammation. *J. Exp. Med.* **2003**, *197*, 1303–1310. [CrossRef] [PubMed]

162. Boswell, K.; Koskelo, E.-K.; Carl, L.; Glaze, S.; Hensen, D.J.; Williams, K.D.; Kyle, D.J. Preclinical evaluation of single-cell oils that are highly enriched with arachidonic acid and docosahexaenoic acid. *Food Chem. Toxicol.* **1996**, *34*, 585–593. [CrossRef]

163. Suarez, A.; del Carmen Ramirez, M.; Faus, M.J.; Gil, A. Dietary long-chain polyunsaturated fatty acids influence tissue fatty acid composition in rats at weaning. *J. Nutr.* **1996**, *126*, 887–897. [PubMed]

164. De la Presa-Owens, S.; Innis, S.M.; Rioux, F.M. Addition of triglycerides with arachidonic acid or docosahexaenoic acid to infant formula has tissue- and lipid class-specific effects on fatty acids and hepatic desaturase activities in formula-fed piglets. *J. Nutr.* **1998**, *128*, 1376–1384. [PubMed]

165. Baur, L.A.; O'Connor, J.; Pan, D.A.; Kriketos, A.D.; Storlien, L.H. The fatty acid composition of skeletal muscle membrane phospholipid: Its relationship with the type of feeding and plasma levels in young children. *Metabolism* **1998**, *47*, 106–112. [CrossRef]

166. Blaauw, B.; Del Piccolo, P.; Rodriguez, L.; Hernandez Gonzales, V.H.; Agata, L.; Solagna, F.; Mammano, F.; Pozzan, T.; Schiaffino, S. No evidence for inositol 1,4,5-triphosphate-dependent Ca^{2+} release in isolated fibers of adult mouse skeletal muscle. *J. Gen. Physiol.* **2012**, *140*, 235–241. [CrossRef] [PubMed]

167. Berthier, C.; Kutchukian, C.; Bouvard, C.; Okamura, Y.; Jacquemond, V. Depression of voltage-activated Ca^{2+} release in skeletal muscle by activation of a voltage-sensing phosphatase. *J. Gen. Physiol.* **2015**, *145*, 315–330. [CrossRef] [PubMed]

168. Ohizumi, Y.; Hirata, Y.; Suzuki, A.; Kobayashi, M. Two novel types of calcium release from skeletal sarcoplasmic reticulum by phosphatidylinositol 4,5 biphosphate. *Can. J. Physiol. Pharmacol.* **1999**, *77*, 276–285. [CrossRef] [PubMed]

169. Sandow, A. Excitation-contraction coupling in muscular response. *Yale J. Biol. Med.* **1952**, *25*, 176–201. [PubMed]

170. Melzer, W.; Herrmann-Frank, A.; Luttgau, H.C. The role of Ca^{2+} ions in excitation-contraction coupling of skeletal muscle fibres. *Biochim. Biophys. Acta* **1995**, *1241*, 59–116. [CrossRef]

171. Kobayashi, M.; Muroyama, A.; Ohizumi, Y. Phosphatidylinositol 4,5-bisphosphate enhances calcium release from sarcoplasmic reticulum of skeletal muscle. *Biochem. Biophys. Res. Commun.* **1989**, *29*, 1487–1491. [CrossRef]

172. Ghigo, A.; Perino, A.; Hirsch, E. Phosphoinositides and cardiac function. In *Phosphoinositides and Disease, Current Topics in Microbiology and Immunology*; Falasca, M., Ed.; Springer Science + Business Media: Dordrecht, The Netherlands, 2012; pp. 43–60.

173. Rodemann, H.P.; Goldberg, A.L. Arachidonic acid, prostaglandin E_2 and $F_{2\alpha}$ influence rates of protein turnover in skeletal and cardiac muscle. *J. Biol. Chem.* **1982**, *25*, 1632–1638.

174. Standley, R.A.; Liu, S.; Jemiolo, B.; Trappe, S.W.; Trappe, T.A. Prostaglandin E_2 induces transcription of skeletal mass regulators interleukin-6 and muscle RING finger-1 in humans. *Prostaglandins Leukot. Essent. Fat. Acids* **2013**, *88*, 361–364. [CrossRef] [PubMed]

175. Kuipers, R.S.; Luxwolda, M.F.; Dijck-Brouwer, J.; Muskiet, F.A.J. Intrauterine, postpartum and adult relationships between arachidonic acid (AA) and docosahexaenoic acid (DHA). *Prostaglandins Leukot. Essent. Fat. Acids* **2011**, *85*, 245–252. [CrossRef] [PubMed]

176. Luxwolda, M.F.; Kuipers, R.S.; Sango, W.S.; Kwesigabo, G.; Dijck-Brouwer, D.A.J.; Muskiet, F.A.J. A maternal erythrocyte DHA content of approximately 6 g% is the DHA status at which intrauterine DHA biomagnifications turns into bioattenuation and postnatal infant DHA equilibrium is reached. *Eur. J. Nutr.* **2012**, *51*, 665–675. [CrossRef] [PubMed]

177. Carlson, S.E.; Werkman, S.H.; Peoples, J.M.; Cooke, R.J.; Tolley, E.A. Arachidonic acid status correlates with first year of growth in preterm infants. *Proc. Natl. Acad. Sci. USA* **1993**, *90*, 1073–1077. [CrossRef] [PubMed]

178. Clandinin, M.T. Brain development and assessing the supply of polyunsaturated fatty acids. *Lipids* **1999**, *34*, 131–137. [CrossRef] [PubMed]

179. Clandinin, M.T.; Chappell, J.E.; Leong, S.; Heim, T.; Sayer, P.R.; Chance, G.W. Intrauterine fatty acid accretion in infant brain: Implications for fatty acid requirements. *Early Hum. Dev.* **1980**, *4*, 121–129. [CrossRef]

180. Cunnane, S. Problems with essential fatty acids: Time for a new paradigm? *Prog. Lipid Res.* **2003**, *42*, 544–568. [CrossRef]

181. Stoffel, W.; Holz, B.; Jenke, B.; Binczek, E.; Günter, R.H.; Kiss, C.; Karakesisoglou, I.; Thevis, M.; Weber, A.A.; Arnhold, S.; *et al.* Δ6-desaturase (FADS2) deficiency unveils role of ω3- and ω6-polyunsaturated fatty acids. *EMBO J.* **2008**, *27*, 2281–2292. [CrossRef] [PubMed]

182. Stroud, C.K.; Nara, T.Y.; Roqueta-Rivera, M.; Radlowski, E.C.; Lawrence, P.; Zhang, Y.; Cho, B.H.; Segre, M.; Hess, R.A.; Brenna, J.T.; *et al.* Disruption of FADS2 gene in mice impairs male reproduction and causes dermal and intestinal ulceration. *J. Lipid Res.* **2009**, *50*, 1870–1880. [CrossRef] [PubMed]

183. Mohrhauer, H.; Holman, R.T. The effect of dose level of essential fatty acids upon fatty acid composition of the rat liver. *J. Lipid Res.* **1963**, *4*, 151–159. [PubMed]

184. Prottey, C. Essential fatty acids and the skin. *Br. J. Dermatol.* **1976**, *94*, 579–587. [CrossRef] [PubMed]

185. Hansen, H.S.; Jensen, B. Essential function of linoleic acid esterified in acylglucosylceramide and acylceramide in maintaining the epiderma; water permeability barrier. Evidence from feeding studies with oleate, linoleate, arachidonate, columbinate and alpha-linolenate. *Biochem. Biophys. Acta* **1985**, *834*, 357–363. [CrossRef]

186. Hartop, P.J.; Prottey, C. Changes in transepidermal water loss and the composition of epidermal lecithin after application of pure fatty acid triglycerides to the skin of essential fatty acid-deficient rats. *Br. J. Dermatol.* **1976**, *95*, 255–264. [CrossRef] [PubMed]

187. Bertram, T.A. Gastrointestinal tract. In *Handbook of Toxicologic Pathology*; Haschek, W.M., Rousseaux, C.G., Wallig, M., Eds.; Academic Press: San Diego, CA, USA, 2002; pp. 121–186.

188. Miller, C.C.; Ziboh, V.A. Induction of epidermal hyperproliferation by topical *n*-3 polyunsaturated fatty acids on guinea pig skin linked to decreased levels of 13-hydroxyoctadecadienoic acid (13-Hode). *J. Investig. Dermatol.* **1990**, *94*, 353–358. [CrossRef] [PubMed]

189. Cho, H.P.; Nakamura, T.; Clarke, S.D. Cloning, expression, and nutritional regulation of the mammalian delta-6 desaturate. *J. Biol. Chem.* **1999**, *274*, 471–477. [CrossRef] [PubMed]

190. Williard, D.E.; Nwankwo, J.O.; Kaduce, T.L.; Harmon, S.D.; Irons, M.; Moser, H.W.; Raymond, G.V.; Spector, A.A. Identification of a fatty acid delta6-desaturase deficiency in human skin fibroblasts. *J. Lipid Res.* **2001**, *42*, 501–508. [PubMed]

191. Fan, Y-Y.; Monk, J.M.; Hou, T.Y.; Callway, E.; Vincent, L.; Weeks, B.; Yang, P.; Chapkin, R.S. Characterization of an arachidonic acid-deficient (Fads1 knockout) mouse model. *J. Lipid Res.* **2012**, *53*, 1287–1295.

192. Hatanaka, E.; Yasuda, H.; Harauma, A.; Watanabe, J.; Konishi, Y.; Nakamura, M.; Salem, N., Jr.; Moriguchi, T. The Effects of Arachidonic Acid and/or Docosahexaenoic Acid on the Brain Development Using Artificial Rearing of Delta-6-Desaturase Knockout Mice. In Proceedings of the Asian Conference of Nutrition, Yokohama, Japan, 14–18 May 2015.

193. Tian, C.; Fan, C.; Liu, X.; Xu, F.; Qi, K. Brain histological changes in young mice submitted to diets with different ratios of *n*-6/*n*-3 polyunsaturated fatty acids during maternal pregnancy and lactation. *Clin. Nutr.* **2011**, *30*, 659–667. [CrossRef] [PubMed]

194. Nguyen, L.N.; Ma, D.; Shui, G.; Wong, P.; Cazenave-Gassiot, A.; Zhang, X.; Wenk, M.R.; Goh, E.L.K.; Silver, D.L. Mfsd2a is a transporter for the essential omega-3 fatty acid docosahexaenoic acid. *Nature* **2014**, *509*, 503–506. [CrossRef] [PubMed]

195. Berger, J.H.; Charron, M.J.; Silver, D.L. Major Facilitator superfamily domain-containing protein 2a (MFSD2A) has roles in body growth, motor function, and lipid metabolism. *PLoS ONE* **2012**, *7*, e50629. [CrossRef] [PubMed]

196. Peterson, L.D.; Jeffrey, N.M.; Sanderson, P.; Newholme, E.A.; Calder, P.C. Eicosapentaenoic and docosahexaenoic acids alter rat spleen leukocyte fatty acid composition and prostaglandin E_2 production but have different effects on lymphocyte functions and cell-mediated immunity. *Lipids* **1998**, *33*, 171–180. [CrossRef] [PubMed]

197. Jolly, C.A.; Jiang, Y.-H.; Chapkin, R.S.; McMurray, D.N. Dietary (*n*-3) polyunsaturated fatty acids suppress murine lymphoproliferation, interleukin-2 secretion, and the formation of diacylglycerol and ceramide. *J. Nutr.* **1997**, *127*, 37–43. [PubMed]

198. Kelley, D.S.; Taylor, P.C.; Nelson, G.J.; Schmidt, P.C.; Mackey, B.E.; Kyle, D. Effects of dietary arachidonic acid on human immune response. *Lipids* **1997**, *32*, 449–456. [CrossRef] [PubMed]

199. Blikslager, A.T.; Moeser, A.J.; Gookin, J.L.; Jones, S.L.; Odle, J. Restoration of barrier function in injured intestinal mucosa. *Physiol. Rev.* **2007**, *87*, 545–564. [CrossRef] [PubMed]

200. Ferrer, R.; Moreno, J.J. Role of eicosanoids on intestinal epithelial homeostatis. *Biochem. Pharmacol.* **2010**, *80*, 431–438. [CrossRef] [PubMed]

201. Jacobi, S.K.; Moeser, A.J.; Corl, B.A.; Harrell, R.J.; Bilksager, A.T. Dietary long-chain PUFA enhances acute repair of ischemia-injured intestine of suckling pigs. *J. Nutr.* **2012**, *142*, 1266–1271. [CrossRef] [PubMed]

202. Le, H.D.; Meisel, J.A.; de Meijer, V.E.; Fallon, E.M.; Gura, K.M.; Nose, V.; Bistrian, B.R.; Puder, M. Docosahexaenoic acid and arachidonic acid prevent essential fatty acid deficiency and hepatic steatosis. *J. Parenter. Enter. Nutr.* **2012**, *36*, 431–441. [CrossRef] [PubMed]

203. Bassaganya-Riera, J.; Guri, A.J.; Noble, A.M.; Reynolds, K.A.; King, J.; Wood, C.M.; Ashby, M.; Rai, D.; Hontecillas, R. Arachidonic acid- and docosahexaenoic acid-enriched formulas modulate antigen-specific T cell responses to influenza virus in neonatal piglets. *Am. J. Clin. Nutr.* **2007**, *85*, 824–836. [PubMed]

204. Weisinger, H.S.; Vingrys, A.J.; Sinclair, A.J. The effect of docosahexaenoic acid on the electroretinogram of the guinea pig. *Lipids* **1996**, *31*, 65–70. [CrossRef] [PubMed]

205. Champoux, M.; Hibbeln, J.R.; Shannon, C.; Majchrzak, S.; Suomi, S.J.; Salem, N., Jr.; Higley, J.D. Fatty acid formula supplementation and neuromotor development in rhesus monkey neonates. *Pediatr. Res.* **2002**, *51*, 273–281. [CrossRef] [PubMed]

206. Ikemoto, A.; Ohishi, M.; Sato, Y.; Hata, N.; Misawa, Y.; Fujii, Y.; Okuyama, H. Reversibility of *n*-3 fatty acid deficiency-induced alterations of learning behavior in the rat: Level of *n*-6 fatty acids as another factor. *J. Lipid Res.* **2001**, *42*, 1655–1663. [PubMed]

207. Wainwright, P.E.; Xing, H.-C.; Mutsaers, L.; McCutcheon, D.; Kyle, D. Arachidonic acid offsets the effects on mouse brain and behavior of a diet with a low (*n*-6):(*n*-3) ratio and very high levels of docosahexaenoic acid. *J. Nutr.* **1997**, *127*, 184–193. [PubMed]

208. Wainwright, P.E.; Xing, H.-C.; Ward, G.R.; Huang, Y.-S.; Bobik, E.; Auestad, N.; Montalto, M. Water maze performance is unaffected in artificially reared rats fed diets supplemented with arachidonic acid and docosahexaenoic acid. *J. Nutr.* **1999**, *129*, 1079–1089. [PubMed]

209. Wainwright, P.E.; Huang, Y.S.; Bulman-Fleming, B.; Dalby, B.; Mills, D.E.; Redden, P.; McCutcheon, D. The effect of dietary *n*-3/*n*-6 ration on brain development in the mouse: A dose response study with long-chain *n*-3 fatty acids. *Lipids* **1992**, *27*, 98–103. [CrossRef] [PubMed]

210. Min, Y.; Lowry, C.; Ghebremeskel, K.; Thomas, B.; Offley-Shore, B.; Crawford, M. Unfavorable effect of type 1 and type 2 diabetes on maternal and fetal essential fatty acid status: A potential marker of fetal insulin resistance. *Am. J. Clin. Nutr.* **2005**, *82*, 1162–1168. [PubMed]

211. Siddappa, A.M.; Georgieff, M.K.; Wewerka, S.; Worwa, C.; Nelson, C.A.; Deregnier, R.A. Iron deficiency alters auditory recognition memory in newborn infants of diabetic mothers. *Pediatr. Res.* **2004**, *55*, 1034–1041. [CrossRef] [PubMed]

212. DeBoer, T.; Wewerka, S.; Bauer, P.J.; Geogieff, M.K.; Nelson, C.A. Explicit memory performance in infants of diabetic mothers at 1 year of age. *Dev. Med. Child Neurol.* **2005**, *47*, 525–531. [CrossRef] [PubMed]

213. Holman, R.T.; Johnson, S.B.; Gerrand, J.M.; Mauer, S.M.; Kupcho-Sandberg, S.; Brown, D.M. Arachidonic acid deficiency in streptozotocin-induced diabetes. *Proc. Natl. Acad. Sci. USA* **1983**, *80*, 1375–2379. [CrossRef]

214. Hadders-Algra, M. Prenatal long-chain polyunsaturated fatty acid status: The importance of a balanced intake of docosahexaenoic acid and arachidonic acid. *J. Perinat. Med.* **2008**, *36*, 101–109. [CrossRef] [PubMed]

215. Clandinin, M.T.; Chappell, J.E.; Leong, S.; Heim, T.; Sayer, P.R.; Chance, G.W. Extrauterine fatty acid accretion in infant brain: Implications for fatty acid requirements. *Early Hum. Dev.* **1980**, *4*, 131–138. [CrossRef]

216. Zhao, J.; Bigio, M.R.; Weiler, H.A. Maternal arachidonic acid supplementation improves neurodevelopment in young adult offspring from rat dams with and without diabetes. *Prostaglandins Leukot Essent. Fat. Acids* **2011**, *84*, 63–70. [CrossRef] [PubMed]

217. Amusquivar, E.; Ruperez, F.J.; Barbas, C.; Herrera, E. Low arachidonic acid rather than α-tocopherol is responsible for the delayed postnatal development of offspring of rats fed fish oil instead of olive oil during pregnancy and lactation. *J. Nutr.* **2000**, *13*, 2855–2865.

218. Haubner, L.; Sullivan, J.; Ashmeade, T.; Saste, M.; Wiener, D.; Carver, J. The effects of maternal dietary docosahexaenoic acid intake on rat pup myelin and the auditory startle response. *Dev. Neurosci.* **2007**, *29*, 460–467. [CrossRef] [PubMed]

219. Elsherbiny, M.E.; Goruk, S.; Monckton, E.A.; Richard, C.; Brun, M.; Emara, M.; Field, C.J.; Godbout, R. Long-term effect of docosahexaenoic acid feeding on lipid composition and brain fatty acid-binding protein expression in rats. *Nutrients* **2015**, *7*, 8802–8817. [CrossRef] [PubMed]

220. Maekawa, M.; Takashima, N.; Matsumata, M.; Ikegami, S.; Kontani, M.; Hara, Y.; Kawashima, H.; Owada, Y.; Kiso, Y.; Yoshikawa, T.; *et al.* Arachidonic acid drives postnatal neurogenesis and elicits a beneficial effect on prepulse inhibition, a biological trait of psychiatric illnesses. *PLoS ONE* **2009**, *4*, e5085. [CrossRef] [PubMed]

221. Fleith, M.; Clandinin, T. Dietary PUFA for preterm and term infants: Review of clinical studies. *Crit. Rev. Food Sci. Nutr.* **2005**, *3*, 205–229. [CrossRef]

222. Jensen, C.L.; Prager, T.C.; Fraley, J.K.; Chen, H.; Anderson, R.E.; Heird, W.C. Effect of dietary linoleic/alpha-linolenic acid ratio on growth and visual function of term infants. *J. Pediatr.* **1997**, *131*, 200–209. [CrossRef]

223. Makrides, M.; Neumann, M.A.; Jeffrey, B.; Lien, E.L.; Gibson, R.A. A randomized trial of different ratios of linoleic to alpha-linolenic acid in the diet of term infants: Effect on visual function and growth. *Am. J. Clin. Nutr.* **2000**, *71*, 120–129. [PubMed]

224. Makrides, M.; Neumann, M.A.; Simmer, K.; Gibson, R.A. Erythrocyte fatty acids of term infants fed either breast milk, standard formula, or formula supplemented with long-chain polyunsaturates. *Lipids* **1995**, *30*, 941–948. [CrossRef] [PubMed]

225. Makrides, M.; Neumann, M.A.; Simmer, K.; Pater, J.; Gibson, R. Are long-chain polyunsaturated fatty acids essential nutrients in infancy? *Lancet* **1995**, *345*, 1463–1468. [CrossRef]

226. Makrides, M.; Neumann, M.A.; Simmer, K.; Gibson, R.A. Dietary long-chain polyunsaturated fatty acids do not influence growth in term infants: A randomized clinical trial. *Pediatrics* **1999**, *104*, 468–475. [CrossRef] [PubMed]

227. Scott, D.T.; Janowsky, J.S.; Carroll, R.E.; Taylor, J.A.; Auestad, N.; Montalto, M.B. Formula supplementation with long-chain polyunsaturated fatty acids: Are there developmental benefits? *Pediatrics* **1998**, *102*, e59. [CrossRef] [PubMed]

228. Gibson, R.A.; Neumann, M.; Makrides, M. The effects of diets rich in docosahexaenoic acid and/or gamma-linolenic acid on plasma fatty acid profiles in term infants. In *Lipids in Infant Nutrition*; Huang, Y.S., Sinclair, A., Eds.; AOCS Press: Champaign, IL, USA, 1998; pp. 19–28.

229. Simmer, K. Longchain polyunsaturated fatty acid supplementation in infants born at term. *Cochrane Database Syst. Rev.* **2001**, *4*. [CrossRef]

230. Uauy, R.D.; Hoffman, D.R.; Birch, E.E.; Birch, D.G.; Jameson, D.M.; Tyson, J.E. Safety and efficacy of omega-3 fatty acids in the nutrition of very low birth weight infants: Soy oil and marine oil supplementation of formula. *J. Pediatr.* **1994**, *124*, 612–620. [CrossRef]

231. Clandinin, M.T.; Van Aerde, J.E.; Parrott, A.; Field, C.J.; Euler, A.R.; Lien, E.L. Assessment of the efficacious dose of arachidonic and docosahexaenoic acids in preterm infant formula: Fatty acid composition of erythrocyte membrane lipids. *Pediatr. Res.* **1997**, *42*, 819–825. [CrossRef] [PubMed]

232. Vanderhoof, J.; Gross, S.; Hegyi, T.; Clandinin, T.; Porcelli, P.; DeCristofaro, J.; Rhodes, T.; Tsang, R.; Shattuck, K.; Cowett, R.; *et al.* Evaluation of a long-chain polyunsaturated fatty acid supplemented formula on growth, tolerance, and plasma lipids in preterm infants up to 48 weeks postconceptional age. *J. Pediatr. Gastr. Nutr.* **1999**, *29*, 318–326. [CrossRef]

233. Vanderhoof, J.; Gross, S.; Hegyi, T. A multicenter long-term safety and efficacy trial of preterm formula with long-chain polyunsaturated fatty acids. *J. Pediatr. Gastr. Nutr.* **2000**, *31*, 121–127. [CrossRef]

234. Food and Drug Administration. *Agency Response Letter. GRAS Notice No. GRN 000041*; U.S. Food and Drug Administration, Department of Health and Human Services: Washington, DC, USA, 2001.

235. Health Canada. Novel Food Decision, DHASCO and ARASCO Oils as Sources of Docosahexaenoic (DHA) and Arachidonic Acid (ARA) in Human Milk Substitutes, 2002. Available online: http://www.novelfoods.gc.ca (accessed on 19 October 2015).

236. Ryan, A.S.; Zeller, S.; Nelson, E.B. Safety evaluation of single cell oils and the regulatory requirements for use as food ingredients. In *Single Cell Oils. Microbial and Algal Oil*, 2nd ed.; Cohen, Z., Ratledge, C., Eds.; AOCS Press: Urbana, IL, USA, 2010; pp. 317–350.

237. Dobbing, J. Vulnerable periods in developing brain. In *Brain, Behavior, and Iron in the Infant Diet*; Dobbing, J., Ed.; Springer-Verlag: London, UK, 1990; pp. 1–25.

238. Uauy, R.D.; Birch, D.G.; Birch, E.E.; Hoffman, D.R.; Tyson, J.E. Effect of dietary essential ω-3 fatty acids on retinal and brain development in premature infants. In *Essential Fatty Acids and Eicosanoids*; Sinclair, A., Gibson, E., Eds.; American Oil Chemists' Society: Champaign, IL, USA, 1992; pp. 197–202.

239. Uauy, R.D.; Treen, M.; Hoffman, D.R. Essential fatty acid metabolism and requirements during development. *Semin. Perinatol.* **1989**, *13*, 118–130. [PubMed]

240. Carlson, S.E.; Crooke, R.J.; Werkman, S.H.; Tolley, E.A. First year growth of preterm infants fed standard compared to marine oil *n*-3 supplemented formula. *Lipids* **1992**, *27*, 901–907. [CrossRef] [PubMed]

241. Carlson, S.E.; Werkman, S.H. A randomized trial of visual attention of preterm infants fed docosahexaenoic acid until two months. *Lipids* **1996**, *31*, 85–90. [CrossRef] [PubMed]

242. Diersen-Schade, D.A.; Hansen, J.W.; Harris, C.L.; Merkel, K.L.; Wisont, K.D.; Boettcher, J.A. Docosahexaenoic acid plus arachidonic acid enhance preterm infant growth. In *Essential Fatty Acids and Eicosanoids: Invited Papers from the Fourth International Congress*; Riemersma, R.A., Armstrona, R., Kelly, W., Wilson, R., Eds.; AOCS Press: Champaign, IL, USA, 1998; pp. 123–127.

243. Ryan, A.S.; Montalto, M.B.; Groh-Wargo, S.; Mimouni, F.; Sentipal-Walerius, J.; Doyle, J.; Siegman, J.; Thomas, A.J. Effect of DHA-containing formula on growth of preterm infants to 59 weeks postmenstrual age. *Am. J. Hum. Biol.* **1999**, *11*, 457–467. [CrossRef]

244. Carlson, S.E.; Werkman, S.H.; Peeples, J.M.; Wilson, W.M. Long-chain fatty acids and early visual and cognitive development of preterm infants. *Eur. J. Clin. Nutr.* **1994**, *48*, S27–S30. [PubMed]

245. Werkman, S.H.; Carlson, S.E. A randomized trial of visual attention of preterm infants fed docosahexaenoic acid until nine months. *Lipids* **1996**, *31*, 91–97. [CrossRef] [PubMed]

246. Carlson, S.E.; Werkman, S.H.; Tolley, E.A. Effect of long-chain *n*-3 fatt acid supplementation on visual acuity and growth of preterm infants with and without bronchopulmonary dysplasia. *Am. J. Clin. Nutr.* **1996**, *63*, 687–697. [PubMed]

247. Root, A.W. Mechanisms of hormone action: General Principals. In *Clinical Pediatric Endocrinology*; Hung, W., Ed.; Mosby-Year Book: St. Louis, MO, USA, 1992; pp. 1–12.

248. Watkins, B.A.; Shen, C.-L.; Allen, K.G.D.; Siefert, M.F. Dietary (*n*-3) and (*n*-6) polyunsaturates and acetylsalicylic acid alter *ex vivo* PGE_2 biosynthesis, tissue IGF-I levels, and bone morphometry in chicks. *J. Bone Miner. Res.* **1996**, *11*, 1321–1332. [CrossRef] [PubMed]

249. Colombo, J.; Carlson, S.E.; Cheatham, C.L.; Fitzgerald-Gust Afson, K.M.; Kepler, A.; Doty, T. Long-chain polyunsaturated fatty acid supplementation in infancy reduces heart rate and positively affects distribution of attention. *Pediatr. Res.* **2011**, *70*, 406–410. [CrossRef] [PubMed]

250. Colombo, J.; Carlson, S.E.; Cheatham, C.L.; Shaddy, D.J.; Kerling, E.H.; Thodosoff, J.M.; Gustafson, K.M.; Brez, C. Long-term effects of LCPUFA supplementation on childhood cognitive outcomes. *Am. J. Clin. Nutr.* **2013**, *98*, 403–412. [CrossRef] [PubMed]

251. Alshweki, A.; Munuzuri, A.P.; Bana, A.M.; de Castro, J.; Andrade, F.; Aldamiz-Echevarria, L.; de Pipaon, M.S.; Fraga, J.M.; Couce, M.L. Effects of different arachidonic acid supplementation on psychomotor development in very preterm infants; a randomized trial. *Nutr. J.* **2015**, *14*, 101. [CrossRef] [PubMed]

252. Beyerlein, A.; Hadders-Algra, M.; Kennedy, K.; Fewtrell, M.; Singhal, A.; Rosenfeld, E.; Lucas, A.; Bouwstra, H.; Koletzko, B.; von Kries, R. Infant formula supplementation with long-chain polyunsaturated fatty acids has no effect on Bayley developmental scores at 18 months of age-IPD meta-analysis of 4 large clinical trials. *J. Pediatr. Gastroenterol. Nutr.* **2010**, *50*, 79–84. [CrossRef] [PubMed]

253. Innis, S.M.; Auestad, N.; Siegman, J.S. Blood lipid docosahexaenoic and arachidonic acid in term gestation infants fed formula with high docosahexaenoic, low eicosapentaenoic acid fish oil. *Lipids* **1996**, *31*, 617–625. [CrossRef] [PubMed]

254. Desci, T.; Keleman, B.; Minda, H.; Burus, I.; Kohn, G. Effect of type of early infant feeding on fatty acid composition of plasma lipid classes in full-term infants during the second 6 months of life. *J. Pediatr. Gastroenterol. Nutr.* **2000**, *30*, 547–551.

255. Hoffman, D.R.; Boettcher, J.A.; Diersen-Schade, D.A. Toward optimizing vision and cognition in term infants by dietary docosahexaenoic and arachidonic acid supplementation: A review of randomized clinical trials. *Prostaglandins Leukot. Essent. Fat. Acids* **2009**, *81*, 151–158. [CrossRef] [PubMed]

256. Ryan, A.S.; Entin, E.K.; Hoffman, J.P.; Kuratko, C.N.; Nelson, E.B. Role of fatty acids in the neurological development of infants. In *Nutrition in Infancy, Volume 2, Nutrition and Health*; Watson, R.R., Ed.; Springer Science + Business Media: New York, NY, USA, 2013; pp. 331–346.

257. Drover, J.R.; Hoffman, D.R.; Casteneda, Y.S.; Morale, S.E.; Garfield, S.; Wheaton, D.H.; Birch, E.E. Cognitive function in 18-month-old term infants of the DIAMOND study: A randomized, controlled trial with multiple dietary levels of docosahexaenoic acid. *Early Hum. Dev.* **2011**, *87*, 223–230. [CrossRef] [PubMed]

258. Makrides, M.; Gibson, R.A.; McPhee, A.J.; Collins, C.T.; Davis, P.G.; Doyle, L.W.; Simmer, K.; Colditz, P.B.; Morris, S.; Smithers, L.G.; et al. Neurodevelopment outcomes of preterm infants fed high-dose docosahexaenoic acid: A randomized controlled trial. *JAMA* **2009**, *301*, 175–182. [CrossRef] [PubMed]

259. Makrides, M.; Gibson, R.A.; McPhee, A.J.; Yelland, L.; Quinlivan, J.; Ryan, P. Effect of DHA supplementation during pregnancy on maternal depression and neurodevelopment of young children: A randomized controlled trial. *JAMA* **2010**, *304*, 1675–1683. [CrossRef] [PubMed]

260. Lucas, A.; Stafford, M.; Morley, R.; Abbott, R.; Stephenson, T.; MacFadyen, U.; Elias-Jones, A.; Clements, H. Efficacy and safety of long-chain polyunsaturated fatty acid supplementation of infant formula milk: A randomized trial. *Lancet* **1999**, *354*, 1948–1954. [CrossRef]

261. Fewtrell, M.S.; Morley, R.; Abbott, R.A.; Singhal, A.; Isaacs, E.B.; Stephenson, T.; MacFadyen, U.; Lucas, A. Double-blind, randomized trial of long-chain polyunsaturated fatty acid supplementation in formula fed to preterm infants. *Pediatrics* **2002**, *110*, 73–82. [CrossRef] [PubMed]

262. Henriksen, C.; Haugholt, K.; Lindgren, M.; Aurvåg, A.K.; Rønnestad, A.; Grønn, M.; Solberg, R.; Moen, A.; Nakstad, B.; Berge, R.K.; et al. Improved cognitive development among preterm infants attributable to early supplementation of human milk with docosahexaenoic acid and arachidonic acid. *Pediatrics* **2008**, *121*, 1137–1145. [CrossRef] [PubMed]

263. Westerberg, A.C.; Schei, R.; Henriksen, C.; Smith, L.; Veierød, M.B.; Drevon, C.A.; Iversen, P.O. Attention among very low birth weight infants following early supplementation with docosahexaenoic acid and arachidonic acid. *Acta Pediatr.* **2011**, *100*, 47–52. [CrossRef] [PubMed]

264. Clandinin, M.T.; Van Aerde, J.E.; Merkel, K.L.; Harris, C.L.; Springer, M.A.; Hansen, J.W.; Diersen-Schade, D.A. Growth and development of preterm infants fed infant formulas containing docosahexaenoic acid and arachidonic acid. *J. Pediatr.* **2005**, *146*, 461–468. [CrossRef] [PubMed]

265. Birch, E.E.; Garfield, S.; Hoffman, D.R.; Uauy, R.; Birch, D.G. A randomized controlled trial of early dietary supply of long-chain polyunsaturated fatty acids and mental development in term infants. *Dev. Med. Child Neurol.* **2000**, *42*, 174–181. [CrossRef] [PubMed]

266. Carlson, S.E.; Montalto, M.B.; Ponder, D.L.; Werkman, S.H.; Korones, S.B. Lower incidence of necrotizing enterocolitis in infants fed a preterm formula with egg phospholipids. *Pediatr. Res.* **1998**, *44*, 491–498. [CrossRef] [PubMed]

267. Seki, H.; Sasaki, T.; Ueda, T.; Arita, M. Resolvins as regulators of the immune system. *Sci. World J.* **2010**, *10*, 18–31. [CrossRef] [PubMed]

268. Das, U.N. Perinatal supplementation of long-chain polyunsaturated fatty acids, immune response and adult diseases. *Med. Sci. Monit.* **2004**, *10*, HY19–HY25. [PubMed]

269. D'Vas, N.; Meldrum, S.J.; Dunstan, J.A.; Lee-Pullen, T.F.; Metcalfe, J.; Holt, B.J.; Serralha, M.; Tulic, M.K.; Mori, T.A.; Prescott, S.L. Fish oil supplementation in early infancy modulates developing infant immune responses. *Clin. Exp. Allergy* **2012**, *42*, 1206–1216.

270. Khader, S.A.; Gaffen, S.L.; Kolls, J.K. Th17 cells at the crossroads of innate and adaptive immunity against infectious diseases at the mucosa. *Mucosal Immunol.* **2009**, *2*, 403–411. [CrossRef] [PubMed]

271. Muc, M.; Kreiner-Moller, E.; Larsen, J.M.; Birch, S.; Brix, S.; Bisgaard, H.; Lauritzen, L. Maternal fatty acid desaturase genotype correlates with infant immune responses at 6 months. *Br. J. Nutr.* **2015**, *114*, 891–898. [CrossRef] [PubMed]

272. Barakat, R.; Abou El-Ela, N.E.; Sharaf, S.; El Sagheer, O.; Selim, S.; Tallima, H.; Bruins, M.J.; Hadley, K.B.; El Ridi, R. Efficacy and safety of arachidonic acid for treatment of school-aged children in *Schistosoma mansoni* high-endemicity regions. *Am. J. Trop. Med. Hyg.* **2015**, *92*, 797–804. [CrossRef] [PubMed]

273. Standl, M.; Lattka, E.; Stach, B.; Koletzko, S.; Bauer, C.P.; von Berg, A.; Berdel, D.; Kramer, U.; Schaaf, B.; Roder, S.; et al. FADS1 FADS2 gene cluster, PUFA intake and blood lipids in children: Results from the GINIplus and LISAplus Study Group. *PLoS ONE* **2012**, *7*, e37780.

274. Makajima, H.; Hirose, K. Role of IL-23 and Th17 cells in airway inflammation in asthma. *Immune Netw.* **2010**, *10*, 1–4. [CrossRef] [PubMed]

275. Dong, C. Regulation and pro-inflammatory function of interleukin-17 family cytokines. *Immunol. Rev.* **2008**, *226*, 80–86. [CrossRef] [PubMed]

276. Sapone, A.; Lammers, K.M.; Casolaro, V.; CAmmarota, M.; Giulano, M.T.; De Rosa, M.; Stefanile, R.; Mazzarella, G.; Tolone, C.; Russo, M.I.; et al. Divergence of gut permeability and mucosal immune gene expression in two gluten-associated conditions: Celiac disease and gluten sensitivity. *BMC Med.* **2011**, *9*, 23. [CrossRef] [PubMed]

277. Pastor, N.; Soler, B.; Mitmesser, S.H.; Ferguson, P.; Lifschitz, C. Infants fed docosahexaenoic acid- and arachidonic acid-supplemented formula have decreased incidence of bronchiolitis/bronchitis the first year of life. *Clin. Pediatr.* **2006**, *45*, 850–855. [CrossRef] [PubMed]

278. Lapillone, A.; Pastor, N.; Zhuang, W.; Scalabrin, D.M.F. Infants fed formula with added long chain polyunsaturated fatty acids have reduced incidence of respiratory illnesses and diarrhea during the first year of life. *BMC Pediatr.* **2014**, *14*, 168. [CrossRef] [PubMed]

279. Birch, E.E.; Carlson, S.E.; Hoffman, D.R.; Fitzgerald-Gustafson, K.M.; Fu, V.L.; Drover, J.R.; Castañeda, Y.S.; Minns, L.; Wheaton, D.K.; Mundy, D.; et al. The DIAMOND (DHA Intake and Measurement of Neural Development) Study: A double-masked, randomized controlled clinical trial of the maturation of infant visual acuity as a function of the dietary level of docosahexaenoic acid. *Am. J. Clin. Nutr.* **2010**, *91*, 848–859. [CrossRef] [PubMed]

280. Foiles, A.M.; Kerling, E.H.; Wick, J.A.; Scalabrin, D.M.; Colombo, J.; Carlson, S.E. Formula with long chain polyunsaturated fatty acids reduces incidence of allergy in early childhood. *Pediatr. Allergy Immunol.* **2015**. [CrossRef] [PubMed]

281. Hindenes, J.O.; Nerdal, W.; Guo, W.; Di, L.; Small, D.M.; Holmsen, H. Physical properties of the transmembrane signal molecule, sn-1-stearoyl-2-arachidonylglycerol. Acyl chain segregation and its biochemical implications. *J. Biol. Chem.* **2000**, *275*, 6857–6867. [CrossRef] [PubMed]

282. Moodley, T.; Vella, C.; Djahanbakhch, O.; Branford-White, C.J.; Crawford, M.A. Arachidonic and docosahexaenoic acid deficits in preterm neonatal mononuclear cell membranes. Implications for the immune response at birth. *Nutr. Health* **2009**, *20*, 167–185. [CrossRef] [PubMed]

283. Van Goor, S.A.; Schaafsma, A.; Erwich, J.J.; Dijck-Brouwer, D.A.; Muskiet, F.A. Mildly abnormal general movement quality in infants is associated with high Mead acid and lower arachidonic acid shows a U-shaped relation with the DHA/AA ratio. *Prostaglandins Leukot. Essent. Fat. Acids* **2010**, *82*, 15–20. [CrossRef] [PubMed]

284. Groen, S.E.; de Blecourt, A.C.; Postema, K.; Hadders-Algra, M. General movements in early infancy predict neuromotor development at 9 to 12 years of age. *Dev. Med. Child Neurol.* **2005**, *47*, 731–738. [CrossRef] [PubMed]

285. Field, C.J.; Thompson, C.A.; Van Aerde, J.E.; Parrott, A.; Euler, A.; Lien, E.; Clandinin, M.T. Lower proportion of CD45R0+ cells and deficient interleukin-10 production by formula-fed infants, compared with human-fed, is correlated with supplementation of long-chain polyunsaturated fatty acids. *J. Pediatr. Gastroenterol. Nutr.* **2000**, *31*, 291–299. [CrossRef] [PubMed]

286. Richardson, A.J.; Calvin, C.M.; Clisby, C.; Schoenheimer, D.R.; Montgomery, P.; Hall, J.A. Fatty acid deficiency signs predict the severity of reading and related difficulties in dyslexic children. *Prostaglandins Leukot. Essent. Fat. Acids* **2000**, *63*, 69–74. [CrossRef] [PubMed]
287. Burgess, J.R.; Stevens, L.; Zhang, W.; Peck, L. Long-chain polyunsaturated fatty acids in children with attention-deficit hyperactivity disorder. *Am. J. Clin. Nutr.* **2000**, *71*, 327S–330S. [PubMed]
288. Chen, J.R.; Hsu, S.F.; Hsu, C.D.; Hwang, L.H.; Yang, S.C. Dietary patterns and blood fatty acid composition in children with attention-deficit hyperactivity disorder in Taiwan. *J. Nutr. Biochem.* **2004**, *15*, 467–472. [CrossRef] [PubMed]
289. Young, G.S.; Maharaj, N.J.; Conquer, J.A. Blood phospholipid fatty acid analysis of adults with and without attention deficit/hyperactivity disorder. *Lipids* **2004**, *39*, 117–123. [PubMed]
290. Morse, N.L. A meta-analysis of blood fatty acids in people with learning disorders with particular interest in arachidonic acid. *Prostaglandins Leukot. Essent. Fat. Acids* **2009**, *81*, 373–389. [CrossRef] [PubMed]
291. Yamada, J.; Banks, A. Evidence for and characteristics of dyslexia among Japanese children. In *Annals of Dyslexia*; Schatschneider, C., Compton, D., Eds.; Springer: New York, NY, USA, 1994; pp. 103–119.
292. FAO. *Dietary Fats and Oils in Human Nutrition*; FAO/WHO: Rome, Italy, 1978.
293. FAO/WHO. *Fats and Oils in Human Nutrition*; Report of a Joint FAO/WHO Expert Consultation, 19 to 26 October 1993; FAO/WHO: Rome, Italy, 1994.
294. FAO. *Fats and Fatty Acids in Human Nutrition*; FAO/WHO: Rome, Italy, 2010.
295. Codex Alimentarius Commission. *Standards for Infant Formula and Formulas for Special Medical Purposes Intended for Infants*; CODEX STAN 72-1981, Last Revised 2007; Codex Alimentarius Commission: Rome, Italy, 2007.
296. Codex Alimentarius Commission. Amendments, 2015. Available online: http://www.fao.org/fao-who-codexalimentarius/en (accessed on 26 January 2016).
297. Infant Formula Act. H.R.6940—An Act to Amend the Federal Food, Drug, and Cosmetic Act to Strengthen the Authority under that Act to Assure the Safety and Nutrition of Infant Formulas, and for Other Purposes. *Fed. Regist.* **1980**, *50*, 45106–45108.
298. European Commission. *Commission Directive 2006/141/EC of 22 December 2006 on Infant Formulae and Follow-on Formulae and Amending Directive 1999/21/EC*; L.401/1; Official Journal of the European Union: Brussels, Belgium, 2008.
299. Koletzko, B.; Boey, C.C.; Campoy, C.; Carlson, S.E.; Chang, N.; Guillermo-Tuazon, M.A.; Joshi, S.; Prell, C.; Quak, S.H.; Sjarif, D.R.; *et al.* Current information and Asian perspectives on long-chain polyunsaturated fatty acids in pregnancy, lactation, and infancy: Systematic review and practice recommendations from an early nutrition academy workshop. *Ann. Nutr. Metab.* **2014**, *65*, 49–80. [CrossRef] [PubMed]
300. Crawford, M.A.; Wang, Y.; Forsyth, S.; Brenna, J.T. The European Food Safety Authority recommendation for polyunsaturated fatty acid composition of infant formula overrules breast milk, puts infants at risk, and should be revised. *Prostaglandins Leukot. Essent. Fat. Acids* **2015**, *102–103*, 1–3. [CrossRef] [PubMed]
301. Leaf, A.A.; Leighfield, M.J.; Costeloe, K.L.; Crawford, M.A. Long chain polyunsaturated fatty acids and fetal growth. *Early Hum. Dev.* **1992**, *30*, 183–191. [CrossRef]
302. Forsyth, J.S.; Willatts, P.; Agostoni, C.; Bissenden, J.; Casaer, P.; Boehm, G. Long chain polyunsaturated fatty acid supplementation in infant formula and blood pressure in later childhood: Follow up of a randomized controlled trial. *Br. Med. J.* **2003**, *326*, 953. [CrossRef] [PubMed]
303. Makrides, M.; Gibson, R.A.; Udell, T.; Ried, K. Supplementation of infant formula with long-chain polyunsaturated fatty acids does not influence the growth of term infants. *Am. J. Clin. Nutr.* **2005**, *81*, 1094–1101. [PubMed]

6

Increased Calcium Supplementation Postpartum is Associated with Breastfeeding among Chinese Mothers: Finding from Two Prospective Cohort Studies

Jian Zhao, Yun Zhao *, Colin W. Binns and Andy H. Lee

School of Public Health, Curtin University, Perth 6102, Australia; jian.zhao@postgrad.curtin.edu.au (J.Z.); c.binns@curtin.edu.au (C.W.B.); andy.lee@curtin.edu.au (A.H.L.)
* Correspondence: y.zhao@curtin.edu.au

Abstract: The calcium supplementation status during the postpartum period among Chinese lactating women is still unclear. The objective of this study is to utilize data from two population-based prospective cohort studies to examine the calcium supplementation status and to identify whether breastfeeding is associated with increased calcium supplementation among Chinese mothers after child birth. Information from 1540 mothers on breastfeeding and calcium supplementation measured at discharge, 1, 3, and 6 months postpartum were extracted to evaluate the association between breastfeeding and calcium supplementation postpartum. A generalized linear mixed model was applied to each study initially to account for the inherent correlation among repeated measurements, adjusting for socio-demographic, obstetric factors and calcium supplementation during pregnancy. In addition, breastfeeding status measured at different follow-up time points was treated as a time dependent variable in the longitudinal analysis. Furthermore, the effect sizes of the two cohort studies were pooled using fixed effect model. Based on the two cohort studies, the pooled likelihood of taking calcium supplementation postpartum among breastfeeding mothers was 4.02 times (95% confidence interval (2.30, 7.03)) higher than that of their non-breastfeeding counterparts. Dietary supplementation intervention programs targeting different subgroups should be promoted in Chinese women, given currently a wide shortage of dietary calcium intake and calcium supplementation postpartum.

Keywords: calcium supplementation; breastfeeding; postpartum; infant; nutrients; generalized linear mixed model; time dependent variable; pooled analysis; China

1. Introduction

The mineral accretion rate of a neonate reaches about 30–40 mg/kg per day, while calcium transfer between mothers and infants is on average 210 mg per day [1–3]. For babies who are breastfed exclusively through the first 6 months, the amount of mineral demand from the mothers is four times greater than that during 9 months of pregnancy [4]. The calcium requirement of mothers during lactation has been the subject of much discussion [5–7]. In 2011, the Institute of Medicine published the calcium dietary reference intakes by life stage, in which Estimated Average Requirement (EAR) of calcium for pregnant and lactating adult women is recommended as 800 mg [8].

Compared to western countries, the lower consumption of dairy products in China results in that most of Chinese residents have calcium intake lower than the adequate intake (AI) [9–11]. In a prospective cohort study of women's health from Shanghai, the median intake of calcium was 485 mg/day, 60% of calcium from plant sources, and only 20% from milk, which was lower than the age group specific AI (800 mg/day for 18–49 years group and 1000 mg/day for over 50 years group) [11,12]. Only 6.25% of perimenopausal women reached the standard of calcium intake in Changsha [13]. The average intake of calcium of Beijing elderly was 505 mg/day, which was about one half of the recommended adequate intake for the elderly [14]. In the National Nutrition and Health Survey of 2002, fewer than 5% reached the adequate intake levels of calcium for all age groups and the prevalence of calcium supplementation during pregnancy was 41.4% [15,16]. Besides cultural preferences, the lower consumption of dairy products in China is attributed to the high rate of lactose intolerance, which is around 80% to 95% [17,18].

The Chinese National Health and Family Planning Commission recommends that pregnant women should have a dietary calcium intake of 1000 mg per day from the second trimester and increase to 1200 mg per day from the third trimester until the end of lactation [19]. However, low dietary calcium intake in lactating women has been reported in different regions of China, as shown in Table 1. This suggests that calcium supplementation for lactating women is an important public health issue to mothers in China based on the current evidence about the benefits of calcium intake during lactation on reducing maternal bone loss [20–23].

Table 1. Dietary calcium intake of lactating women in different regions of China.

Study Location	Study Design	Study Period	Average Daily Dietary Calcium Intake (Postpartum)
Guangzhou [24]	Prospective cohort	2002	786.45 mg (12 weeks)
Hunan [25]	Cross-sectional	2011–2012	426 mg
Beijing, Suzhou & Guangzhou [26]	Cross-sectional	2011–2012	401.4 mg (0–1 month) 585.3 mg (1–2 months) 591.2 mg (2–4 months) 649.0 mg (4–8 months)
Fujian [27]	Prospective cohort	2012	428 mg (2 days) 454 mg (7 days) 595 mg (30 days) 544 mg (90 days)
Shanghai [28]	Prospective cohort	2014–2015	749.3 mg (1–3 days) 781.1 mg (7–9 days) 762.3 mg (14–17 days) 768.4 mg (25–27 days) 678.5 mg (39–41 days)

The calcium supplementation status during postpartum period among Chinese lactating women is still unclear. The objective of the present study is to utilize data from two population-based prospective cohort studies to examine the calcium supplementation status and to identify whether breastfeeding is associated with increased calcium supplementation among Chinese mothers after child birth.

2. Materials and Methods

2.1. Study Participants

Two prospective cohort studies were conducted in an urban area, Chengdu (capital city) and a rural area, Jiangyou (county-level city), Sichuan Province, China between 2010 and 2012. Mothers who gave birth to a healthy singleton infant were invited to participate before discharge. These two studies used the same methodology based on same questionnaires, which had been used in Australia and China [29–31] previously, to interview all consented women face-to-face at discharge, and followed up the participants at one, three and six months postpartum by telephone interviews. The baseline interview collected detailed information on mothers and newborns, including socio-demographic, obstetric characteristics and dietary supplements during pregnancy. The follow-up interviews collected detailed information on lactation patterns and durations and dietary supplements during the postpartum period. The World Health Organization (WHO) standard definition of any breastfeeding was used in these two studies; 'Any breastfeeding' is defined as the infant has received breast milk (direct from the breast or expressed) with or without other drink, formula or other infant food [32].

2.2. Ethical Approval

The two cohort studies were approved by the Human Research Ethics Committee of Curtin University, Perth, Western Australia (approval numbers: HR169/2009 and HR168/2009, respectively). The present study was also approved by the Human Research Ethics Committee of Curtin University (approval number: RDHS-101-15). The data used in this study were de-identified.

2.3. Statistical Analysis

The outcome of the present study is maternal calcium supplementation status (yes or no) measured longitudinally during three different postpartum periods (from discharge to 1 month, from 1 month to 3 months, and from 3 months to 6 months, respectively) at three follow-up time points (namely, 1 month, 3 months and 6 months postpartum). The main variable of interest, any breastfeeding status, was measured longitudinally at three different postpartum time points (discharge, 1 month and 3 months postpartum). Descriptive statistics of mothers' socio-demographic status, obstetric characteristics, calcium supplementation during pregnancy and the three postpartum periods, and any breastfeeding status at the three postpartum time points were obtained and reported. Chi-square test was conducted to compare the calcium supplementation rates between breastfeeding group and non-breastfeeding group at the different follow-up time points. Generalized linear mixed model (GLMM) was used to examine the effect of breastfeeding on calcium supplementation postpartum taking into account inherent correlations among repeated measurements. Furthermore, the breastfeeding status was included as a time-dependent variable in the longitudinal analysis. Random intercept model without covariates (Model I) was run initially to test random intercept effect, and then any breastfeeding status at the different time points and an indicator variable of measurement times were added into the above Model I to be a Model II. Furthermore, subject level socio-demographic covariates such as household annual income, maternal age and maternal education were then added into and adjusted in the Model II to formulate a Model III. Finally, obstetric characteristics such as parity, gravidity, infant gender, infant birth weight and infant gestational week, together with calcium supplementation during pregnancy, were further adjusted in the Model III to become the final Model IV. The above regression analysis was carried out for data set extracted from each cohort study separately, and the results of Model II and final Model IV were reported. In addition, a pooled effect size was calculated using a fixed effect model given that the heterogeneity between the two studies was tested being statistically nonsignificant. All statistical analyses were performed by using SAS 9.4 (SAS Institute Inc., Cary, NC, USA).

3. Results

3.1. Characteristics of Participants

For each cohort, mothers' baseline socio-demographic status, obstetric characteristics and calcium supplementation during pregnancy are presented in Table 2. In the Jiangyou study, 695 mothers were interviewed at baseline, and 648 and 620 mothers remained in the study at 1 month and 3 months postpartum, respectively. Any breastfeeding rate dropped slightly from 93.53% at discharge to 91.05% at 1 month postpartum then continuously to 83.71% at 3 months postpartum. In the other cohort conducted in Chengdu, 845 mothers were interviewed at baseline and 760 mothers were followed up until six months postpartum. Any breastfeeding rate declined from 93.02% at discharge to 87.89% at 1 month postpartum then substantially to 73.42% at 3 months postpartum.

Table 2. Characteristics of participants at baseline by breastfeeding status.

Variable	Cohort in Jiangyou (n = 695)		Cohort in Chengdu (n = 845)	
	BF	Non-BF	BF	Non-BF
Number of participants	650 (93.5)	45 (6.5)	786 (93.0)	59 (7.0)
Household annual income (Chinese yuan)				
<2000	186 (31.0)	9 (23.1)	1 (0.2)	0 (0.0)
2000–5000	309 (51.4)	23 (59.0)	155 (23.5)	12 (24.0)
>5000	106 (17.6)	7 (17.9)	503 (76.3)	38 (76.0)
Maternal age (years)				
<25	373 (57.4)	26 (57.8)	156 (19.9)	5 (8.5)
25–29	163 (25.1)	13 (28.9)	372 (47.3)	28 (47.5)
>29	114 (17.5)	6 (13.3)	258 (32.8)	26 (44.0)
Maternal education				
Secondary school or lower	355 (54.6)	25 (55.6)	90 (11.5)	11 (18.6)
Senior school	215 (33.1)	18 (40.0)	165 (21.0)	11 (18.6)
University or higher	80 (12.3)	2 (4.4)	531 (67.5)	37 (62.8)
Parity				
Primiparous	518 (79.7)	37 (82.2)	700 (89.1)	51 (86.4)
Multiparous	132 (20.3)	8 (17.8)	86 (10.9)	8 (13.6)
Gravidity				
Primigravida	249 (38.3)	18 (40.0)	430 (54.7)	26 (44.1)
Multigravida	401 (61.7)	27 (60.0)	356 (45.3)	33 (55.9)
Infant gender				
Male	328 (50.5)	26 (57.8)	412 (52.4)	34 (57.6)
Female	322 (49.5)	19 (42.2)	374 (47.6)	25 (42.4)
Infant birth weight (g)				
<2500	10 (1.5)	2 (4.4)	13 (1.7)	0 (0.0)
≥2500	640 (98.5)	43 (95.6)	773 (98.3)	59 (100.0)
Infant gestational week				
<37	8 (1.2)	3 (6.8)	9 (1.2)	2 (3.4)
≥37	640 (98.8)	41 (93.2)	777 (98.8)	57 (96.6)
Calcium supplementation during pregnancy				
Yes	410 (63.1)	25 (55.6)	627 (79.8)	47 (79.7)
No	240 (36.9)	20 (44.4)	159 (20.2)	12 (20.3)

Data are presented as n (%); BF: any breastfeeding; Non-BF: non-breastfeeding.

3.2. Calcium Supplementation Status during Postpartum Period

Overall, among mothers in the Jiangyou cohort, an inverted U shape of calcium supplementation rates at three different postpartum periods was observed, which corresponded to 13.4%, 19.4% and 17.7%, respectively. While in the Chengdu cohort, a constant decline trend was recorded with 22.5%, 22.2% and 12.0% reported at the three postpartum periods. When considering separately for breastfeeding and non-breastfeeding groups, as shown in Figures 1 and 2, the calcium supplementation rate in the breastfeeding group was statistically significantly higher than that in the non-breastfeeding group for all the different postpartum periods, except between discharge and 1 month in the Jiangyou cohort ($p = 0.36$). In the Jiangyou cohort, calcium supplementation rates ranged from 13.7% to 21.2% for breastfeeding mothers, and ranged from 1.7% to 8.9% for non-breastfeeding mothers. In the Chengdu cohort, calcium supplementation rates reduced from around 23% in the first 3 months postpartum to 14.5% between 3 months and 6 months in breastfeeding mothers, and ranged from 5.0% to 14.1% in non-breastfeeding mothers.

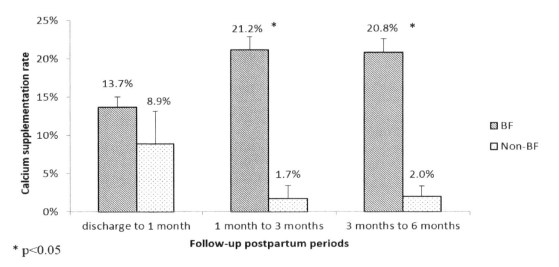

Figure 1. Calcium supplementation postpartum in Jiangyou.

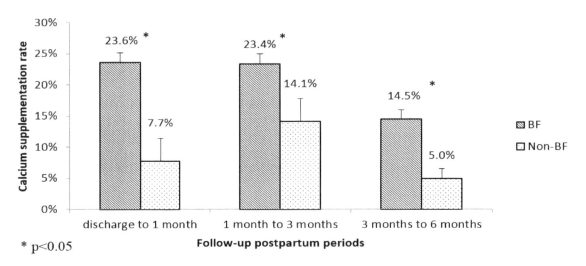

Figure 2. Calcium supplementation postpartum in Chengdu.

3.3. The Association between Breastfeeding and Calcium Supplementation Postpartum

In Model I (without any covariates) for both cohorts, subject random effect was found to be statistically significant. Hence, both the primary variables of interest (i.e., breastfeeding status and the indicator variable of measurement times) were subsequently added into the Model I for examining the association between breastfeeding and calcium supplementation postpartum. As shown in Table 3, the likelihood of calcium supplementation in breastfeeding mothers were 5.85 times (95% confidence interval (CI) (2.50, 13.72)) and 2.88 times (95% CI (1.50, 5.54)) higher of that in non-breastfeeding mothers in Jiangyou and Chengdu, respectively. After adjusting for socio-demographic and obstetric factors as well as calcium supplementation during pregnancy, the odds ratios (ORs) and its 95% CI had changed appreciably to 6.95 and (2.68, 18.04) in the Jiangyou study, and 3.03 and (1.52, 6.02) in the Chengdu study, respectively. The heterogeneity between these two studies was not significant ($I^2 = 0.479$, $p = 0.17$) statistically, therefore a fixed effect model was used to pool the ORs of the two studies. The pooled analysis of these two cohort studies revealed that calcium supplementation postpartum was significantly positively associated with breastfeeding with an adjusted OR = 4.02 with a 95% CI of (2.30, 7.03).

Table 3. Association between breastfeeding status and calcium supplementation postpartum.

Variable	Model II	Model IV
	Crude ORs (95% CI)	Adjusted ORs (95% CI)
Jiangyou Cohort		
Measurement times *		
At discharge (ref)	1	1
1 month	1.72 (1.24, 2.38)	1.90 (1.33, 2.70)
3 months	1.57 (1.12, 2.20)	1.69 (1.18, 2.44)
Breastfeeding status *		
Non-breastfeeding (ref)	1	1
Any breastfeeding	5.85 (2.50, 13.72)	6.95 (2.68, 18.04)
Chengdu Cohort		
Measurement times *		
At discharge (ref)	1	1
1 month	1.02 (0.74, 1.43)	1.02 (0.72, 1.45)
3 months	0.31 (0.21, 0.46)	0.30 (0.20, 0.45)
Breastfeeding status *		
Non-breastfeeding (ref)	1	1
Any breastfeeding	2.88 (1.50, 5.54)	3.03 (1.52, 6.02)
Pooled effect size of two studies		
Non-breastfeeding (ref)	-	1
Any breastfeeding	-	4.02 (2.30, 7.03)

Crude ORs (obtained from Model II): Model included breastfeeding status and the indicator variable of measurement times; Adjusted ORs (obtained from the final Model IV): Model adjusted for socio-demographics variables (household annual income, maternal age and maternal education); obstetric factors (parity, gravidity, infant gender, infant birth weight and infant gestational week); and calcium supplementation during pregnancy; * $p < 0.05$; ref: reference category.

4. Discussion

To our knowledge, the present study is the first population-based study that determines the longitudinal trend of calcium supplementation by Chinese women from discharge to 6 months postpartum and the effect of breastfeeding on calcium supplementation. A relatively low level of calcium supplementation (less than 23%) was observed throughout the postpartum period in either breastfeeding mothers or non-breastfeeding mothers. The pooled effect size after adjusting for socio-demographics variables (household annual income, maternal age and maternal education); obstetric factors (parity, gravidity, infant gender, infant birth weight and infant gestational week); and calcium supplementation during pregnancy reveals that mothers who breastfed their babies were 4.02 times more likely to take calcium supplements compared to their non-breastfeeding counterparts during postpartum. The present result is consistent with previous findings that breastfeeding mothers consumed more calcium than non-breastfeeding counterparts [33–35]. One reason leading to the higher calcium supplementation in breastfeeding mothers may be the general belief that adequate calcium intake is beneficial to breast milk production, and mothers' special attention to infants' calcium intake under the context of wide shortage of calcium intake for Chinese women, in spite of recent evidence demonstrating that calcium supplementation in lactation has no significant effect on increasing calcium content in breast milk [36–38]. The other reason might be mothers' perception of the beneficial effect of calcium supplementation on maternal bone loss during lactating. Some studies found little benefits of calcium supplementation on maternal bone loss during lactating [36,39,40], whereas other studies carried out in the U.S. and Brazil suggested that higher calcium intake during early lactation could minimize the bone loss for the mothers who had daily calcium intake less than 500 mg [20,21]. Further investigation on the factors contributing to difference of calcium supplementation between breastfeeding mothers and non-breastfeeding mothers as well as the effect of calcium supplementation on reducing maternal bone loss during lactation or enhancing maternal skeleton remodeling and remineralization after weaning of breastfeeding is recommended.

Given the habitually lower calcium dietary intake and relatively high lactose intolerance rate in the general Chinese population [12,15,17], calcium supplementation plays an important role on bone health, especially for exclusive breastfeeding women who provide around 300 mg of calcium per day to their babies via breast milk which accompany maternal bone calcium turnover [41].

This study had several strengths. We utilized data from two cohort studies to investigate the longitudinal trends of calcium supplementation at three different postpartum time points (i.e., 1 month, 3 months and 6 months postpartum) and conducted random effect regression modelling accounting for inherent dependency between the repeated measurements. Moreover, since the breastfeeding status was measured longitudinally as well in two cohorts, it was treated as a time-dependent variable in the analysis to account for possible feedback effects between the breastfeeding status and calcium supplementation at different times. In addition, our pooled analysis based on the two individual studies yielded the combined effect size with a larger sample size and higher statistical power. Moreover, calcium supplementation during pregnancy was adjusted in the modelling to control for the consequent effect of calcium intake during pregnancy on calcium supplementation during lactation.

A caveat of this study was that both cohort studies were carried out in Sichuan Province, which may limit the results being able to generalize to other regions of China. Sichuan Basin has special geographic characteristics, where the number of cloudy or rainy days is substantially larger than that in other regions in China, which may lead to a relatively lower level of vitamin D synthesis and calcium deficiency consequently [42]. However, to the best of our knowledge, no data were available currently on calcium supplementation during postpartum in other regions of China for comparison purpose.

5. Conclusions

In conclusion, calcium supplementation during postpartum in Sichuan is variable at different times postpartum with a relatively low level (less than 23%). Although breastfeeding has a substantive effect on calcium supplementation postpartum, dietary supplementation intervention programs and health education targeting different subgroups (e.g., breastfeeding mothers and bottle feeding mothers) should be promoted in Chinese women, given currently a wide shortage of dietary calcium intake and calcium supplementation during postpartum.

Acknowledgments: We would like to thank Li Tang and Chuan Yu from West China Hospital, Sichuan University for providing the two datasets. Jian Zhao would like to acknowledge China Scholarship Council (CSC) for their financial support for his doctoral studies.

Author Contributions: J.Z., Y.Z. and C.W.B. designed the research; J.Z. performed statistical analyses and Y.Z., C.W.B. and A.H.L. provided theoretical and methodological guidance; J.Z., Y.Z. and A.H.L. wrote the manuscript. All authors read and approved the final version of the manuscript.

References

1. Trotter, M.; Hixon, B.B. Sequential changes in weight, density, and percentage ash weight of human skeletons from an early fetal period through old age. *Anat. Rec.* **1974**, *179*, 1–18. [CrossRef] [PubMed]
2. Olausson, H.; Goldberg, G.R.; Laskey, M.A.; Schoenmakers, I.; Jarjou, L.M.; Prentice, A. Calcium economy in human pregnancy and lactation. *Nutr. Res. Rev.* **2012**, *25*, 40–67. [CrossRef] [PubMed]
3. Kalkwarf, H.J.; Specker, B.L.; Ho, M. Effects of calcium supplementation on calcium homeostasis and bone turnover in lactating women. *J. Clin. Endocrinol. Metab.* **1999**, *84*, 464–470. [CrossRef] [PubMed]
4. Kovacs, C.S.; Ralston, S.H. Presentation and management of osteoporosis presenting in association with pregnancy or lactation. *Osteoporos. Int.* **2015**, *26*, 2223–2241. [CrossRef] [PubMed]
5. Thomas, M.; Weisman, S.M. Calcium supplementation during pregnancy and lactation: Effects on the mother and the fetus. *Am. J. Obstet. Gynecol.* **2006**, *194*, 937–945. [CrossRef] [PubMed]

6.   Prentice, A. Calcium in pregnancy and lactation. *Annu. Rev. Nutr.* **2000**, *20*, 249–272. [CrossRef] [PubMed]

7.   Kovacs, C.S. Calcium and bone metabolism disorders during pregnancy and lactation. *Endocrinol. Metab. Clin. N. Am.* **2011**, *40*, 795–826. [CrossRef] [PubMed]

8.   Institute of Medicine. *Dietary Reference Intakes for Calcium and Vitamin D*; National Academies Press: Washington, DC, USA, 2011.

9.   Chen, Y.M.; Teucher, B.; Tang, X.Y.; Dainty, J.R.; Lee, K.K.; Woo, J.L.; Ho, S.C. Calcium absorption in postmenopausal Chinese women: A randomized crossover intervention study. *Br. J. Nutr.* **2007**, *97*, 160–166. [CrossRef] [PubMed]

10. Ma, G.; Li, Y.; Jin, Y.; Zhai, F.; Kok, F.J.; Yang, X. Phytate intake and molar ratios of phytate to zinc, iron and calcium in the diets of people in China. *Eur. J. Clin. Nutr.* **2007**, *61*, 368–374. [CrossRef] [PubMed]

11. Wang, Y.; Li, S. Worldwide trends in dairy production and consumption and calcium intake: Is promoting consumption of dairy products a sustainable solution for inadequate calcium intake? *Food Nutr. Bull.* **2008**, *29*, 172–185. [CrossRef] [PubMed]

12. Shin, A.; Li, H.; Shu, X.O.; Yang, G.; Gao, Y.T.; Zheng, W. Dietary intake of calcium, fiber and other micronutrients in relation to colorectal cancer risk: Results from the Shanghai Women's Health Study. *Int. J. Cancer* **2006**, *119*, 2938–2942. [CrossRef] [PubMed]

13. Deng, J.; Huang, Y.M.; Lin, Q. Main sources of dietary calcium in perimenopausal women in Changsha. *Zhong Nan Da Xue Xue Bao Yi Xue Ban* **2008**, *33*, 875–879. [PubMed]

14. Liu, X.; Zhao, X.; Xu, L. Food sources of calcium and iron in the diet of Beijing elderly. *Wei Sheng Yan Jiu* **2004**, *33*, 336–338. [PubMed]

15. He, Y.; Zhai, F.; Wang, Z.; Hu, Y. Status of dietary calcium intake of Chinese residents. *Wei Sheng Yan Jiu* **2007**, *36*, 600–602. [PubMed]

16. Lai, J.; Yin, S.; Ma, G.; Piao, J.; Yang, X. The nutrition and health survery of pregnant women in China. *Acta Nutr. Sin.* **2007**, *29*, 4–8.

17. De Vrese, M.; Stegelmann, A.; Richter, B.; Fenselau, S.; Laue, C.; Schrezenmeir, J. Probiotics—Compensation for lactase insufficiency. *Am. J. Clin. Nutr.* **2001**, *73*, 421S–429S. [PubMed]

18. Wang, Y.G.; Yan, Y.S.; Xu, J.J.; Du, R.F.; Flatz, S.D.; Kuhnau, W.; Flatz, G. Prevalence of primary adult lactose malabsorption in three populations of northern China. *Hum. Genet.* **1984**, *67*, 103–106. [PubMed]

19. National Health and Family Planning Commission of the People's Republic of China. Maternal and Child Health Basic Knowledge and Skills (Trial Version). Available online: http://www.nhfpc.gov.cn/fys/kpxc/201405/0065ee2071204f0c9b52f7cdcbb392f2.shtml (accessed on 5 July 2016).

20. O'Brien, K.O.; Donangelo, C.M.; Ritchie, L.D.; Gildengorin, G.; Abrams, S.; King, J.C. Serum 1,25-dihydroxyvitamin D and calcium intake affect rates of bone calcium deposition during pregnancy and the early postpartum period. *Am. J. Clin. Nutr.* **2012**, *96*, 64–72. [CrossRef] [PubMed]

21. O'Brien, K.O.; Donangelo, C.M.; Zapata, C.L.; Abrams, S.A.; Spencer, E.M.; King, J.C. Bone calcium turnover during pregnancy and lactation in women with low calcium diets is associated with calcium intake and circulating insulin-like growth factor 1 concentrations. *Am. J. Clin. Nutr.* **2006**, *83*, 317–323. [PubMed]

22. Chan, G.M.; McMurry, M.; Westover, K.; Engelbert-Fenton, K.; Thomas, M.R. Effects of increased dietary calcium intake upon the calcium and bone mineral status of lactating adolescent and adult women. *Am. J. Clin. Nutr.* **1987**, *46*, 319–323. [PubMed]

23. Yoneyama, K.; Ikeda, J. The effects of increased dietary calcium intake on bone mineral density in long-term lactating women, and recovery of bone loss caused by long-term lactation with low calcium diet. *Nihon Koshu Eisei Zasshi* **2004**, *51*, 1008–1017. [PubMed]

24. Li, Y.; Liao, D.; Miao, L.; Qian, X. Analysis on dietary investigation of pregnant and lactating women. *Chin. Prim. Health Care* **2004**, *18*, 27–28.

25. Huang, Z. The Dietary Status of 269 Lactating Women and the Content of Minerals in Breast Milk. Master's Thesis, Central South University, Changsha, China, 2014.

26. Yang, T.; Zhang, Y.; Ma, D.; Li, W.; Yang, X.; Wang, P. Survey on the nutrients intake of lactating women in three cities of China. *Acta Nutr. Sin.* **2014**, *36*, 84–86.

27. Chen, H.; Wang, P.; Han, Y.; Ma, J.; Troy, F.A., II; Wang, B. Evaluation of dietary intake of lactating women in China and its potential impact on the health of mothers and infants. *BMC Women's Health* **2012**, *12*, 18. [CrossRef] [PubMed]

28. Kong, X.; Fei, J.; Zhai, Y.; Feng, Y.; Li, J. Dietary survey of lactating mothers during the puerperal state. *China Med. Her.* **2016**, *13*, 49–68.

29. Qiu, L.; Zhao, Y.; Binns, C.W.; Lee, A.H.; Xie, X. A cohort study of infant feeding practices in city, suburban and rural areas in Zhejiang Province, PR China. *Int. Breastfeed. J.* **2008**, *3*, 4. [CrossRef] [PubMed]

30. Xu, F.; Liu, X.; Binns, C.W.; Xiao, C.; Wu, J.; Lee, A.H. A decade of change in breastfeeding in China's far north-west. *Int. Breastfeed. J.* **2006**, *1*, 22. [CrossRef] [PubMed]

31. Scott, J.A.; Landers, M.C.; Hughes, R.M.; Binns, C.W. Factors associated with breastfeeding at discharge and duration of breastfeeding. *J. Paediatr. Child Health* **2001**, *37*, 254–261. [CrossRef] [PubMed]

32. World Health Organization. Indicators for assessing infant and young child feeding practices: Part 1: Definitions. In Proceedings of the Conclusions of a Consensus Meeting, Washington, DC, USA, 6–8 November 2007.

33. Chan, S.M.; Nelson, E.A.; Leung, S.S.; Cheng, J.C. Bone mineral density and calcium metabolism of Hong Kong Chinese postpartum women—A 1-y longitudinal study. *Eur. J. Clin. Nutr.* **2005**, *59*, 868–876. [CrossRef] [PubMed]

34. Laskey, M.A.; Prentice, A.; Hanratty, L.A.; Jarjou, L.M.; Dibba, B.; Beavan, S.R.; Cole, T.J. Bone changes after 3 mo of lactation: Influence of calcium intake, breast-milk output, and vitamin D-receptor genotype. *Am. J. Clin. Nutr.* **1998**, *67*, 685–692. [PubMed]

35. Lopez, J.M.; Gonzalez, G.; Reyes, V.; Campino, C.; Diaz, S. Bone turnover and density in healthy women during breastfeeding and after weaning. *Osteoporos. Int.* **1996**, *6*, 153–159. [CrossRef] [PubMed]

36. Kalkwarf, H.J.; Specker, B.L.; Bianchi, D.C.; Ranz, J.; Ho, M. The effect of calcium supplementation on bone density during lactation and after weaning. *N. Engl. J. Med.* **1997**, *337*, 523–528. [CrossRef] [PubMed]

37. Prentice, A.; Jarjou, L.M.; Cole, T.J.; Stirling, D.M.; Dibba, B.; Fairweather-Tait, S. Calcium requirements of lactating Gambian mothers: Effects of a calcium supplement on breast-milk calcium concentration, maternal bone mineral content, and urinary calcium excretion. *Am. J. Clin. Nutr.* **1995**, *62*, 58–67. [PubMed]

38. Jarjou, L.M.; Prentice, A.; Sawo, Y.; Laskey, M.A.; Bennett, J.; Goldberg, G.R.; Cole, T.J. Randomized, placebo-controlled, calcium supplementation study in pregnant Gambian women: Effects on breast-milk calcium concentrations and infant birth weight, growth, and bone mineral accretion in the first year of life. *Am. J. Clin. Nutr.* **2006**, *83*, 657–666. [PubMed]

39. Zhang, Z.Q.; Chen, Y.M.; Wang, R.Q.; Huang, Z.W.; Yang, X.G.; Su, Y.X. The effects of different levels of calcium supplementation on the bone mineral status of postpartum lactating Chinese women: A 12-month randomised, double-blinded, controlled trial. *Br. J. Nutr.* **2016**, *115*, 24–31. [CrossRef] [PubMed]

40. Cross, N.A.; Hillman, L.S.; Allen, S.H.; Krause, G.F. Changes in bone mineral density and markers of bone remodeling during lactation and postweaning in women consuming high amounts of calcium. *J. Bone Miner. Res.* **1995**, *10*, 1312–1320. [CrossRef] [PubMed]

41. Kovacs, C.S. Maternal mineral and bone metabolism during pregnancy, lactation, and post-weaning recovery. *Physiol. Rev.* **2016**, *96*, 449–547. [PubMed]

42. Wang, J.; Yang, F.; Mao, M.; Liu, D.H.; Yang, H.M.; Yang, S.F. High prevalence of vitamin D and calcium deficiency among pregnant women and their newborns in Chengdu, China. *World J. Pediatr. WJP* **2010**, *6*, 265–267. [CrossRef] [PubMed]

7

Comparison of a Powdered, Acidified Liquid and Non-Acidified Liquid Human Milk Fortifier on Clinical Outcomes in Premature Infants

Melissa Thoene [1,*], Elizabeth Lyden [2], Kara Weishaar [3], Elizabeth Elliott [3], Ruomei Wu [3], Katelyn White [3], Hayley Timm [3] and Ann Anderson-Berry [3]

[1] Newborn Intensive Care Unit, Nebraska Medicine, 981200 Nebraska Medical Center, Omaha, NE 68198, USA
[2] College of Public Health, University of Nebraska Medical Center, 984375 Nebraska Medical Center, Omaha, NE 68198-4375, USA; elyden@unmc.edu
[3] Department of Pediatrics, University of Nebraska Medical Center, 981205 Nebraska Medical Center, Omaha, NE 68198-1205, USA; kara.weishaar@unmc.edu (K.W.); elizabeth.elliott@unmc.edu (E.E.); Ruomei.Wu@Creighton.edu (R.W.); katelyn.white@huskers.unl.edu (K.W.); hayley.timm@grmep.com (H.T.); alanders@unmc.edu (A.A.-B.)
* Correspondence: mthoene@nebraskamed.com

Abstract: We previously compared infant outcomes between a powdered human milk fortifier (P-HMF) vs. acidified liquid HMF (AL-HMF). A non-acidified liquid HMF (NAL-HMF) is now commercially available. The purpose of this study is to compare growth and outcomes of premature infants receiving P-HMF, AL-HMF or NAL-HMF. An Institutional Review Board (IRB) approved retrospective chart review compared infant outcomes (born < 2000 g) who received one of three HMF. Growth, enteral nutrition, laboratory and demographic data were compared. 120 infants were included (P-HMF = 46, AL-HMF = 23, NAL-HMF = 51). AL-HMF infants grew slower in g/day (median 23.66 vs. P-HMF 31.27, NAL-HMF 31.74 ($p < 0.05$)) and in g/kg/day, median 10.59 vs. 15.37, 14.03 ($p < 0.0001$). AL-HMF vs. NAL-HMF infants were smaller at 36 weeks gestational age (median 2046 vs. 2404 g, $p < 0.05$). However AL-HMF infants received more daily calories ($p = 0.21$) and protein ($p < 0.0001$), mean 129 cal/kg, 4.2 g protein/kg vs. P-HMF 117 cal/kg, 3.7 g protein/kg , NAL-HMF 120 cal/kg, 4.0 g protein/kg. AL-HMF infants exhibited lower carbon dioxide levels after day of life 14 and 30 ($p < 0.0001$, $p = 0.0038$). Three AL-HMF infants (13%) developed necrotizing enterocolitis (NEC) vs. no infants in the remaining groups ($p = 0.0056$). A NAL-HMF is the most optimal choice for premature human milk-fed infants in a high acuity neonatal intensive care unit (NICU).

Keywords: human milk; fortifier; premature infant; enteral nutrition; growth; acidosis; necrotizing enterocolitis

1. Introduction

Premature infants have significantly increased nutrient needs compared to those born at term [1]. Nutrition-related goals for these infants must aim at promoting similar nutrient provision and growth as that achieved in utero. Providing human milk remains a preferable nutrient source over customized premature infant formulas, but alone remains inadequate to meet the high nutritional needs for rapid growth and development. Long term provision of unfortified human milk has been linked to suboptimal growth, poor bone mineralization, and multiple nutrient deficiencies of vitamins, minerals, and trace elements [1]. As a result, human milk fortifiers (HMF) are used to significantly enhance calorie, protein, vitamin, and mineral intake of the human milk fed premature infant.

Enteral macronutrient recommendations for premature infants vary according to size. The American Academy of Pediatrics on nutrition suggests 130–150 calories/kilogram (kg) and 3.8–4.4 g protein/kg/day for infants weighing <1000 g, and 110–130 calories/kg and 3.4–4.2 g protein/kg/day for infants weighing between 1000 and 1500 g [2]. Protein is highly emphasized as high adequate provision has been correlated with improved growth and neurodevelopment [3–6]. To achieve enteral protein goals, powdered or liquid protein modulars may be added alongside HMF to optimize overall nutrition.

Human milk fortifiers are available in many different compositions, specifically varying in protein type, protein amount, and form (powder vs. liquid). However if available, the Food and Drug Administration strongly recommends the use of liquid products over powder in the neonatal intensive care unit (NICU) setting in an effort to reduce contamination and infection risk [7]. Our unit originally used a powdered HMF, but transitioned to liquid form when they became commercially available. Previously, we published a study comparing two HMF used in our unit, one being a powder (P-HMF) and one being an acidified liquid (AL-HMF) [8]. Our results demonstrated that the acidified product, though sterile, caused more metabolic acidosis and poor growth in our population of premature infants. Infants receiving the AL-HMF also had a higher incidence of necrotizing enterocolitis (NEC), though we were not powered to find this. Our unit has now transitioned to using a non-acidified liquid fortifier (NAL-HMF). The purpose of this study is compare growth and clinical outcomes of infants receiving this new HMF to the previous two fortifier groups.

2. Patients and Methods

2.1. Participants and Data Collection

The institutional review board at the University of Nebraska Medical Center (Omaha, NE, USA) approved this study. Data was retrospectively collected from inpatient electronic medical records of all infants admitted to the NICU between August 2012 and July 2014 if they met the following criteria; birth weight (BW) < 2000 g, received at least 25% of enteral feedings as fortified human milk (with the NAL-HMF) during their NICU stay, and remained in the NICU at least 14 days. Exclusion criteria included infants with congenital abnormalities or conditions that inhibited growth, such as Trisomy 13. No infants were excluded based on clinical acuity, intrauterine growth restriction, APGAR score, or ventilator requirements.

Data on the P-HMF and AL-HMF groups was previously collected for infants admitted to the NICU between October 2009 and July 2011. The AL-HMF group contained a lower number of included infants due to this HMF being used for a limited time period. Six investigators familiar with the electronic medical record obtained all data for the NAL-HMF group in a similar manner as the original groups. Data was reviewed closely for accuracy and corrected if an electronic error occurred. Available data on each infant was included in the analysis and is displayed in the tables.

2.2. Demographics and Clinical Outcomes

Demographic information was collected for all infants including gender, gestational age at birth and discharge, and day of life (DOL) at discharge. Additional clinical outcomes were collected as available including presence of bronchopulmonary dysplasia (BPD) defined as oxygen requirement at 36 weeks estimated gestational age (EGA), retinopathy of prematurity (ROP) Stage 2 or greater, Grade 3 or 4 intraventricular hemorrhage (IVH), NEC, and death. Treatment requirements were also analyzed including need for intraventricular shunt, ROP procedure, and Dexamethasone use.

2.3. Growth and Nutrition

Infants were weighed daily on a gram (g) scale, and length and head circumference measurements (cm = centimeters) were taken weekly using a measuring tape by nursing staff. Percentile rankings from the Fenton growth chart were electronically plotted for each documented measurement. Weight, length, and head circumference measurements were recorded for infants at birth and 36 weeks EGA if still hospitalized. An EGA of 36 weeks was empirically selected as an equivalent point of analysis for growth prior to discharge.

Enteral feeding data collected included DOL enteral feedings were initiated and DOL full enteral feedings were reached. Full enteral feedings was defined as the infant receiving at least 140 milliliters (mL)/kilogram (kg)/day of fortified enteral feedings and no parenteral nutrition. Average calorie and protein intake measured in per kg/day was analyzed for infants who received at least 50% of their feedings as fortified human milk during NICU stay. Intake was analyzed from the start of full feedings until the HMF was discontinued or the infant received <50% of feedings as fortified milk. Growth as measured in g/day and g/kg/day was calculated for infants during the time of reaching full enteral feedings until they received <50% of feedings as fortified milk. Maximum caloric density of feedings was recorded for each infant. Number of days on caloric densities higher than the standard 24 calories/ounce was collected for infants requiring more to maintain growth chart percentiles for weight. Nutrient provision was captured by an electronic medical system (Intuacare), which contained protein references based on the caloric density of specified formulas or fortified human milk. Nursing staff recorded daily intake (in mL) of specified feedings, and daily calorie and protein per kilogram was electronically calculated using the daily recorded weight. The electronic system also calculated the percentage of human milk vs. infant formula received according to nursing documentation.

2.4. Comparison and Use of Human Milk Fortifiers

Comparison of ingredients and key HMF nutrients are listed in Table 1 according to online nutritional references [9–11].

Table 1. Comparison of primary nutrients and ingredients of the powdered, acidified liquid, and non-acidified liquid HMF.

24-Calorie-Per-Ounce Fortified Human Milk [9–11]			
Per 100 mL	**P-HMF**	**AL-HMF**	**NAL-HMF**
Protein (g)	2.35 g	3.2 g	2.34 g
Iron (mg)	0.46 mg	1.85 mg	0.46
Calcium (mg)	138 mg	141 mg	138
Phosphorus (mg)	78 mg	78 mg	77
Vitamin D (IU)	119 IU	200 IU	118
pH	—	4.7	—
Osmolality (mOsm/kg water)	385	326	385
Primary Fortifier Macronutrient Ingredients	nonfat milk, whey protein concentrate, corn syrup solids, medium-chain triglycerides (MCT oil)	water, whey protein isolate hydrolysate (milk), medium chain triglycerides (MCT oil), vegetable oil (soy and high oleic sunflower oils)	water, nonfat milk, corn syrup solids, medium-chain triglycerides (MCT oil), whey protein concentrate

– Information not available. P-HMF, powdered human milk fortifier; AL-HMF, acidified liquid HMF; NAL-HMF, non-acidified liquid HMF.

Enteral feeding are initiated in this NICU as soon as able following birth, within the first one to three days of life using maternal breast milk (MBM) as available or donor human milk (from the Milk Bank of Austin, Texas) at 20 mL/kg/day. Trophic feedings are continued for three to five days at the discretion of the attending neonatologist. Feedings are then advanced by 20 mL/kg/day and HMF is added when enteral volumes feedings reach 80–100 mL/kg. A protein modular is also added once caloric densities reach 24 calories/ounce to optimize protein intake to approximately 4 g/kg/day. The calories provided from the protein modular are accounted for in the calorie-per-ounce estimates. The P-HMF group received a powdered protein modular and the NAL-HMF group received a liquid protein modular. No additional protein modular was provided to infants receiving the AL-HMF due to higher protein content of the fortifier. All infants are transitioned off of donor human milk to 24 calorie/ounce high protein (3.5 g protein per 100 calories) premature infant formula at 14 days of life if a supplement to MBM is needed. We did not analyze differences in donor human milk use between groups because it is only used for a short period after birth and is provided to all infants in a similar manner. There were no other nutrition practice changes during the periods of different fortifier use. Our unit follows a written feeding protocol, so nutrition is managed closely and remains consistent among providers.

2.5. Laboratory Measurements

Lowest carbon dioxide (CO_2) lab values were collected after DOL 14 and 30 for all infants, if available. Values were not collected prior to eliminate values reflective of parenteral nutrition support and unfortified enteral feedings. Maximum blood urea nitrogen (BUN) while on full enteral feedings was additionally collected.

2.6. Data Analysis

The Kruskal Wallis test was used to compare continuous data between the three HMF groups. If the overall p-value was significant, indicating a significant difference between at least two of the three groups, the Dunn's post hoc test for three pair wise comparisons (i.e., Group 1 vs. 2, Group 1 vs. 3, Group 2 vs. 3) was performed. Associations of categorical variables were assessed with the Fisher's exact test. Time to weaning off oxygen distributions were estimated using the method of Kaplan and Meier and were compared using the log-rank test. A p-value < 0.05 was considered statistically significant.

To assess the difference in growth patterns between infants, a mixed effects model was used. We included random slopes and intercepts for each subject to capture individual growth pattern as well as fixed effects for group and day and a group day interaction term. A significant interacting of day and group indicated differing growth patterns based on group. Growth Velocity (GV) was calculated using the following equation [12]:

$$GV = [1000 \times \ln(W_n/W_1)]/(D_n - D_1) \tag{1}$$

Where W_n refers to the weight on the last evaluated day; W_1 refers to the first weight; D_n refers to the last day of the time period evaluated and; D_1 refers to the first day of the time period evaluated.

3. Results

There were 46 infants in the P-HMF, 23 in the AL-HMF, and 51 in the NAL-HMF groups. There were no significant differences in gender ($p = 0.6$) or baseline characteristics as shown in Table 2. Clinical outcomes are displayed in Table 3. Laboratory, growth, and nutrition data are displayed in Table 4.

Table 2. Baseline characteristics of subjects by group.

Variable	P-HMF (Group 1)		AL-HMF (Group 2)		NAL-HMF (Group 3)		Overall p-Value
	n	Median	n	Median	n	Median	
EGA at Birth	46	29.15	22	31.00	51	29.60	0.15
Birth Weight (g)	46	1305	22	1481	51	1340	0.21
Weight at 36 Weeks EGA (g)	44	2179	18	2046	50	2404	0.0092 Group 2 vs. 3 $p < 0.05$
Birth Length (cm)	46	39	22	41	51	39	0.14
Length at 36 Weeks EGA (cm)	42	44.5	18	43.5	47	44	0.38
Birth HC (cm)	46	27	22	27.75	51	27.5	0.53
HC at 36 Weeks EGA (cm)	42	32.5	18	31.75	47	32.2	0.55

EGA = Estimated Gestational Age; HC = Head Circumference.

Table 3. Clinical outcomes of subjects by group.

Variable	P-HMF (Group 1) $n = 46$	AL-HMF (Group 2) $n = 23$	NAL-HMF (Group 3) $n = 51$	Overall p-Value
	n (%)	n (%)	n (%)	
NEC	0	3 (13%)	0	0.0056
ROP	16 (35%)	3 (13%)	4 (8%)	0.0030 Group 1 vs. 3, $p = 0.006$
ROP Procedure	3 (7%)	2 (9%)	1 (2%)	0.24
IVH (Grade 3 or 4)	3 (7%)	1 (5%)	4 (8%)	1.00
Intraventricular Shunt	0	0	0	N/A
Dexamethasone Treatment	9 (20%)	1 (5%)	7 (14%)	0.29
Death	0	0	1 (2%)	1.00
BPD	10/40 (25%)	4/18 (22%)	16/49 (33%)	0.65

Table 4. Laboratory, growth, and enteral nutrition data.

Variable	P-HMF (Group 1)		AL-HMF (Group 2)		NAL-HMF (Group 3)		Overall p-Value
	n	Median	n	Median	n	Median	
Mean Daily Calorie Provision (per kg)	42	117	18	129	48	120	0.21
Mean Daily Protein Provision (g/kg)	42	3.7	18	4.2	48	4.0	0.0001 Group 1 vs. 2 and Group 2 vs. 3, p <0.05
Day of Life Feedings Started	46	1	22	1	51	1	0.0019 Group 1 vs. 3 p < 0.05
Day of Life Full Feedings Achieved	46	12	22	10	51	9	0.0007 Group 1 vs. 3 p < 0.05
Growth on HMF (g/day)	45	31.27	21	23.66	49	31.74	0.0001 Group 1 vs. 2 and Group 2 vs. 3, p < 0.05
Growth on HMF (g/kg/day)	45	15.37	21	10.59	49	14.03	<0.0001 Group 1 vs. 2 and Group 2 vs. 3, p < 0.05
BUN Maximum on Full Feedings	33	17	17	19	47	16	0.43
CO_2 Minimum after DOL 14	33	23	17	19	32	27	<0.0001 Group 1 vs. 3 and Group 2 vs. 3, 0.05
CO_2 Minimum after DOL 30	23	25	9	20	18	25.5	0.0038 Group 1 vs. 2 and Group 2 vs. 3, p < 0.05

3.1. Clinical Outcomes

All laboratory data analyzed for this study was collected for clinical purposes. Median lowest C02 levels while on full enteral feedings were significantly lower in the AL-HMF group compared to the other two groups after both DOL 14 and DOL 30 ($p < 0.0001$, $p = 0.0038$). Maximum BUN levels on full enteral feedings were similar among all groups and were not statistically significant.

The incidence of NEC was significantly higher in the AL-HMF group compared to the P-HMF and NAL-HMF groups (13% vs. 0% and 0%, $p = 0.0056$), though we were not powered to evaluate this variable. Incidence of ROP was significantly higher among the P-HMF than the NAL-HMF group (35% vs. 8%, $p = 0.003$). There were no differences in rates of BPD or IVH (Grade 3 or 4) among all groups.

3.2. Enteral Growth and Nutrition

Growth, as measured in both g/day and g/kg/day, was statistically significant between groups. More specifically, infants in the AL-HMF group grew slower than infants in the P-HMF and NAL-HMF groups. Median growth in g/day from start of full enteral feedings until 36 weeks EGA was 23.66, compared to 31.27 in the P-HMF and 31.74 in the NA-LHMF group ($p = 0.0001$). Median growth in g/kg/day was 10.59 in the AL-HMF group, compared to 15.37 and 14.03 respectively ($p < 0.0001$). Infants in the AL-HMF group were smaller at 36 weeks EGA compared to the NAL-HMF group (median 2046 g vs. 2404 g, $p = 0.0092$), though there were no differences in length or head circumference. There were no differences in Dexamethasone use among groups ($p = 0.15$) that may account for reduced growth. Infants in the NAL-HMF group started enteral feedings and achieved full enteral feedings faster than the P-HMF group ($p = 0.0019$, $p = 0.0007$), but these infants achieved similar growth.

Among infants receiving >50% of their feedings during NICU stay as fortified human milk , infants in the AL-HMF group received more protein at mean 4.2 g/kg/day compared to 3.7 and 4.0 g/kg/day in the P-HMF and NAL-HMF groups ($p < 0.0001$). These infants also received a higher mean calorie intake at 129 calories/kg, compared to 117 and 120 calories/kg, respectively, though this was not significant ($p = 0.21$).

There were no differences in maximum caloric density of enteral feedings ($p = 0.6$) or the number of days on feedings >24 calories/ounce ($p = 0.21$). Noted however, is that 48% of infants in the AL-HMF group received enteral feedings >24 calorie/ounce compared to 26% in the P-HMF group and 35% in the NAL-HMF group.

4. Discussion

Our previous research analyzing the P-HMF and AL-HMF suggested the P-HMF was the more optimal choice in promoting best clinical outcomes [8]. Now comparing data among all three fortifier groups, the NAL-HMF appears to be the most successful fortifier for use in a high acuity NICU population. Despite achieving adequate similar growth, the NAL-HMF is more desirable than the P-HMF due to its composition as a sterile liquid. When compared to the AL-HMF, the NAL-HMF promoted greater growth and was not associated with metabolic acidosis or NEC.

4.1. Growth and Enteral Nutrition

Appropriate growth was best achieved among the NAL-HMF and P-HMF groups when comparing both g/day and g/kg/day weight gain. Infants receiving the NAL-HMF attained the highest weight among all three groups at 36 weeks EGA, demonstrating most significance when compared to the AL-HMF group (median 2046 g vs. 2404 g, $p < 0.0092$). In further comparison of this, the median length and head circumference for both the acidified and non-acidified liquid group at this point plotted between the 25%–30% on the Fenton growth chart. By comparison of median weights at 36 weeks, the NAL-HMF group plotted around the 18% and the AL-HMF group plotted at the 5th. This demonstrates that infants receiving the NAL-HMF were able to achieve a more proportional weight-for-length ratio. Though we did not directly assess infant acuity level between groups, we do not suspect this to be a significant factor for decreased growth given the AL-HMF group having similar baseline characteristics as the other groups.

As growth remains a high priority, infants with suboptimal growth were fed enteral feedings with caloric densities >24 calories/ounce. Suboptimal growth was determined by clinical evaluation when an infant was unable to maintain growth percentiles for weight. Despite decreased growth, more infants in the AL-HMF (48%) group required increased caloric density of feedings compared to the P-HMF (26%) and NAL-HMF (35%) groups, $p = 0.6$. The AL-HMF group also received higher mean calorie intake compared to the other two groups. Had no infants been advanced to increased caloric densities, it is likely that the discrepancy of growth between the AL-HMF and the remaining two groups would have been of even greater significance. It may be theorized that additional enteral additives and higher caloric densities contributed to a higher incidence of NEC in the AL-HMF group. However, our previously low recorded rate of NEC at 3% is reflective of similar fortification practices to achieve desired growth [13]. Despite individual theories for these NEC occurrences, we must address why the additional additives were required in the first place to achieve adequate growth.

In additional to increased calories, infants in the AL-HMF group also received a higher mean protein intake compared to the other groups. Higher protein provisions have been linked to improved growth, yet these infants exhibited poor weight gain. We hypothesize that the acidification of the AL-HMF may be the explanatory factor in this conundrum. A study by Erickson et al. concluded that acidifying human milk resulted in 14% decrease in protein and a 56% decrease in lipase activity [14]. This may result in partial fat malabsorption and resulting poor energy intake. A recent study by Cibulskis and Armbrecht comparing infants receiving an acidified vs. powdered HMF did not report significant growth differences in weight, length, or head circumference between birth and discharge [15]. However, growth measured in g/day while on the HMF approached significance as infants receiving the acidified HMF grew slower (22.3 vs. 19.2 g/day, $p = 0.08$). In comparison, Moya et al. reported no discrepancies in weight gain when comparing infants $\leqslant 1250$ g receiving either an acidified or powdered HMF, and further reported that infants receiving the acidified HMF had improved linear growth [16]. Limitations of this study, however, include that protein modulars were used infrequently among infants, so baseline protein provisions were higher in the acidified HMF group. This study also excluded infants with low APGAR scores and higher respiratory requirements so may not be applicable to the most fragile infants.

4.2. NEC

The only infants who developed NEC received the AL-HMF. Though not statistically powered to find NEC, the results raise concern from a clinical standpoint. Our feeding practices have remained consistent outside of which HMF was used, and we have documented low baseline rates of NEC on these feeding practices [13]. Feeding initiation and advancement remained fairly consistent across all three groups. While infants in the NAL-HMF group achieved full feedings more quickly, none developed NEC. Formula was utilized equally in all groups when MBM was limited and donor human milk was weaned.

The primary differences in enteral feedings between all fortifier groups are the acidity, high protein, and high iron content of the AL-HMF. Theoretically, infants receiving the AL-HMF had a reduced risk for cross-contamination due to the HMF composition as a sterile liquid and because additional enteral substrates (protein modular, iron) were not required. These infants also received lower osmolality feedings at baseline, and furthermore as additional supplements were not required due to the high iron and protein in the AL-HMF. A study by *Chan* suggests that a high iron-containing HMF compared to a low iron-containing HMF negates the antimicrobial effects of human milk against the growth of *E. coli*, Staphylococcus, Enterobacter, and Streptococcus [17]. Erickson et al. also noted a reduced white cell count by 76% in human milk acidified to a pH of 4.5, questioning if this decreases an infant's host defense [14]. The AL-HMF used in our study acidifies milk similarly to a pH of 4.7. We must consider if the protective effects of human milk were compromised in infants receiving the AL-HMF, making them more susceptible to infections. A limitation to this theory is that we did not analyze the incidence of sepsis between groups. As the cause of these NEC occurrences remains unknown, we can neither confirm nor exclude use of the AL-HMF as a primary contributor.

4.3. Acidosis

There was a higher incidence of metabolic acidosis in the AL-HMF group compared to the other two groups. As discussed in our previous study, premature infants are at risk for developing metabolic acidosis secondary to immature renal and metabolic processes [8]. There were no significant differences in baseline characteristics such as birth weight or gestational age to suggest any of the three groups included infants that were smaller or born more prematurely, and therefore more obviously susceptible to acidosis. We do not suspect protein provision as a contributor to acidosis. While infants receiving the AL-HMF received higher daily protein ($p < 0.001$), mean values remained within the reference ranges for very low birth weight infants of 3.4–4.4 g protein/kg/day [2]. BUN levels also remained similar among groups.

While the P-HMF and NAL-HMF do not have defined pH values as shown in Table 1, we suspect they have limited effects on the final pH of fortified milk, unlike the AL-HMF. Considering a similar baseline of other characteristics, we again hypothesize that the acidification of the AL-HMF contributed to this metabolic imbalance. Our results are concurrent with Cibulskis and Armbrecht who reported a higher incidence of metabolic acidosis (54% vs. 10%) in infants <32 weeks EGA or <1500 g receiving an acidified vs. powdered HMF [15]. Moya et al. also reported a lower pH at day of life 14 ($p = 0.004$) and lower carbon dioxide levels at both day of life 14 ($p < 0.001$) and 30 ($p = 0.021$) in infants ⩽1250 g receiving an acidified HMF [16].

Development of metabolic acidosis may also contribute to altered weight gain and poor nutritional consequences. A small study by Rochow et al. reported lower weight gain (median 9 vs. 21 g/kg/day, $p < 0.01$) in infants <34 weeks EGA who developed metabolic acidosis compared to those who remained unaffected [18]. It was also reported that infants who developed metabolic acidosis had a lower bone density at discharge. Likewise, an early study by Kalhoff et al. analyzed urinary excretion of minerals in premature infants, concluding that a higher amount of calcium and phosphorus is excreted during metabolic acidosis [19]. Resultantly, we suggest using a NAL-HMF to provide appropriate growth, without increasing risk for metabolic acidosis and suboptimal nutrient accretion.

4.4. Strengths and Limitations

This study is the first to quantify nutrition and growth outcomes of three HMF in a Level IIIc NICU. We did not exclude infants based on acuity, such as presence of IVH, need for high ventilatory settings, or low APGAR scores. Our high inclusion is more reflective of a standard NICU population, and therefore provides genuine outcomes for both high and moderate acuity infants. This is both relevant and applicable to current NICU settings. Nutrition is managed closely and consistently in our unit, and our current nutrition practices have been published demonstrating excellent growth and low baseline rates of NEC [13]. Additionally unique to our study is the use of protein modulars to provide infants similar protein provisions at baseline (approximately 4 g protein/kg/day when receiving 120 calories/kg/day), and reducing this as a significant confounding factor across fortifier groups.

Limitations of this study include that it is retrospective, and there is a limited number of subjects in the AL-HMF group due to its short term use. Additionally included is our reliance on electronic documentation for data collection, as we cannot quantify unrecorded or misrecorded data. However, the system does allow for review of daily entered data for each subject if needed. Evaluation of head circumference and length measurements may vary among nursing staff due to differences in measuring tape placement. Additionally, growth measurements were unavailable for infants discharged prior to 36 weeks EGA. Growth at 36 weeks EGA may also be partially reflective of formula use if MBM was no longer available. However, it may also provide indication of early growth failure while on MBM if growth percentiles are low or fall drastically from those at birth. The calculated provision for calories and protein in fortified human milk were estimated according to manufacturer information for each HMF. These may only serve as general estimates for our comparisons as the composition of human milk varies continuously. While standard NICU practices remain consistent, feedings may be advanced differently based on each infant's clinical status. Length of trophic feedings may also impact the day of life to achieving full enteral feedings. As in our previous study of the original two fortifiers, NEC was statistically significant despite our limited power to find this.

5. Conclusions

The NAL-HMF is an appropriate choice for use in a high level NICU. Caution should be taken when using an acidified HMF due to its potential effects on growth, tolerance, and metabolic acidosis.

Author Contributions: M.T. and A.A.-B. conceived and designed the study; M.T., K.W., E.E., R.W., K.W., and H.T. performed all required data collection for the study experiment; E.L. analyzed the data; M.T. and A.A.B. wrote the paper.

References

1. Groh-Wargo, S.; Thompson, M.; Hovasi Cox, J.H. *Nutritional Care for High.-Risk Newborns*, 3rd ed.; Hartline, J.V., Ed.; Precept Press, Inc.: Chicago, IL, USA, 2000.

2. American Academy of Pediatrics. *Pediatric Nutrition Handbook*, 6th ed.; American Academy of Pediatrics: Washington, DC, USA, 2009; pp. 79–81.

3. Wagner, J.; Hanson, C.; Anderson-Berry, A. Considerations in meeting protein needs of the human milk-fed preterm infant. *Adv. Neonatal Care* **2014**, *14*, 281–289. [CrossRef] [PubMed]

4. Fenton, T.R.; Premji, S.S.; Al-Wassia, H.; Sauve, R.S. Higher versus lower protein intake in formula-fed low birth weight infants. *Cochrane Database Syst. Rev.* **2014**, *4*, CD003959. [CrossRef] [PubMed]

5. Ramel, S.E.; Gray, H.L.; Christiansen, E.; Boys, C.; Georgieff, M.K.; Demerath, E.W. Greater early gains in fat-free mass, but not fat mass, are associated with improved neurodevelopment at 1 year corrected age for prematurity in very low birth weight preterm infants. *J. Pediatr.* **2016**, *173*, 105–115. [CrossRef] [PubMed]

6. Yang, J.; Chang, S.S.; Poon, W.B. Relationship between amino acid and energy intake and long-term growth and neurodevelopmental outcomes in very low-birth-weight infants. *JPEN J. Parenter. Enter. Nutr.* **2016**, *40*, 820–826. [CrossRef] [PubMed]

7. Taylor, C.J. Health Professionals Letter on *Enterobacter sakazakii* Infections Associated With Use of Powdered (Dry) Infant Formulas in Neonatal Intensive Care Units. US Department of Health and Human Services, 2002. Available online: http://www.fda.gov/Food/RecallsOutbreaksEmergencies/SafetyAlertsAdvisories/ucm111299.htm (accessed on 24 May 2016).

8. Thoene, M.; Hanson, C.; Lyden, E.; Dugick, L.; Ruybal, L.; Anderson-Berry, A. Comparison of the effect of two human milk fortifiers on clinical outcomes in premature infants. *J. Nutr.* **2014**, *6*, 261–275. [CrossRef] [PubMed]

9. Abbott Nutrition Similac Human Milk Fortifier. Available online: http://abbottnutrition.com/brands/products/similac-human-milk-fortifier (accessed on 29 January 2015).

10. Enfamil Human Milk Fortifier Acidified Liquid. Available online: http://www.enfamil.com/products/enfamil-human-milk-fortifier-acidified-liquid (accessed on 29 January 2015).

11. Abbott Nutrition Similac Human Milk Fortifier Concentrated Liquid. Available online: http://abbottnutrition.com/brands/products/similac-human-milk-fortifier-concentrated-liquid (accessed on 29 January 2015).

12. Patel, A.L.; Engstrom, J.L.; Meier, P.P.; Kimura, R.E. Accuracy of methods for calculating postnatal growth velocity for extremely low birth weight infants. *Pediatrics* **2005**, *116*, 1466–1473. [CrossRef] [PubMed]

13. Hanson, C.; Sundermeier, J.; Dugick, L.; Lyden, E.; Anderson-Berry, A.L. Implementation, process, and outcomes of nutrition best practices for infants <1500 g. *Nutr. Clin. Pract.* **2001**, *26*, 614–624.

14. Erickson, T.; Gill, G.; Chan, G.M. The effects of acidification on human milk's cellular and nutritional content. *J. Perinatol.* **2013**, *3*, 371–373. [CrossRef] [PubMed]

15. Cibulskis, C.C.; Armbrecht, E. Association of metabolic acidosis with bovine milk-based human milk fortifiers. *J. Perinatol.* **2015**, *35*, 115–119. [CrossRef] [PubMed]

16. Moya, F.; Sisk, P.M.; Walsh, K.R.; Berseth, C.L. A new liquid human milk fortifier and linear growth in preterm infants. *J. Pediatr.* **2012**, *130*, 928–935. [CrossRef] [PubMed]

17. Chan, G.M. Effects of powdered human milk fortifiers on the antibacterial actions of human milk. *J. Perinatol.* **2003**, *23*, 620–623. [CrossRef] [PubMed]

18. Rochow, N.; Jochum, F.; Redlich, A.; Korinekova, Z.; Linnemann, K.; Weitmann, K.; Boehm, G.; Müller, H.; Kalhoff, H.; Topp, H.; et al. Fortification of breast milk in VLBW infants: Metabolic acidosis is linked to the composition of fortifiers and alters weight gain and bone mineralization. *J. Clin. Nutr.* **2011**, *30*, 99–105. [CrossRef] [PubMed]

19. Kalhoff, H.; Diekmann, L.; Rudloff, S.; Manz, F. Renal excretion of calcium and phosphorus in premature infants with incipient late metabolic acidosis. *J. Pediatr. Gastroenterol. Nutr.* **2001**, *33*, 565–569. [CrossRef] [PubMed]

8

Probiotics and Time to Achieve Full Enteral Feeding in Human Milk-Fed and Formula-Fed Preterm Infants

Arianna Aceti [1,2], Davide Gori [2,3], Giovanni Barone [2,4], Maria Luisa Callegari [2,5], Maria Pia Fantini [2,3], Flavia Indrio [2,6,7], Luca Maggio [2,4,7], Fabio Meneghin [2,8], Lorenzo Morelli [2,5], Gianvincenzo Zuccotti [2,9] and Luigi Corvaglia [1,2,7,*]

[1] Neonatology and Neonatal Intensive Care Unit, Department of Medical and Surgical Sciences (DIMEC), University of Bologna, S.Orsola-Malpighi Hospital, Bologna 40138, Italy; arianna.aceti2@unibo.it

[2] Task Force on Probiotics of the Italian Society of Neonatology, Milan 20126, Italy; dedegori27@gmail.com (D.G.); gbarone85@yahoo.it (G.B.); marialuisa.callegari@unicatt.it (M.L.C.); mariapia.fantini@unibo.it (M.P.F.); f.indrio@alice.it (F.I.); luca.maggio@fastwebnet.it (L.Ma.); fabio.meneghin@asst-fbf-sacco.it (F.M.); lorenzo.morelli@unicatt.it (L.Mo.); gianvincenzo.zuccotti@unimi.it (G.Z.)

[3] Department of Biomedical and Neuromotor Sciences (DIBINEM), University of Bologna, Bologna 40138, Italy

[4] Neonatal Unit, Catholic University, Rome 00168, Italy

[5] Institute of Microbiology, UCSC, Piacenza 29122, Italy

[6] Department of Pediatrics, Aldo Moro University, Bari 70124, Italy

[7] Study Group of Neonatal Gastroenterology and Nutrition of the Italian Society of Neonatology, Milan 20126, Italy

[8] Division of Neonatology, Children Hospital V. Buzzi, ICP, Milan 20154, Italy

[9] Department of Pediatrics, Children Hospital V. Buzzi, University of Milan, Milan 20154, Italy

* Correspondence: luigi.corvaglia@unibo.it

Abstract: Probiotics have been linked to a reduction in the incidence of necrotizing enterocolitis and late-onset sepsis in preterm infants. Recently, probiotics have also proved to reduce time to achieve full enteral feeding (FEF). However, the relationship between FEF achievement and type of feeding in infants treated with probiotics has not been explored yet. The aim of this systematic review and meta-analysis was to evaluate the effect of probiotics in reducing time to achieve FEF in preterm infants, according to type of feeding (exclusive human milk (HM) vs. formula). Randomized-controlled trials involving preterm infants receiving probiotics, and reporting on time to reach FEF were included in the systematic review. Trials reporting on outcome according to type of feeding (exclusive HM vs. formula) were included in the meta-analysis. Fixed-effect or random-effects models were used as appropriate. Results were expressed as mean difference (MD) with 95% confidence interval (CI). Twenty-five studies were included in the systematic review. In the five studies recruiting exclusively HM-fed preterm infants, those treated with probiotics reached FEF approximately 3 days before controls (MD -3.15 days (95% CI $-5.25/-1.05$), $p = 0.003$). None of the two studies reporting on exclusively formula-fed infants showed any difference between infants receiving probiotics and controls in terms of FEF achievement. The limited number of included studies did not allow testing for other subgroup differences between HM and formula-fed infants. However, if confirmed in further studies, the 3-days reduction in time to achieve FEF in exclusively HM-fed preterm infants might have significant implications for their clinical management.

Keywords: probiotics; preterm infants; human milk; full enteral feeding; systematic review

1. Introduction

Nutrition during critical time windows in early life can affect long-term health [1]. Early provision of optimal enteral nutrition to preterm infants might improve neurodevelopmental outcome by decreasing the rate of several complications of prematurity, such as extrauterine growth restriction, necrotizing enterocolitis (NEC), sepsis, bronchopulmonary dysplasia, and retinopathy of prematurity [2].

Late introduction and slow advancement of enteral feeding may alter gastrointestinal motility and disrupt microbial colonization [3], leading to a delay in establishing full enteral feeding (FEF). The consequent prolonged need for parenteral nutrition can have serious infectious and metabolic complications, which might prolong hospital stay, increase morbidity and mortality, and affect growth and development [4].

Several clinical variables and interventions have been proposed as predictors of the time to FEF achievement in preterm and very-low-birth-weight (VLBW) infants. Among these variables, the influence of type of feeding was also documented, as FEF achievement was delayed in formula-fed infants compared to human milk (HM)-fed infants [5].

Recently, probiotic use has been associated with a reduced time to achieve FEF and better feeding tolerance [6], as well as a reduction of NEC [7,8] and late-onset sepsis [9]. Probiotics are live microorganisms which, when ingested in adequate amounts, confer a health benefit to the host, by modifying the composition and function of gut microbiota and the immunological responses in the host [10]. The role of probiotics in attaining a more rapid achievement of FEF could be related to their favorable effect on the physiological intestinal dysbiosis of preterm infants [11], which is the result of the exposure to a unique environment and to several iatrogenic manipulations, such as broad spectrum antibiotics [12]. It is well known that gut microbiota in HM-fed infants is different compared to formula-fed infants [13]; data from an observational study also suggest a feeding-dependent effect of probiotics, as in that study NEC incidence was reduced in infants treated with probiotics and receiving HM, but not in those exclusively formula-fed [14]. However, the relationship between probiotics and type of feeding in attaining a more rapid achievement of FEF has not been explored yet, even in the most recent meta-analysis on this topic [6].

Thus, the aim of the present paper was to evaluate the effect of probiotics on time to FEF achievement according to type of feeding (exclusive HM vs. formula), by performing a systematic review and meta-analysis of currently available literature on this topic.

2. Materials and Methods

2.1. Literature Search

The study protocol was designed by the members of the Task Force on Probiotics of the Italian Society of Neonatology. PRISMA guidelines [15] were followed in order to perform a systematic review of published studies reporting the relationship between probiotic use and time to FEF achievement in preterm infants according to type of feeding.

In order to be included in the meta-analysis, studies had to meet the following inclusion criteria: randomized or quasi-randomized clinical trials involving preterm infants (gestational age (GA) <37 weeks) who received, within one month of age, any probiotic compared to placebo or no treatment, and reporting on type of feeding. The outcome of interest was time for FEF achievement (any definition). Only English-written studies and studies involving humans were included in the meta-analysis.

A search was conducted for studies published before 2 March 2016 in PubMed [16], the Cochrane Library [17], and Embase [18]. The following search string was used for the PubMed search: ((preterm infant OR pre-term infant) OR (preterm infants OR pre-term infants) OR (preterm neonate OR pre-term neonate) OR (preterm neonates OR pre-term neonates) OR (preterm newborn OR pre-term newborn) OR (preterm newborns OR pre-term newborns) OR (premature infant OR premature infants) OR (premature neonate OR premature neonates) OR (premature newborn OR premature newborns)

OR infant, extremely premature (MeSH Heading (MH)) OR premature birth (MH) OR infant, low birth weight (MH) OR infant, very low birth weight (MH)) AND (full enteral* OR feed*) AND (probiotic OR probiotics OR pro-biotic OR pro-biotics OR probio*)) NOT (animals (MH) NOT humans (MH).

The string was built up by combining all the terms related to probiotics and FEF achievement: PubMed MeSH terms, free-text words, and their combinations obtained through the most proper Boolean operators were used. The same criteria were used for searching the Cochrane Library and Embase.

Arianna Aceti and Luigi Corvaglia performed the literature search: relevant studies were identified from the abstract; full-texts of relevant studies were examined, as well as their reference lists in order to identify additional studies.

2.2. Data Extraction and Meta-Analysis

Study details (population, characteristics of probiotic and placebo, type of feeding, and outcome assessment) were evaluated independently by Arianna Aceti and Luigi Corvaglia, and checked by Davide Gori. Study quality was evaluated independently by Arianna Aceti and Davide Gori using the risk of bias tool as proposed by the Cochrane collaboration (Chapter 8 of the Cochrane Handbook of Systematic Reviews) [19].

The corresponding authors of the studies in which days to FEF achievement were not reported as mean ± standard deviation (SD) were contacted by email. When data were not provided, the study was not included in the meta-analysis.

The association between probiotic use and FEF achievement according to type of feeding was evaluated by a meta-analysis conducted by AA and DG using the RevMan software (Cochrane Informatics and Knowledge Management Department, version 5.3.5) downloaded from the Cochrane website [20]. Mean difference (MD) in days to achieve FEF between infants receiving probiotics and those receiving placebo or no treatment was calculated using the inverse variance method, and reported with 95% confidence interval (CI).

For the analysis, we planned to use at first a fixed effect model. Heterogeneity was measured using the I^2 test: if significant heterogeneity was present ($p < 0.05$ from the χ^2 test) and/or the number of studies was ⩽5, a random-effects model was used instead.

3. Results

Literature Search

Overall, 372 papers were identified through the literature search, 155 in PubMed [16], 73 in the Cochrane Library [17], and 144 in Embase [18].

As shown in Figure 1, 35 studies met the inclusion criteria [21–55]. Fourteen additional papers were identified from the reference lists of included studies or by "snowballing" techniques [52,56–68].

Twenty-four studies were excluded after examining the full-texts [28,29,31–33,35,42–47,51,53–55,57–59, 62,63,65,69]. Twenty-five studies were then suitable for inclusion in the systematic review (Table 1) [21–27, 30,34,36–41,48–50,56,60,61,64,66,68,70].

Among them, only eight studies reported FEF achievement according to type of feeding: infants were fed exclusively HM, either own mother's (OMM) or donor human milk (DHM), in six studies [22,38,50,56,60,70], while two studies reported FEF in exclusively formula-fed infants [41,61].

The corresponding authors of four of these papers were contacted by email, as data for FEF achievement were not suitable for inclusion in the meta-analysis: mean ± SD of days for FEF achievement were provided for one study [22], while data were unavailable for three studies [41,61,70]; these three studies were thus excluded from the meta-analysis.

Overall, five studies were included in the meta-analysis: in all these studies, infants were fed exclusively HM, either OMM or DHM (Figure 1) [22,38,50,56,60].

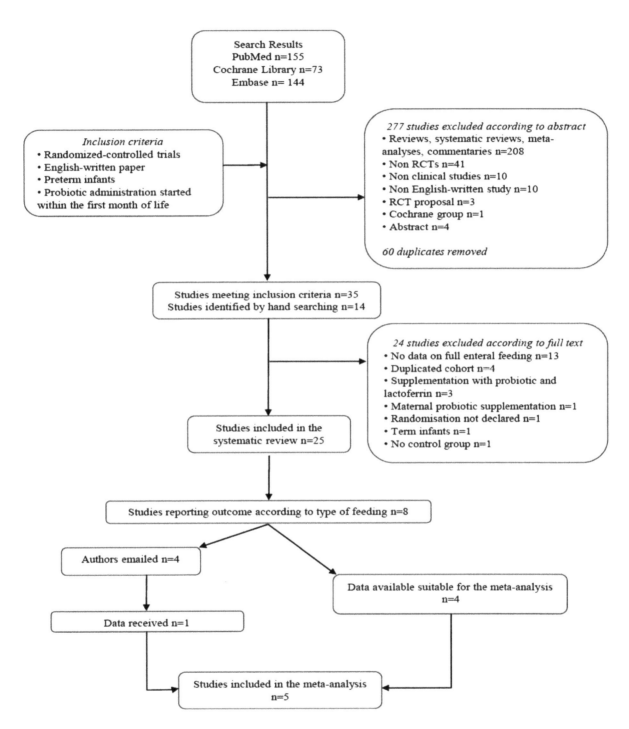

Figure 1. Flow chart of the search strategy used for the systematic review. The relevant number of papers at each point is given.

Table 1. Studies included in the systematic review.

Author, Year	Study Details	Study Population	Intervention Specie / Dose (D) / Start of Treatment (S) / End of Treatment (E)	Milk	Placebo	FEF Definition
Bin-Nun, 2005 [40]	P, B, R, C	Preterm infants with BW <1500 g, who began enteral feeding on a weekday	*B. infantis, Str. thermophilus, B. bifidus* D: 0.35×10^9 CFU each, OD S: start of enteral feeding E: 36 w postconceptual age	OMM, PFM	HM or FM	100 mL/kg/day
Braga, 2011 [60]	P, DB, R, C	Inborn infants with BW 750–1499 g	*L. casei, B. Breve* D: 3.5×10^7 CFU to 3.5×10^9 CFU OD S: day 2 E: day 30, NEC diagnosis, discharge, death, whichever occurred first	HM ($\pm$ PFM from w3)	Extra HM	150 mL/kg/day
Costalos, 2003 [41]	P, R, C	GA 28–32 w; No major GI problem; Not receiving antibiotics; Not receiving breast milk	*Saccharomyces boulardii* D: 1×10^9 CFU BD S: non-specified Median duration of probiotic supplementation: 30 days	PFM	MDX	Not defined
Costeloe, 2015 [64]	P, DB, R, C, Multic.	Preterm infants with GA 23–30 + 6 weeks, without any lethal malformation or any malformation of the GI tract	*Bifidobacterium breve BBG-001* D: $8 \cdot 3$–$8 \cdot 8 \log_{10}$ CFU/day S: as soon as possible after randomisation E: 36 w PMA or discharge if sooner	OMM, DHM, FM	Corn starch powder	150 mL/kg/day
Demirel, 2013 [27]	P, B, R, C	Preterm infants with GA ≤ 32 weeks and BW ≤ 1500 g, who survived to feed enterally	*S. boulardii* D: 5×10^9 CFU OD S: first feed E: discharge	HM, FM	None	Not defined
Dilli, 2015 [49]	P, DB, R, C, Multic.	Preterm infants with GA < 32 weeks and BW <1500 g, born at or transferred to the NICU within the first week of life and fed enterally before inclusion	*B. lactis* D: 5×10^9 CFU S: beyond d7 after birth E: death or discharge (max 8 weeks)	HM, FM	MDX powder	100 mL/kg/day (FEF for hydration) 150 mL/kg/day (FEF for growth)

Table 1. *Cont.*

Author, Year	Study Details	Study Population	Intervention Specie — Dose (D) / Start of Treatment (S) / End of Treatment (E)	Milk	Placebo	FEF Definition
Fernández-Carrocera, 2013 [30]	P	Preterm infants with	$L.\ acidophilus$ 1 × 10^9 CFU/g, $L.\ rhamnosus$ 4.4 × 10^8 CFU/g, $L.\ casei$ 1 × 10^9 CFU/g, $L.\ plantarum$ 1.76 × 10^8 CFU/g, $B.\ infantis$ 2.76 × 10^7 CFU/g, $Str.\ thermophilus$ 6.6 × 10^5 CFU/g	OMM, PFM	None	Not defined
	DB	BW < 1500 g	Total D: 1 g powder OD			
	R	Infants with NEC stage IA and stage IB were excluded	S: start of enteral feeding			
	C		E: non specified			
Hays, 2014 [66]	P	Preterm infants with GA 25–31 weeks, BW 700–1600 g, AGA, enteral feeding initiated before day 5	Probiotic group composed of 3 subgroups:	OMM, DM or PFM	MDX	Not defined
	DB		P1 $B.\ lactis$			
	R	Infants with NEC stage ≥ IB, malformations or severe medical or surgical conditions were excluded	P2 $B.\ longum$			
	C		P3 $B.\ lactis$ + $longum$			
	Multic.		D: 1 × 10^9 CFU each probiotic daily; Duration: 4 weeks for infants ≥29 w/6 weeks for infants ≤28 w GA			
Hikaru, 2010 [68]	P	Extremely low birth weight and very low birth weight infants	$B.\ breve$	OMM, PFM	None	Not defined
	DB		D: 0.5 × 10^9 CFU BD			
	R		S: birth			
	C		E: discharge from NICU			
Jacobs, 2013 [25]	P	Preterm infants with GA <32 weeks and BW <1500 g	$B.\ infantis$ BB-02 300 CFU × 10^6, $Str.\ thermophilus$ Th-4 350 CFU × 10^6, $B.\ lactis$ BB-12 350 CFU × 10^6	HM, FM	MDX powder	Enteral feeds of 120 mL/kg for ≥3 days
	DB		Total D: 1 × 10^9 CFU × 1.5 g MDX powder OD			
	R		S: enteral feed ≥ 1 mL every 4 h			
	C		E: discharge or term corrected age			
	Multic.					

Table 1. *Cont.*

Author, Year	Study Details	Study Population	Intervention Specie — Dose (D) / Start of Treatment (S) / End of Treatment (E)	Milk	Placebo	FEF Definition
Lin, 2008 [39]	P, B, R, C, Multic.	Preterm infants with GA < 34 weeks and BW ≤ 1500 g, who survived to feed enterally	*L. acidophilus* NCDO 1746, *B. bifidum* NCDO 1453 10^9 CFU; D: 1×10^9 CFU each probiotic (= 125 mg/kg) BD; S: day 2 of age; Duration: 6 weeks	HM, FM	None	Oral intake of 100 mL/kg/day
Manzoni, 2006 [56]	P, DB, R, C	Infants with BW < 1500 g, ≥3 day of life, who started enteral feeding with HM	*L. casei* subspecies *rhamnosus* LGG; D: 6×10^9 CFU/day; S: day 3 of life; E: end of the 6th week or discharge	OMM, DM	None	Not defined
Mihatsch, 2010 [36]	P, R, C	Preterm infants with GA < 30 weeks and BW ≤ 1500 g	*B. lactis* BB12; D: 2×10^9 CFU/kg 6 times a day; S: start of enteral feeding; E: non specified	OMM, PFM	Indistinguishable powder	150 mL/kg/day
Oncel, 2014 [24]	P, DB, R, C	Preterm infants with GA ≤ 32 weeks and BW ≤ 1500 g, who survived to feed enterally	*L. reuteri* DSM 17938; D: 1×10^8 CFU OD; S: first feed; E: death or discharge	HM, FM	Oil base	Not defined
Patole, 2014 [23]	P, DB, R, C	Preterm infants with GA < 33 weeks and BW < 1500 g	*B. breve*; D: 3×10^9 CFU OD (1.5×10^9 CFU OD for newborn ≤ 27 w until they reached 50 mL/kg/day enteral feeds); S: start of enteral feed; E: corrected age of 37 w	HM, FM	Dextrin	150 mL/kg/day enteral feeding
Rougé, 2009 [37]	P, DB, R, C, Bic.	Preterm infants with GA < 32 weeks and BW < 1500 g, ≤2 weeks of age, without any disease other than those linked to prematurity, who started enteral feeding before inclusion	*B. longum* BB536, *L. rhamnosus* GG BB536-LGG; Total D: 1×108 CFU/day; S: start of enteral feeding; E: discharge	OMM, DM or PFM	MDX	Not defined

Table 1. Cont.

Author, Year	Study Details	Study Population	Intervention Specie — Dose (D) / Start of Treatment (S) / End of Treatment (E)	Milk	Placebo	FEF Definition
Roy, 2014 [50]	P	Preterm infants (GA < 37 weeks) and BW < 2500 g, with stable enteral feeding within 72 h of birth	L. acidophilus 1.25×10^9 CFU $\times$ 1 g, B. longum 0.125×10^9 CFU $\times$ 1 g, B. bifidum 0.125×10^9 CFU $\times$ 1 g, B. lactis 1×10^9 CFU $\times$ 1 g	HM	Sterile water	120 mL/kg/day for $\geq$3 d
	DB		D: half a 1 g sachet			
	R		S: from 72 h of life			
	C		E: after 6 w or at discharge			
Saengtawesin, 2014 [48]	P	Preterm infants with GA $\leqslant$ 34 weeks and BW $\leqslant$ 1500 g	L. acidophilus 1×10^9 CFU, B. bifidum 1×10^9 CFU	HM, PFM	None	150 mL/kg/day
	R		D: 125 mg/kg BD			
	C		S: start of feeding			
			E: 6 w of age or discharge.			
Samanta, 2008 [38]	P	Preterm infants with GA < 32 weeks and BW < 1500 g, who started enteral feeding and survived beyond 48 h of age	B. infantis, B. bifidum, B. longum, L. acidophilus	HM	None	Not defined
	DB		D: 2.5×10^9 CFU each probiotic, BD			
	R		S: start of enteral feeding			
	C		E: discharge			
Sari, 2011 [34]	P	Preterm infants with GA < 32 weeks or BW < 1500 g, who survived to feed enterally	L. sporogenes	HM, FM	None	Not defined
	B		D: 0.35×10^9 CFU OD			
	R		S: first feed			
	C		E: discharge			
Serce, 2013 [26]	P	Preterm infants with GA $\leqslant$ 32 weeks and BW $\leqslant$ 1500 g, who survived to feed enterally	S. boulardii	HM, FM	Distilled water	100 mL/kg/day enteral feeding
	M		D: 0.5×10^9 CFU/kg BD			
	R		S: non specified			
	C		E: non specified			
Stratiki, 2007 [61]	P	Preterm infants with GA 27–32 weeks, formula-fed, without major congenital anomalies	Bifidobacterium lactis	FM	None	150 mL/kg/day
	B		D: 2×10^7 CFU/g of milk powder			
	R		S: start of enteral feeding			
	C		E: not specified			

Table 1. *Cont.*

Author, Year	Study Details	Study Population	Intervention Specie Dose (D) Start of Treatment (S) End of Treatment (E)	Milk	Placebo	FEF Definition
Tewari, 2015 [70]	P	Preterm infants with GA <34 weeks	*Bacillus clausii*	OMM, DHM	Sterile water	180 mL/kg/day
	DB	Excluded if: NEC, congenital anomaly, outborn and >10 days of with sepsis	D: 2.4×10^9 CFU/day			
	R	Stratified as extreme preterm (GA 27–30 + 6) and very preterm (GA 31–33 + 6)	S: by day 5 in asymptomatic and by day 10 in symptomatic infants			
	C		E: 6 weeks of age, discharge or death (whichever occurred first)			
Totsu, 2014 [21]	P	Infants with BW <1500 g	*B. bifidum*	HM, FM	Dextrin	Postnatal day at which the amount of enteral feeding exceeded 100 mL/kg/day
	DB		D: 2.5×10^9 CFU, divided in two doses			
	CLR		S: within 48 h after birth			
	C		E: body weight 2000 g			
	Multic.					
Van Niekerk, 2014 [22]	P	Preterm infants with GA <34 weeks and BW <1250 g, exposed and non-exposed to HIV (only infants unexposed to HIV are included in the meta-analysis)	*L. rhamnosus*, *B. infantis*	HM	MCT oil	"when infants no longer required the use of IV fluids"
	DB		D: 0.35×10^9 CFU each probiotic			
	R		S: start of enteral feeding			
	C		E: day 28 postconceptual age			

P: prospective; B: blinded; R: randomized; C: controlled; DB: double-blinded; Multic: multicentric; M: masked; CLR: cluster-randomized; BW: birth weight; GA: gestational age; HM: human milk; L.: Lactobacillus; B.: Bifidobacterium; Str.: Streptococcus; S.: Saccharomyces; CFU: colony forming unit; OD: once daily; NEC: necrotizing enterocolitis; BD: twice daily; OMM: own mother's milk; PFM: preterm formula; FM: formula; MDX: maltodextrin; PMA: postmenstrual age; AGA: appropriate for gestational age.

Data from 359 infants in the probiotic group and 360 infants in the control group were evaluated: probiotic use was associated with a reduction in the time for FEF achievement (MD −3.15 days (95% CI −5.25/−1.05), p = 0.003; Figure 2a). The funnel plot did not show any clear asymmetry (Figure 2b).

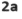

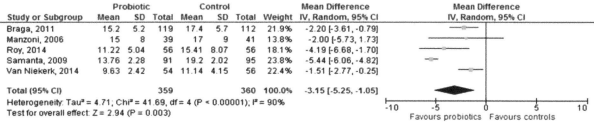

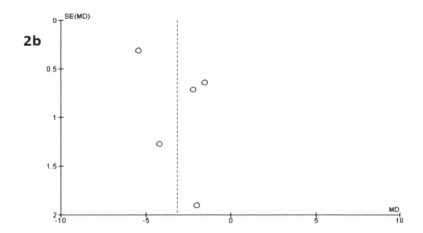

Figure 2. Forest plot (**2a**) and funnel plot (**2b**) showing the association between the use of probiotics and achievement of full enteral feeding in exclusively human milk-fed preterm infants. IV: inverse variance method.

Three studies were not included in the meta-analysis because data on FEF were not available as mean ± SD [41,61,70]. One study reported the use of *Bacillus clausii* in preterm infants with GA < 34 weeks, fed expressed breast milk or DHM [70] and stratified as extreme preterm (GA 27–30 + 6 weeks) and very preterm (GA 31–33 + 6 weeks). In both groups, probiotic use was associated with a reduced time to achieve FEF (risk ratio 0.82 (95% CI 0.74–0.88) and 0.67 (95% CI 0.32–0.77), respectively).

The other two studies reported probiotic use in exclusively formula-fed infants: in the study by Costalos et al., infants born at 28–32 weeks gestation and fed exclusively preterm formula received *Saccharomyces boulardii* or placebo for approximately 30 days [41]. In the study by Stratiki et al., formula-fed infants with a similar gestational age (27–32 weeks) received *Bifidobacterium lactis* vs. no treatment [61]. Neither of these two studies reported any significant difference between groups in terms of time to FEF achievement.

All the studies included in the meta-analysis, except one [50], recruited exclusively infants with birth weight <1500 g. The study by Roy et al. [50] reported specific data for extremely low birth weight (ELBW) infants: time to reach FEF in ELBW infants treated with probiotics was significantly lower than in controls (mean ± SD 13.22 ± 5.04 vs. 17.41 ± 8.07, respectively, p = 0.014). None of the studies included in the meta-analysis reported separate data on intrauterine growth restricted (IUGR) infants.

In all the studies, except one [56], a probiotic mix was used: the meta-analysis performed after the exclusion of the study by Manzoni et al., where a single-strain product containing Lactobacillus GG was used, confirmed the results of the overall analysis (MD −3.33 days (95% CI −5.63/−1.04), $p \leqslant 0.004$).

4. Methodological Study Quality

Evaluation of the quality of the studies included in the meta-analysis according to the risk of bias tool as proposed by the Cochrane Collaboration [19] is shown in Table 2.

Table 2. Evaluation of the quality of the studies included in the meta-analysis according to the risk of bias tool as proposed by the Cochrane collaboration.

Study	Random Sequence Generation	Allocation Concealment	Blinding	Incomplete Outcome Data	Selective Outcome Reporting	Other Sources of Bias
Braga, 2011 [60]	Low	Low	Low	Low	Unclear	Low
Manzoni, 2006 [56]	Low	Low	Low	Unclear	Unclear	Low
Roy, 2014 [50]	Low	Unclear	Low	Low	Unclear	Unclear
Samanta, 2008 [38]	Low	Low	Low	Unclear	Unclear	Unclear
Van Niekerk, 2014 [22]	Low	Unclear	Low	Unclear	Unclear	Unclear

5. Discussion

The present meta-analysis shows that the use of probiotics in preterm, VLBW infants fed exclusively HM is associated with 3-days reduction in the time to FEF achievement. The only two studies included in the present systematic review in which infants were exclusively formula-fed did not report any difference between the probiotic and the control group.

The single previous meta-analysis investigating FEF as primary outcome showed an overall smaller reduction in the time to FEF achievement, but did not report separate data for HM-fed and formula-fed infants [6]. The studies included in the meta-analysis by Athalye-Jape et al. are almost the same as those included in our systematic review; quite surprisingly, in the majority of the studies included in these two reviews, both HM and formula-fed infants were recruited, but no detailed information on the relationship between type of feeding and outcome was provided.

Type of feeding might modulate the relationship between probiotics and neonatal clinical outcome [14]. It has been previously shown that HM feeding is associated with shorter time to achieve FEF compared to formula feeding [5]. Our meta-analysis, which included only studies where infants were exclusively HM-fed, showed a significant reduction in the time to achieve FEF attributable to probiotics. Despite the limitation given by the small number of studies, a probiotic-related 3-days reduction in time to achieve FEF in preterm infants fed exclusively HM has strong clinical implications and deserves further consideration. When OMM is not available or contraindicated, the use of pasteurized DHM is recommended for preterm infants: pasteurization inactivates most viral and bacterial agents, but at the same time affects some nutritional and immunological properties of HM, including endogenous probiotics [71]. It can be speculated that the beneficial effect of probiotics documented in exclusively HM-fed infants could be attributed to a synergic action exerted by the prebiotic components of HM and the exogenous probiotic, which partially restores the symbiotic properties of naïve HM [72]. In the present meta-analysis, no separate data for OMM-fed and DHM-fed infants were available; for this reason, it is not possible to clarify whether the beneficial effect of HM on FEF achievement applies both to OMM and to DHM.

Heterogeneity among included studies was high; however, given the small number of papers, our ability to explore sources of heterogeneity was limited. In the five included studies, different probiotic strains were used. We aimed to perform strain-specific sub-meta-analyses, in order to clarify whether there was any probiotic product showing a significant benefit in terms of reduction in the time to achieve FEF. However, such analyses were not feasible, as none of the studies used the same probiotic strain or mix. Similarly, it was not possible to explore additional sources of heterogeneity, such as the characteristics of probiotic administration (dose, duration, infant age at probiotic initiation, etc.). In addition, we were unable to test for subgroup differences between HM-fed and formula-fed infants, which might have partially explained the different results in terms of FEF achievement.

Apparently, studies were homogeneous in terms of included populations, as almost all of them recruited only VLBW infants. However, few data on "high-risk" infants, such as ELBW and IUGR infants, could be extrapolated from the main results of the included studies.

The use of probiotics should be weighed against their potential side effects. There are some reports about the occurrence of sepsis in preterm newborns, potentially linked to probiotic administration [73].

However, none of the studies included in the systematic review reported any side effect related to the use of probiotics.

6. Conclusions

According to the results of the present meta-analysis, the use of probiotics is linked to 3-days reduction in time to achieve FEF in preterm VLBW infants fed exclusively HM. If confirmed in further studies, this reduction might have strong clinical implications for this high-risk population.

Acknowledgments: No funding was received to produce the present paper.

Author Contributions: Each author listed on the manuscript has seen and approved the submission of this version of the manuscript and takes full responsibility for the manuscript. Specifically, all the authors, as part of the Task Force on Probiotics of the Italian Society of Neonatology, conceived and designed the study protocol. A.A. and L.C. performed the literature search and assessed study details, which were checked by D.G. A.A. and D.G. evaluated study quality and performed the meta-analyses. A.A. and L.C. wrote the first draft of the paper, which was critically revised by all the other authors.

References

1. Faldella, G.; Aceti, A.; Corvaglia, L. Formula milk and neurodevelopmental and cognitive outcomes: Where are we now? *Early Hum. Dev.* **2011**, *87S*, S5–S8. [CrossRef] [PubMed]

2. Hsiao, C.-C.; Tsai, M.-L.; Chen, C.-C.; Lin, H.-C. Early optimal nutrition improves neurodevelopmental outcomes for very preterm infants. *Nutr. Rev.* **2014**, *72*, 532–540. [CrossRef] [PubMed]

3. Berrington, J.E.; Stewart, C.J.; Embleton, N.D.; Cummings, S.P. Gut microbiota in preterm infants: Assessment and relevance to health and disease. *Arch. Dis. Child. Fetal Neonatal Ed.* **2013**, *98*, F286–F290. [CrossRef] [PubMed]

4. The SIFT Investigators Group. Early enteral feeding strategies for very preterm infants: Current evidence from Cochrane reviews. *Arch. Dis. Child. Fetal Neonatal Ed.* **2013**, *98*, F470–F472.

5. Corvaglia, L.; Fantini, M.P.; Aceti, A.; Gibertoni, D.; Rucci, P.; Baronciani, D.; Faldella, G. Predictors of full enteral feeding achievement in very low birth weight infants. *PLoS ONE* **2014**, *9*. [CrossRef] [PubMed]

6. Athalye-Jape, G.; Deshpande, G.; Rao, S.; Patole, S. Benefits of probiotics on enteral nutrition in preterm neonates: a systematic review. *Am. J. Clin. Nutr.* **2014**, *100*, 1508–1519. [CrossRef] [PubMed]

7. Aceti, A.; Gori, D.; Barone, G.; Callegari, M.L.; Di Mauro, A.; Fantini, M.P.; Indrio, F.; Maggio, L.; Meneghin, F.; Morelli, L.; et al. Probiotics for prevention of necrotizing enterocolitis in preterm infants: Systematic review and meta-analysis. *Ital. J. Pediatr.* **2015**, *41*, 89. [CrossRef] [PubMed]

8. Alfaleh, K.; Anabrees, J.; Bassler, D. Probiotics for prevention of necrotizing enterocolitis in preterm infants. *Cochrane Database Syst. Rev.* **2014**, CD005496. [CrossRef] [PubMed]

9. Rao, S.C.; Athalye-jape, G.K.; Deshpande, G.C.; Simmer, K.N.; Patole, S.K. Probiotic supplementation and late-onset sepsis in preterm infants: A meta-analysis. *Pediatrics* **2016**, *137*, e20153684. [CrossRef] [PubMed]

10. Sanders, M.E.; Guarner, F.; Guerrant, R.; Holt, P.R.; Quigley, E.M.M.; Sartor, R.B.; Sherman, P.M.; Mayer, E.A. An update on the use and investigation of probiotics in health and disease. *Gut* **2013**, *62*, 787–796. [CrossRef] [PubMed]

11. Murguía-Peniche, T.; Mihatsch, W.A.; Zegarra, J.; Supapannachart, S.; Ding, Z.-Y.; Neu, J. Intestinal mucosal defense system, Part 2. Probiotics and prebiotics. *J. Pediatr.* **2013**, *162*, S64–S71. [CrossRef] [PubMed]

12. Martin, C.R.; Walker, W.A. Probiotics: Role in pathophysiology and prevention in necrotizing enterocolitis. *Semin. Perinatol.* **2008**, *32*, 127–137. [CrossRef] [PubMed]

13. Carlisle, E.M.; Morowitz, M.J. The intestinal microbiome and necrotizing enterocolitis. *Curr. Opin. Pediatr.* **2013**, *25*, 382–387. [CrossRef] [PubMed]

14. Repa, A.; Thanhaeuser, M.; Endress, D.; Weber, M.; Kreissl, A.; Binder, C.; Berger, A.; Haiden, N. Probiotics (*Lactobacillus acidophilus and Bifidobacterium bifidum*) prevent NEC in VLBW infants fed breast milk but not formula. *Pediatr. Res.* **2015**, *77*, 381–388. [CrossRef] [PubMed]

15. Moher, D.; Liberati, A.; Tetzlaff, J.; Altman, D.G. Preferred reporting items for systematic reviews and meta-analyses: The PRISMA statement. *PLoS Med.* **2009**, *6*, e1000097. [CrossRef] [PubMed]

16. PubMed. Available online: http://www.ncbi.nlm.nih.gov/pubmed (accessed on 28 July 2016).

17. Cochrane Library. Available online: http://www.cochranelibrary.com/ (accessed on 28 July 2016).

18. Embase. Available online: http://store.elsevier.com/en_US/info/30800006 (accessed on 28 July 2016).

19. Higgins, J.P.; Green, S. *Cochrane Handbook for Systematic Reviews of Interventions*; The Cochrane Collaboration: London, UK, 2011.

20. RevMan Software. Available online: http://tech.cochrane.org/revman/download (accessed on 28 July 2016).

21. Totsu, S.; Yamasaki, C.; Terahara, M.; Uchiyama, A.; Kusuda, S. Bifidobacterium and enteral feeding in preterm infants: Cluster-randomized trial. *Pediatr. Int.* **2014**, *56*, 714–719. [CrossRef] [PubMed]

22. Van Niekerk, E.; Kirsten, G.F.; Nel, D.G.; Blaauw, R. Probiotics, feeding tolerance, and growth: A comparison between HIV-exposed and unexposed very low birth weight infants. *Nutrition* **2014**, *30*, 645–653. [CrossRef] [PubMed]

23. Patole, S.; Keil, A.D.; Chang, A.; Nathan, E.; Doherty, D.; Simmer, K.; Esvaran, M.; Conway, P. Effect of Bifidobacterium breve M-16V supplementation on fecal bifidobacteria in preterm neonates—A randomised double blind placebo controlled trial. *PLoS ONE* **2014**, *9*, e89511. [CrossRef] [PubMed]

24. Oncel, M.Y.; Sari, F.N.; Arayici, S.; Guzoglu, N.; Erdeve, O.; Uras, N.; Oguz, S.S.; Dilmen, U. Lactobacillus Reuteri for the prevention of necrotising enterocolitis in very low birthweight infants: A randomised controlled trial. *Arch. Dis. Child. Fetal Neonatal Ed.* **2014**, *99*, F110–F115. [CrossRef] [PubMed]

25. Jacobs, S.E.; Tobin, J.M.; Opie, G.F.; Donath, S.; Tabrizi, S.N.; Pirotta, M.; Morley, C.J.; Garland, S.M. Probiotic effects on late-onset sepsis in very preterm infants: A randomized controlled trial. *Pediatrics* **2013**, *132*, 1055–1062. [CrossRef] [PubMed]

26. Serce, O.; Benzer, D.; Gursoy, T.; Karatekin, G.; Ovali, F. Efficacy of saccharomyces boulardii on necrotizing enterocolitis or sepsis in very low birth weight infants: A randomised controlled trial. *Early Hum. Dev.* **2013**, *89*, 1033–1036. [CrossRef] [PubMed]

27. Demirel, G.; Erdeve, O.; Celik, I.H.; Dilmen, U. Saccharomyces boulardii for prevention of necrotizing enterocolitis in preterm infants: A randomized, controlled study. *Acta Paediatr.* **2013**, *102*, 560–565. [CrossRef] [PubMed]

28. Rojas, M.A.; Lozano, J.M.; Rojas, M.X.; Rodriguez, V.A.; Rondon, M.A.; Bastidas, J.A.; Perez, L.A.; Rojas, C.; Ovalle, O.; Garcia-Harker, J.E.; et al. Prophylactic probiotics to prevent death and nosocomial infection in preterm infants. *Pediatrics* **2012**, *130*, e1113–e1120. [CrossRef] [PubMed]

29. Sari, F.N.; Eras, Z.; Dizdar, E.A.; Erdeve, O.; Oguz, S.S.; Uras, N.; Dilmen, U. Do oral probiotics affect growth and neurodevelopmental outcomes in very low-birth-weight preterm infants? *Am. J. Perinatol.* **2012**, *29*, 579–586. [CrossRef] [PubMed]

30. Fernández-Carrocera, L.A.; Solis-Herrera, A.; Cabanillas-Ayón, M.; Gallardo-Sarmiento, R.B.; García-Pérez, C.S.; Montaño-Rodríguez, R.; Echániz-Aviles, M.O.L. Double-blind, randomised clinical assay to evaluate the efficacy of probiotics in preterm newborns weighing less than 1500 g in the prevention of necrotising enterocolitis. *Arch. Dis. Child. Fetal Neonatal Ed.* **2013**, *98*, F5–F9. [CrossRef] [PubMed]

31. Havranek, T.; Al-Hosni, M.; Armbrecht, E. Probiotics supplementation increases intestinal blood flow velocity in extremely low birth weight preterm infants. *J. Perinatol.* **2013**, *33*, 40–44. [CrossRef] [PubMed]

32. Chrzanowska-Liszewska, D.; Seliga-Siwecka, J.; Kornacka, M.K. The effect of Lactobacillus rhamnosus GG supplemented enteral feeding on the microbiotic flora of preterm infants-double blinded randomized control trial. *Early Hum. Dev.* **2012**, *88*, 57–60. [CrossRef] [PubMed]

33. Campeotto, F.; Suau, A.; Kapel, N.; Magne, F.; Viallon, V.; Ferraris, L.; Waligora-Dupriet, A.-J.; Soulaines, P.; Leroux, B.; Kalach, N.; Dupont, C.; Butel, M.-J. A fermented formula in pre-term infants: Clinical tolerance, gut microbiota, down-regulation of faecal calprotectin and up-regulation of faecal secretory IgA. *Br. J. Nutr.* **2011**, *105*, 1843–1851. [CrossRef] [PubMed]

34. Sari, F.N.; Dizdar, E.A.; Oguz, S.; Erdeve, O.; Uras, N.; Dilmen, U. Oral probiotics: Lactobacillus sporogenes for prevention of necrotizing enterocolitis in very low-birth weight infants: A randomized, controlled trial. *Eur. J. Clin. Nutr.* **2011**, *65*, 434–439. [CrossRef] [PubMed]

35. Indrio, F.; Riezzo, G.; Raimondi, F.; Bisceglia, M.; Cavallo, L.; Francavilla, R. Effects of probiotic and prebiotic on gastrointestinal motility in newborns. *J. Physiol. Pharmacol.* **2009**, *60*, 27–31. [PubMed]

36. Mihatsch, W.A.; Vossbeck, S.; Eikmanns, B.; Hoegel, J.; Pohlandt, F. Effect of Bifidobacterium lactis on the incidence of nosocomial infections in very-low-birth-weight infants: A randomized controlled trial. *Neonatology* **2010**, *98*, 156–163. [CrossRef] [PubMed]

37. Rougé, C.; Piloquet, H.; Butel, M.-J.; Berger, B.; Rochat, F.; Ferraris, L.; Des Robert, C.; Legrand, A.; de la Cochetiere, M.-F.; N'Guyen, J.-M.; et al. Oral supplementation with probiotics in very-low-birth-weight preterm infants: A randomized, double-blind, placebo-controlled trial. *Am. J. Clin. Nutr.* **2009**, *89*, 1828–1835. [CrossRef] [PubMed]

38. Samanta, M.; Sarkar, M.; Ghosh, P.; Ghosh, J.K.; Sinha, M.K.; Chatterjee, S. Prophylactic probiotics for prevention of necrotizing enterocolitis in very low birth weight newborns. *J. Trop. Pediatr.* **2008**, *55*, 128–131. [CrossRef] [PubMed]

39. Lin, H.-C.; Hsu, C.-H.; Chen, H.-L.; Chung, M.-Y.; Hsu, J.-F.; Lien, R.; Tsao, L.-Y.; Chen, C.-H.; Su, B.-H. Oral probiotics prevent necrotizing enterocolitis in very low birth weight preterm infants: A multicenter, randomized, controlled trial. *Pediatrics* **2008**, *122*, 693–700. [CrossRef] [PubMed]

40. Bin-Nun, A.; Bromiker, R.; Wilschanski, M.; Kaplan, M.; Rudensky, B.; Caplan, M.; Hammerman, C. Oral probiotics prevent necrotizing enterocolitis in very low birth weight neonates. *J. Pediatr.* **2005**, *147*, 192–196. [CrossRef] [PubMed]

41. Costalos, C.; Skouteri, V.; Gounaris, A.; Sevastiadou, S.; Triandafilidou, A.; Ekonomidou, C.; Kontaxaki, F.; Petrochilou, V. Enteral feeding of premature infants with *Saccharomyces boulardii*. *Early Hum. Dev.* **2003**, *74*, 89–96. [CrossRef]

42. Dani, C.; Biadaioli, R.; Bertini, G.; Martelli, E.; Rubaltelli, F.F. Probiotics feeding in prevention of urinary tract infection, bacterial sepsis and necrotizing enterocolitis in preterm infants. *Biol. Neonate* **2002**, *82*, 103–108. [CrossRef] [PubMed]

43. Stansbridge, E.M.; Walker, V.; Hall, M.A.; Smith, S.L.; Millar, M.R.; Bacon, C.; Chen, S. Effects of feeding premature infants with Lactobacillus GG on gut fermentation. *Arch. Dis. Child.* **1993**, *69*, 488–492. [CrossRef] [PubMed]

44. Millar, M.R.; Bacon, C.; Smith, S.L.; Walker, V.; Hall, M.A. Enteral feeding of premature infants with Lactobacillus GG. *Arch. Dis. Child.* **1993**, *69*, 483–487. [CrossRef] [PubMed]

45. Indrio, F.; Riezzo, G.; Raimondi, F.; Bisceglia, M.; Cavallo, L.; Francavilla, R. The effects of probiotics on feeding tolerance, bowel habits, and gastrointestinal motility in preterm newborns. *J. Pediatr.* **2008**, *152*, 801–806. [CrossRef] [PubMed]

46. Al-Hosni, M.; Duenas, M.; Hawk, M.; Stewart, L.A.; Borghese, R.A.; Cahoon, M.; Atwood, L.; Howard, D.; Ferrelli, K.; Soll, R. Probiotics-supplemented feeding in extremely low-birth-weight infants. *J. Perinatol.* **2012**, *32*, 253–259. [CrossRef] [PubMed]

47. Savino, F.; Ceratto, S.; Poggi, E.; Cartosio, M.E.; Cordero di Montezemolo, L.; Giannattasio, A. Preventive effects of oral probiotic on infantile colic: A prospective, randomised, blinded, controlled trial using Lactobacillus reuteri DSM 17938. *Benef. Microbes* **2014**. [CrossRef]

48. Saengtawesin, V.; Tangpolkaiwalsak, R.; Kanjanapattankul, W. Effect of oral probiotics supplementation in the prevention of necrotizing enterocolitis among very low birth weight preterm infants. *J. Med. Assoc. Thail.* **2014**, *97*, S20–S25.

49. Dilli, D.; Aydin, B.; Fettah, N.; Özyazıcı, E.; Beken, S.; Zenciroğlu, A.; Okumuş, N.; Özyurt, B.; İpek, M.; Akdağ, A.; et al. The propre-save study: Effects of probiotics and prebiotics alone or combined on necrotizing enterocolitis in very low birth weight infants. *J. Pediatr.* **2015**, *28*, 1537–1541. [CrossRef] [PubMed]

50. Roy, A.; Chaudhuri, J.; Sarkar, D.; Ghosh, P.; Chakraborty, S. Role of enteric supplementation of Probiotics on late-onset sepsis by Candida species in preterm low birth weight neonates: A randomized, double blind, placebo-controlled trial. *N. Am. J. Med. Sci.* **2014**, *6*, 50–57. [PubMed]

51. Oncel, M.Y.; Arayici, S.; Sari, F.N.; Simsek, G.K.; Yurttutan, S.; Erdeve, O.; Saygan, S.; Uras, N.; Oguz, S.S.; Dilmen, U. Comparison of Lactobacillus reuteri and nystatin prophylaxis on Candida colonization and infection in very low birth weight infants. *J. Matern. Neonatal Med.* **2014**, 1–5. [CrossRef]

52.   Millar, M.; Wilks, M.; Fleming, P.; Costeloe, K. Should the use of probiotics in the preterm be routine? *Arch. Dis. Child. Fetal Neonatal Ed.* **2012**, *97*, F70–F74. [CrossRef] [PubMed]

53.   Rinaldi, M.; Manzoni, P.; Meyer, M.; Casa, E.D.; Pugni, L.; Mosca, F.; Stolfi, I.; Messner, H.; Memo, L.; Laforgia, N.; et al. Bovine lactoferrin supplementation for prevention of necrotising enterocolitis in preterm very-low-birth-weight neonates: A randomised trial. *Early Hum. Dev.* **2012**, *88*, S102. [CrossRef]

54.   Manzoni, P.; Meyer, M.; Stolfi, I.; Rinaldi, M.; Cattani, S.; Pugni, L.; Romeo, M.G.; Messner, H.; Decembrino, L.; Laforgia, N.; et al. Bovine lactoferrin supplementation for prevention of necrotizing enterocolitis in very-low-birth-weight neonates: A randomized clinical trial. *Early Hum. Dev.* **2014**, *90*, S60–S65. [CrossRef]

55.   Benor, S.; Marom, R.; Tov, A.B.; Domany, K.A.; Zaidenberg-Israeli, G.; Dollberg, S. Probiotic supplementation in mothers of very low birth weight infants. *Am. J. Perinatol.* **2014**, *31*, 497–504. [PubMed]

56.   Manzoni, P.; Mostert, M.; Leonessa, M.L.; Priolo, C.; Farina, D.; Monetti, C.; Latino, M.A.; Gomirato, G. Oral supplementation with Lactobacillus casei subspecies rhamnosus prevents enteric colonization by Candida species in preterm neonates: A randomized study. *Clin. Infect. Dis.* **2006**, *42*, 1735–1742. [CrossRef] [PubMed]

57.   Kitajima, H.; Sumida, Y.; Tanaka, R.; Yuki, N.; Takayama, H.; Fujimura, M. Early administration of Bifidobacterium breve to preterm infants: Randomised controlled trial. *Arch. Dis. Child. Fetal Neonatal Ed.* **1997**, *76*, F101–F107. [CrossRef] [PubMed]

58.   Mohan, R.; Koebnick, C.; Schildt, J.; Schmidt, S.; Mueller, M.; Possner, M.; Radke, M.; Blaut, M. Effects of Bifidobacterium lactis Bb12 supplementation on intestinal microbiota of preterm infants: A double-blind, placebo-controlled, randomized study. *J. Clin. Microbiol.* **2006**, *44*, 4025–4031. [CrossRef] [PubMed]

59.   Lin, H.-C.; Su, B.-H.; Chen, A.-C.; Lin, T.-W.; Tsai, C.-H.; Yeh, T.-F.; Oh, W. Oral probiotics reduce the incidence and severity of necrotizing enterocolitis in very low birth weight infants. *Pediatrics* **2005**, *115*, 1–4. [PubMed]

60.   Braga, T.D.; da Silva, G.A.P.; de Lira, P.I.; de Carvalho Lima, M. Efficacy of Bifidobacterium breve and Lactobacillus casei oral supplementation on necrotizing enterocolitis in very-low-birth-weight preterm infants: A double-blind, randomized, controlled trial. *Am. J. Clin. Nutr.* **2011**, *93*, 81–86. [CrossRef] [PubMed]

61.   Stratiki, Z.; Costalos, C.; Sevastiadou, S.; Kastanidou, O.; Skouroliakou, M.; Giakoumatou, A.; Petrohilou, V. The effect of a bifidobacter supplemented bovine milk on intestinal permeability of preterm infants. *Early Hum. Dev.* **2007**, *83*, 575–579. [CrossRef] [PubMed]

62.   Manzoni, P.; Rinaldi, M.; Cattani, S.; Pugni, L.; Romeo, M.G.; Messner, H. Bovine lactoferrin supplementation for prevention of late-onset sepsis in very low-birth-weight neonates. *JAMA* **2009**, *302*, 1421–1428. [CrossRef] [PubMed]

63.   Li, Y.; Shimizu, T.; Hosaka, A.; Kaneko, N.; Ohtsuka, Y.; Yamashiro, Y. Effects of bifidobacterium breve supplementation on intestinal flora of low birth weight infants. *Pediatr. Int.* **2004**, *46*, 509–515. [CrossRef] [PubMed]

64.   Costeloe, K.; Hardy, P.; Juszczak, E.; Wilks, M.; Millar, M.R. Bifidobacterium breve BBG-001 in very preterm infants: A randomised controlled phase 3 trial. *Lancet* **2015**, *387*, 649–660. [CrossRef]

65.   Dutta, S.; Ray, P.; Narang, A. Comparison of stool colonization in premature infants by three dose regimes of a probiotic combination: A randomized controlled trial. *Am. J. Perinatol.* **2015**, *32*, 733–740. [PubMed]

66.   Hays, S.; Jacquot, A.; Gauthier, H.; Kempf, C.; Beissel, A.; Pidoux, O.; Jumas-Bilak, E.; Decullier, E.; Lachambre, E.; Beck, L.; et al. Probiotics and growth in preterm infants: A randomized controlled trial, PREMAPRO study. *Clin. Nutr.* **2014**. [CrossRef] [PubMed]

67.   Romeo, M.G.; Romeo, D.M.; Trovato, L.; Oliveri, S.; Palermo, F.; Cota, F.; Betta, P. Role of probiotics in the prevention of the enteric colonization by Candida in preterm newborns: Incidence of late-onset sepsis and neurological outcome. *J. Perinatol.* **2011**, *31*, 63–69. [CrossRef] [PubMed]

68.   Hikaru, U.; Koichi, S.; Yayoi, S.; Hiromici, S.; Hiroaki, S.; Yoshkazu, O.; Seigo, A.; Satoru, N.; Toshiaki, S.; Yuichiro, Y. Bifidobacteria prevents preterm infants from developing infection and sepsis. *Int. J. Probiotics Prebiotics* **2010**, *5*, 33–36.

69.   Patole, S.K.; Keil, A.D.; Nathan, E.; Doherty, D.; Esvaran, M.; Simmer, K.N.; Conway, P. Effect of *Bifidobacterium breve* M-16V supplementation on fecal bifidobacteria in growth restricted very preterm infants -analysis from a randomised trial. *J. Matern. Fetal Neonatal Med.* **2016**. [CrossRef] [PubMed]

70. Tewari, V.V.; Dubey, S.K.; Gupta, G. Bacillus clausii for prevention of late-onset sepsis in preterm infants: A randomized controlled trial. *J. Trop. Pediatr.* **2015**, *61*, 377–385. [CrossRef] [PubMed]
71. Bertino, E.; Giuliani, F.; Baricco, M.; Di Nicola, P.; Peila, C.; Vassia, C.; Chiale, F.; Pirra, A.; Cresi, F.; Martano, C.; Coscia, A. Benefits of donor milk in the feeding of preterm infants. *Early Hum. Dev.* **2013**, *89*, S3–S6. [CrossRef] [PubMed]
72. Zivkovic, A.M.; German, J.B.; Lebrilla, C.B.; Mills, D.A. Human milk glycobiome and its impact on the infant gastrointestinal microbiota. *Proc. Natl. Acad. Sci. USA* **2011**, *108*, 4653–4658. [CrossRef] [PubMed]
73. Bertelli, C.; Pillonel, T.; Torregrossa, A.; Prod'hom, G.; Fischer, C.J.; Greub, G.; Giannoni, E. Bifidobacterium longum bacteremia in preterm infants receiving probiotics. *Clin. Infect. Dis.* **2015**, *60*, 924–927. [CrossRef] [PubMed]

9

Temporal Changes of Human Breast Milk Lipids of Chinese Mothers

Francesca Giuffrida [1,*], **Cristina Cruz-Hernandez** [1], **Emmanuelle Bertschy** [1], **Patric Fontannaz** [1], **Isabelle Masserey Elmelegy** [1], **Isabelle Tavazzi** [1], **Cynthia Marmet** [1], **Belén Sanchez-Bridge** [1], **Sagar K. Thakkar** [1], **Carlos Antonio De Castro** [1], **Gerard Vinyes-Pares** [2], **Yumei Zhang** [3] and **Peiyu Wang** [4]

[1] Nestlé Research Center, Nestec Ltd., Vers-chez-les-Blanc, P.O. Box 44, 1000 Lausanne 26, Switzerland; cristina.cruz-hernandez@rdls.nestle.com (C.C.-H.); emmanuelle.bertschy@rdls.nestle.com (E.B.); patric.fontannaz@rdls.nestle.com (P.F.); isabelle.masserey-elmlegy@rdls.nestle.com (I.M.E.); isabelle.tavazzi@rdls.nestle.com (I.T.); cynthia.marmet@rdls.nestle.com (C.M.); belen.sanchez-bridge@rdls.nestle.com (B.S.-B.); sagar.thakkar@rdls.nestle.com (S.K.T.); carlosantonio.decastro@rdls.nestle.com (C.A.D.C.)

[2] Nestlé Research Center Beijing, Building E-F, No. 5 Dijin Road, Haidian District, Beijing 100091, China; gerard.vinyespares@nestle.com

[3] Department of Nutrition and Food Hygiene, School of Public Health, Peking University Health Science Center, Beijing 100191, China; zhangyumei@bjmu.edu.cn

[4] Department of Social Medicine and Health Education, School of Public Health, Peking University Health Science Center, Beijing 100191, China; wpeiyu@bjmu.edu.cn

* Correspondance: francesca.giuffrida@rdls.nestle.com

Abstract: Fatty acids (FA), phospholipids (PL), and gangliosides (GD) play a central role in infant growth, immune and inflammatory responses. The aim of this study was to determine FA, PL, and GD compositional changes in human milk (HM) during lactation in a large group of Chinese lactating mothers (540 volunteers) residing in Beijing, Guangzhou, and Suzhou. HM samples were collected after full expression from one breast and while the baby was fed on the other breast. FA were assessed by direct methylation followed by gas chromatography (GC) analysis. PL and GD were extracted using chloroform and methanol. A methodology employing liquid chromatography coupled with an evaporative light scattering detector (ELSD) and with time of flight (TOF) mass spectrometry was used to quantify PL and GD classes in HM, respectively. Saturated FA (SFA), mono-unsaturated FA (MUFA), and PL content decreased during lactation, while polyunsaturated FA (PUFA) and GD content increased. Among different cities, over the lactation time, HM from Beijing showed the highest SFA content, HM from Guangzhou the highest MUFA content and HM from Suzhou the highest n-3PUFA content. The highest total PL and GD contents were observed in HM from Suzhou. In order to investigate the influence of the diet on maternal milk composition, a careful analyses of dietary habits of these population needs to be performed in the future.

Keywords: FA; phospholipids; gangliosides; breast milk; chromatography

1. Introduction

Human milk (HM) is considered the optimal form of nourishment for infants during the first six months of life [1] and among its macronutrients, the lipid fraction is crucial, representing approximately 50% of the energy supplied to the newborn infant [2]. Lipids (2%–5%) occur in milk in the form of fat globules mainly composed of triacylglycerols (TAG) (~98% of total lipids) surrounded by a structural membrane composed of phospholipids (PL) (0.8%), cholesterol (0.5%), enzymes, proteins, glycosphingolipids (e.g., gangliosides (GD)), and glycoproteins [3,4].

The majority of fatty acids (FA), approximately 98%, are esterified to a glycerol backbone to form TAG and about 0.2%–2% is found in molecules, such as cholesterol, PL, and GD. In HM, saturated FA (SFA) content ranges from 20% to 70% of total FA, mono-unsaturated FA (MUFA) from 23% to 55%, polyunsaturated FA (PUFA) from 6% to 36%, and long chain polyunsaturated FA (LCPUFA) from 0.3% to 8%. Among PUFA, linoleic (LA, 18:2n-6) and alpha linolenic acids (ALA, 18:3n-3) are essential because they are not synthesized in the human body and they are precursors of arachidonic (ARA, 20:4n-6) and docosahexaenoic (DHA, 22:6n-3) FA that are associated with normal brain development, especially in early life [5].

PL are mainly distributed into five classes: phosphatydylinositol (PtdIns), phosphatydylethanolamine (PtdEtn), phosphatydylserine (PtdSer), phosphatidylcholine (PtdCho), and sphingomyelin (CerPCho). Ptdlns, PtdEtn, PtdSer, and PtdCho consist of a glycerol esterified with FA in the sn-1 and sn-2 positions. A phosphate residue with different organic groups (inositol, serine, ethanolamine, or choline) is present in the sn-3 position. CerPCho consists of a sphingoid base backbone to which an amide-linked long-chain FA can be attached, leading to the ceramides (N-acyl-sphingoid bases) [6]. In the case of CerPCho the primary hydroxyl group of the sphingoid base is linked to phosphorylcholine. Therefore, PL are a source of FA and choline, the precursors of the neurotransmitter acetylcholine, which acts by regulating the transduction signal and serves as a source of methyl groups in intermediate metabolism, being considered essential for optimum development of the brain [7,8].

GD are glycosphingolipids formed by a hydrophobic ceramide and a hydrophilic oligosaccharide chain. This chain may contain N-acetylneuraminic acid (sialic acid) or, less commonly, N-glycoloylneuraminic acid (Neu5Gc), where a glycol group is bound to the C5 amino group. It has been reported that sialic acid is involved in many biological and pathological phenomena, either recognizing or masking the recognition of several ligands, such as selectins or pathogens [9]. Recently, Gurnida et al. [10] concluded that nutritional supplementation with a milk lipid preparation rich in GD appears to have beneficial effects on cognitive development in healthy infants aged 0–6 months.

Traditionally, lactation has been viewed in three stages: colostrum (day 1–5 postpartum), transitional milk (day 6–15 postpartum), and mature milk (after day 15 postpartum). It has been showed that FA, PL, and GD content in HM change during lactation stages [4,11–19] and factors, such as maternal diet. may influence HM short chain FA [20,21], PUFA composition [22–24], and gangliosides content [25].

The objective of this study was to determine, for the first time, the FA, PL, and GD content in HM of Chinese mothers, follow its temporal change along lactation, and evaluate if the geographical region within China would affect HM lipid composition. This study is part of the larger initiative: the Maternal Infant Nutrition Growth (MING) study [26].

2. Materials and Methods

2.1. Subjects

This study was part of MING, a cross-sectional study designed to investigate the dietary and nutritional status of pregnant women, lactating mothers, and young children aged from birth up to three years living in urban areas of China [26]. In addition, the HM composition of Chinese lactating mothers was characterized. The study was conducted between October 2011 and February 2012. A multi-stage milk sampling from lactating mothers in three cities (Beijing, Suzhou, and Guangzhou) was performed for breast milk characterization. In each city, two hospitals with maternal and child care units were selected and, at each site, mothers at lactation period 0–240 days were randomly selected based on eligibility criteria. Subjects included in the period 0–5 days were recruited at the hospital, whereas the other subjects were requested by phone to join the study; if participation was dismissed a replacement was made. The response rate was 52%. Recruitment and milk, as well as baseline data collection, were done in separate days. A stratified milk sampling of 540 lactating mothers in six lactation periods of 0–4, 5–11, and 12–30 days, and 1–2, 2–4, and 4–8 months was obtained in the MING study.

2.2. Inclusion and Exclusion Criteria

Eligibility criteria included women between 18–45 years of age giving birth to a single, healthy, full-term infant and exclusive breastfeeding at least until four months of age. Exclusion criteria included gestational diabetes, hypertension, cardiac diseases, acute communicable diseases, and postpartum depression. Lactating women who had nipple or lacteal gland diseases, who had been receiving hormonal therapy during the three months preceding recruitment, or who had insufficient skills to understand study questionnaires were also excluded.

2.3. Ethical and Legal Considerations

The study was conducted according to the guidelines in the Declaration of Helsinki. All of the procedures involving human subjects were approved by the Medical Ethics Research Board of Peking University (No. IRB00001052-11042). Written informed consent was obtained from all subjects participating in the study. The study was also registered in ClinicalTrials.gov with the number identifier NCT01971671.

2.4. Data Collection

All subjects responded to a general questionnaire including socio-economic and lifestyle aspects of the mother. Self-reported weight at delivery, number of gestational weeks at delivery, and delivery method were also recorded. Additionally, a physical examination evaluated basic anthropometric parameters (height, weight, mid-arm circumference) blood pressure, and hemoglobin. Data collection was done through face-to-face interviews the day of HM sample collection. In addition, the date of birth and gender information of the baby was collected after the data collection, since the data was not included in the initial questionnaires. Subjects were contacted by phone and were asked to clarify these two aspects retrospectively.

2.5. HM Sampling

Breast milk sampling was standardized for all subjects and an electric pump (Horigen HNR/X-2108ZB, Xinhe Electrical Apparatuses Co., Ltd., Beijing, China) was used to sample the milk. Samples were collected at the second feeding in the morning (9:00–11:00 a.m.) to avoid circadian influence on the outcomes. A single full breast was emptied and aliquots of 10 mL for colostrum and 40 mL for the remaining time points was secured for characterization purposes. The rest of the milk was returned to the mother for feeding to the infant. Each sample was distributed in freezing tubes, labelled with subject number, and stored at −80 °C until analysis. Figure 1 shows the study flowchart for the subjects' recruitment.

2.6. Analytical Methods

2.6.1. FA Quantification

FA profile was determined by preparing the methyl esters of FA (FAMEs). A direct transesterification of HM was performed with methanolic chloridric acid solution, as described by Cruz-Hernandez et al. [27]. Briefly, into a 10 mL screw cap glass test tube, milk (250 μL) was added and mixed with 300 μL of internal standard FAME 11:0 solution (3 mg/mL) and 300 μL of internal standard TAG 13:0 solution (3 mg/mL). After addition of 2 mL of methanol, 2 mL of methanolic chloridric acid (3 N), and 1 mL of hexane, the tubes were heated at 100 °C for 90 min. To stop the reaction 2 mL of water were added and after centrifugation (1200× g for 5 min) the upper phase (hexane) was transferred into gas chromatography vials. The analysis of FAMEs was performed by GC using a CP-Sil 88 capillary column (100 m, 0.25 mm i.d. 0.25 μm film thickness) and their identification by comparison of retention time with authentic standards (GC standard Nestlé 36 from NuCheck-Prep, Elysan, MN, USA).

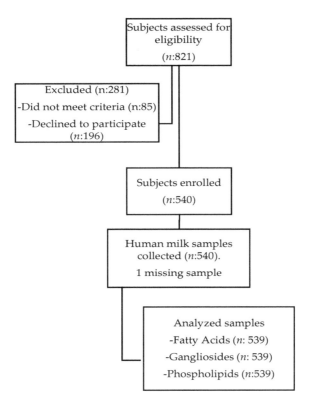

Figure 1. Study flowchart for subject recruitment.

2.6.2. Phospholipid Quantification

PL were quantified as previously described by Giuffrida et al. [28]. Briefly, 250 mg of maternal milk was mixed with 250 mg of water and 9.5 mL of chloroform/methanol (2/1 v/v). After addition of 10 μL of phosphatydilglycerol internal standard solution (5 mg/mL), the sample solution was put into an ultrasonic bath at 40 °C for 15 min. After centrifugation (1000 relative centrifugal force (RCF), for 10 min), the sample solution was filtered through 0.2 μm PTFE filters; the filtrate was mixed with 2 mL of potassium chloride solution (8.8 g/L) and centrifuged (1000 RCF for 10 min). The organic phases were evaporated to dryness and the residual lipids were redissolved in 150 μL of chloroform/methanol (9/1 v/v), filtered through 4 mm polyvinylidene fluoride (PVDF) membrane filters analyzed by high performance liquid chromatography coupled with evaporative light scattering detector (HPLC-ELSD). PL classes were separated by normal-phase HPLC using 2 Nucleosil 50-5, 250 × 3 mm, 5 μm (Macherey-Nagel, Easton, PA, USA) equipped with pre-column Nucleosil 50-5, 8 × 3 mm, 5 μm (Macherey-Nagel, Easton, PA, USA). All chromatography was performed at 55 °C. Solvent A contained ammonium formiate 3 g/L and solvent B of acetonitrile/methanol (100/3 v/v). Gradient conditions for PL analysis were as follows: time = 0 min 1% solvent A; time = 19 min 30% solvent A; time = 21 min 30% solvent A; time = 24 min 1% solvent A; with a flow rate 1 mL/min. Injection volume was 0.01 mL. The best signal and resolution was achieved at the following ELSD conditions: evap. = 90 °C; neb = 40 °C, flow rate of N_2 = 1 L/min.

2.6.3. Gangliosides Quantification

GD were quantified as previously described by Giuffrida et al. [2]. Briefly, HM (0.2 mL) was dissolved in water (1 mL) and mixed with 4 mL methanol/chloroform (2/1). After centrifugation

(3000× *g*, for 10 min), the upper liquid phase was quantitatively transferred into a 15 mL centrifuge tube. The residue was mixed with water (1 mL), 2 mL of methanol/chloroform (2/1), shaken, put into an ultrasonic bath at 25 °C for 10 min, centrifuged (3000× *g*, for 10 min), and upper liquid phases polled together; the volume was adjusted to 12 mL with methanol 60% and pH to 9.2 by adding Na2HPO4 30 mmol/L (0.2 mL). The extract solution was loaded on an Oasis HLB VAC RC SPE cartridges (30 mg, 15 mL, Waters) previously conditioned with methanol (2 mL) and methanol 60% (2 mL). The sample was passed through the cartridge at maximum flow rate 2–3 mL /min. The sorbent was washed with 2 mL of methanol 60% and dried by vacuum suction for a few seconds; the analyte was eluted with methanol (2 mL). Solvent was evaporated to dryness under a nitrogen flow at 30 °C and the residual lipids were re-dissolved in 0.2 mL of methanol 70% and analysed by liquid chromatography (LC) coupled with quadrupole time of flight (QTOF), using an Aquity BEH C18 column (1.7 µm; 150 × 2.1 mm i.d.; Waters). All chromatography was performed at 50 °C. Solvent A was composed of water/methanol/ammonium acetate (1 mmol/L) (90/10/0.1 *v/v/v*) and solvent B of methanol/ammonium acetate (1 mmol/L) (100/0.1 *v/v*). Gradient conditions were as follows: time = 0 min 10% solvent A; time = 0.2 min 10% solvent A; time = 8.2 min 5% solvent A; time = 12.2 min 5% solvent A; time = 12.4 min 0% solvent A; time = 18.4 min 0% solvent A; time = 18.6 min 10% solvent A; time = 21 min 10% solvent A. Flow rate was 0.2 mL/min. Injection volume was 0.01 mL for GD3 and 0.005 mL for GM3. The mass spectrometer was equipped with an electrospray ionization (ESI) ion source. The ESI mass spectra were recorded in the negative ion mode under the following conditions: ion spray voltage (IS) −4000 V, temperature of the source 400 °C, declustering potential (DP) −40 V, ion source gases one and two at 40 and 35 psi, respectively, curtain gas at 15 psi, collision energy −40 V. GD3 and GM3, were monitored by transitions of the precursor ions to the *m/z* 290. Quantification was performed by the standard addition method.

3. Results

3.1. Demographics and Anthropometrics of Study Subjects

In the current study we analyzed HM from 539 mothers (Figure 1), collected in a cross-sectional design over eight months postpartum. Milk obtained for analyses was a single, whole breast milk sample to have a comprehensive view on nutrient content. The details of the demographics and anthropometrics of the study subjects are outlined in Table 1. Groups of mothers, which delivered either a male or a female infant, were comparable for their age and anthropometric and demographic characteristics. Gestational age at birth (average 39 weeks) were also comparable between groups. The details of demographics and anthropometrics of the study subjects for the time period 0–4 days are not available.

Table 1. Maternal descriptive characteristics.

| | 5–11 Days | 12–30 Days | 1–2 Months | 2–4 Months | 4–8 Months |
	(*n* = 90)	(*n* = 90)	(*n* = 90)	(*n* = 90)	(*n* = 90)
Mother					
Age (years), Mean ± SD	27 ± 4	27 ± 3	28 ± 4	27 ± 4	26 ± 4
Natural delivery	27 ± 4	27 ± 3	28 ± 5	26 ± 4	26 ± 4
Caesarean delivery	28 ± 3	27 ± 4	29 ± 4	28 ± 4	27 ± 4
Height (cm), Mean ± SD	160 ± 4	160 ± 5	161 ± 5	161 ± 5	159 ± 5
Weight (kg), Mean ± SD	60.7 ± 8.7	60.8 ± 7.9	61.9 ± 8.9	58.4 ± 8.3	56.2 ± 8.1
BMI (kg/m²), Mean ± SD	23.7 ± 3.3	23.7 ± 2.8	23.9 ± 3.1	22.5 ± 2.9	22.2 ± 3.1
Gestational weight gain(kg), Mean ± SD	16.7 ± 7.4	16.2 ± 6.0	15.9 ± 5.7	15.9 ± 5.9	14.9 ± 7.6
Postpartum weight loss (kg), Mean ± SD	9.1 ± 6.1	8.6 ± 5.3	9.8 ± 4.0	10.0 ± 6.2	10.6 ± 5.9
Gestational age at birth (weeks), Mean ± SD	39.3 ± 1.2	39.2± 1.3	39.2 ± 1.6	39.4 ± 1.3	39.5 ± 1.5

SD: standard deviation.

3.2. FA

FA were determined by gas chromatography coupled with flame ionization detector (GC-FID), as previously described by Cruz-Hernandez et al. [27] and the results are listed in Table 2.

In our study total SFA content increased significantly from colostrum (35.7% of total FA) to transitional milk (38.9% of total FA) and decreased in mature milk (36.2% of total FA), with palmitic acid (16:0) being the most abundant FA and decreasing significantly ($p < 0.05$) from 23.2% in colostrum to 19.8% of total FA in mature milk (Table 2). Stearic acid (18:0) content was constant along the lactation period, i.e., colostrum, transitional, and mature milk, at about 5% of total FA, and medium-chain (MC) FA (10:0–14:0) content was low in colostrum (6.8% of total FA) compared to transitional (13.1% of total FA), and mature milk (11.0% of total FA) (Table 2). Arachidic (20:0) and lignoceric acids (24:0) were constant along the lactation time at about 0.2 and 0.1% of total FA, respectively. No significant differences ($p > 0.05$) on total SFA content were observed among cities in colostrum, and transitional milk (Table 2). SFA content was significant lower ($p < 0.05$) in mature milk from Suzhou (34.5% of total FA). Palmitic (22.5%, 19.4%, and 18.5% of total FA in colostrum, transitional, and mature milk, respectively) and stearic (4.9%, 4.5%, and 4.8% of total FA in colostrum, transitional and mature milk, respectively) FA also showed the lowest content in mature milk from Suzhou.

In the total population the MUFA content of HM decreased from 40.7% in colostrum to 36.9% of total FA in mature milk, with oleic acid (18:1n-9) being the most abundant FA and decreasing along the lactation time from 34.2% in colostrum to 31.9% of total FA in transitional and mature milk. Other MUFA (i.e., 17:1n-7, 20:1n-9, 22:1n-9. and 24:1n-9) also decreased over the lactation period (Table 2). The highest level of total MUFA content was found in colostrum (43.1% of total FA), transitional (39.3% of total FA), and mature milk (38.3% of total FA) from Guangzhou (Table 2). The lowest level of total MUFA content was found in colostrum (38.4% of total FA), transitional (34.7% of total FA), and mature milk (34.3% of total FA) from Beijing (Table 2). HM samples obtained from mothers in Guangzhou contained the highest level of Oleic acid whereas milk obtained from mothers in Beijing contained the lowest level, respectively: colostrum (37.1% vs. 32.6% of total FA), transitional (34.0% vs. 30.3% of total FA), and mature milk (33.4% vs. 30.1% of total FA).

In the total population, total PUFA n-6 increased from 21.7% in colostrum to 24.1% of total FA in mature milk with linoleic acid (18:2n-6) being the most abundant FA and increasing along the lactation time from 18.9% in colostrum to 22.8% of total FA in mature milk. ARA (20:4n-6) content decreased from 0.9% to 0.5% of total FA from colostrum to mature milk. Beijing and Suzhou showed higher total PUFAn-6 content in colostrum (23.3% and 22.8% of total FA, respectively), transitional (22.5% and 22.9% of total FA, respectively), and mature milk (26.6% and 25.3% of total FA, respectively) than Guangzhou (Table 2).

Total PUFA n-3 in HM from total population slightly increased from 1.4% in colostrum to 1.9% of total FA in mature milk with linolenic acid (18:3n-3) being the most abundant and increasing along the lactation time from 0.9% in colostrum to 1.5% of total FA in mature milk. DHA (22:6n-3) slightly decreased over lactation period from 0.5% in colostrum to 0.3% of total FA in mature milk, and EPA (20:5n-3) was present in a small amount (<0.1% of total FA in colostrum, transitional, and mature milk). The highest level of total PUFA n-3 content was found in colostrum (1.8% of total FA), transitional (2.1% of total FA), and mature milk (2.4% of total FA) from Suzhou (Table 2), which, as a consequence, showed the lowest n-6 to n-3 ratio (12.7% in colostrum, 10.9%in transitional milk, and 10.5% of total FA in mature milk).

Table 2. Median fatty acid composition of HM expressed as g/100 g of total FA.

FA (g/100 g)	Total Population			Guangzhou			Beijing			Suzhou		
	Colostrum (0–5 Days) $n = 113$	Transitional (6–15 Days) $n = 81$	Mature (16 Days–8 Months) $n = 345$	Colostrum (0–5 Days) $n = 38$	Transitional (6–15 Days) $n = 22$	Mature (16 Days–8 Months) $n = 120$	Colostrum (0–5 Days) $n = 45$	Transitional (6–15 Days) $n = 21$	Mature (16 Days–8 Months) $n = 113$	Colostrum (0–5 Days) $n = 30$	Transitional (6–15 Days) $n = 38$	Mature (16 Days–8 Months) $n = 112$
10:0	0.5 ± 0.4	1.5 ± 0.5 †	1.6 ± 0.4 ‡	0.4 ± 0.4	1.4 ± 0.5	1.5 ± 0.5	0.6 ± 0.5	1.5 ± 0.4	1.6 ± 0.4	0.5 ± 0.4	1.6 ± 0.5	1.6 ± 0.4
12:0	2.6 ± 1.6	6.1 ± 2.3 †	5.2 ± 1.9	2.3 ± 1.5	5.5 ± 2.1	5.0 ± 2.1	2.6 ± 1.7	6.5 ± 1.7	5.3 ± 1.6	2.7 ± 1.7	6.3 ± 2.6	5.3 ± 1.9
14:0	3.8 ± 1.7	5.5 ± 2.2 †	4.2 ± 1.7 ‡	3.6 ± 1.8	5.2 ± 1.9	4.1 ± 2.0	3.8 ± 1.7	5.8 ± 1.4	4.3 ± 1.4	4.0 ± 1.7	5.2 ± 2.7	4.0 ± 1.7
16:0	23.2 ± 1.9	20.5 ± 2.3 †	19.8 ± 2.6 ‡	23.9 ± 1.9	21.5 ± 2.1	20.6 ± 2.6	22.8 ± 2.2	21.5 ± 2.2	19.8 ± 2.2	22.5 ± 1.3	19.4 ± 2.2	18.5 ± 2.6
16:1n-7	2.0 ± 0.8	2.2 ± 0.7 †	2.0 ± 0.6	1.7 ± 1.0	2.4 ± 0.8	2.2 ± 0.7	2.2 ± 0.6	1.7 ± 0.6	2.0 ± 0.5	1.8 ± 0.8	2.2 ± 0.5	2.0 ± 0.6
18:0	5.2 ± 1.0	5.0 ± 0.8	5.1 ± 1.1	5.5 ± 1.2	5.3 ± 0.7	5.4 ± 1.2	5.1 ± 0.9	5.4 ± 0.7	5.1 ± 1.0	4.9 ± 0.9	4.5 ± 0.8	4.8 ± 1.0
18:1n-9	34.2 ± 3.2	31.9 ± 3.6 †	31.9 ± 3.6	37.1 ± 2.8	34.0 ± 2.2	33.4 ± 3.3	32.6 ± 2.9	30.3 ± 2.9	30.1 ± 2.9	34.0 ± 2.5	31.0 ± 4.1	31.7 ± 3.7
18:1n-7	2.5 ± 0.4	2.2 ± 0.5 †	1.9 ± 0.3 ‡	2.7 ± 0.5	2.2 ± 0.4	2.0 ± 0.3	2.3 ± 0.4	2.0 ± 0.3	1.7 ± 0.2	2.4 ± 0.3	2.3 ± 0.6	1.9 ± 0.3
18:2n-6	18.9 ± 3.6	19.7 ± 3.8 †	22.8 ± 4.9 ‡	15.7 ± 2.8	18.0 ± 3.4	19.7 ± 4.3	20.2 ± 3.5	20.2 ± 3.6	25.1 ± 3.9	19.9 ± 3.0	21.0 ± 3.9	23.8 ± 5.2
18:3n-3	0.9 ± 0.4	1.4 ± 0.6 †	1.5 ± 0.9 ‡	0.7 ± 0.3	1.0 ± 0.5	1.0 ± 0.6	0.9 ± 0.4	1.1 ± 0.7	1.6 ± 1.1	1.2 ± 0.3	1.7 ± 0.6	2.0 ± 0.8
18:3n-6	0.05 ± 0.07	0.09 ± 0.06 †	0.14 ± 0.06 ‡	<0.05	0.1 ± 0.1	0.1 ± 0.1	0.1 ± 0.1	0.1 ± 0.1	0.2 ± 0.1	<0.05	0.1 ± 0.1	0.1 ± 0.1
20:0	0.2 ± 0.1	0.2 ± 0.05	0.2 ± 0.1	0.2 ± 0.1	0.2 ± 0.1	0.2 ± 0.1	0.2 ± 0.1	0.2 ± 0.1	0.2 ± 0.1	0.2 ± 0.1	0.1 ± 0.1	0.2 ± 0.1
20:1n-9	0.9 ± 0.3	0.5 ± 0.2 †	0.4 ± 0.2	1.0 ± 0.3	0.5 ± 0.2	0.4 ± 0.1	0.7 ± 0.3	0.5 ± 0.1	0.3 ± 0.1	0.9 ± 0.2	0.5 ± 0.2	0.6 ± 0.3
20:2n-6	1.2 ± 0.4	0.6 ± 0.3 †	0.4 ± 0.1 ‡	1.1 ± 0.4	0.5 ± 0.3	0.4 ± 0.1	1.1 ± 0.4	0.8 ± 0.3	0.4 ± 0.1	1.3 ± 0.4	0.6 ± 0.2	0.4 ± 0.1
20:3n-6	0.7 ± 0.2	0.5 ± 0.2 †	0.4 ± 0.1 ‡	0.6 ± 0.2	0.4 ± 0.1	0.3 ± 0.2	0.8 ± 0.3	0.6 ± 0.2	0.4 ± 0.1	0.7 ± 0.2	0.5 ± 0.1	0.4 ± 0.1
20:5n-3	0.04 ± 0.05	0.05 ± 0.06 †	0.05 ± 0.07	<0.05	0.10 ± 0.1	<0.05	<0.05	<0.05	0.1 ± 0.1	0.1 ± 0.1	<0.05	0.1 ± 0.1
22:1n-9	0.2 ± 0.2	0.1 ± 0.1	0.1 ± 0.3	0.2 ± 0.1	0.1 ± 0.1	0.10 ± 0.1	1.1 ± 0.4	0.1 ± 0.1	0.1 ± 0.1	0.3 ± 0.3	0.1 ± 0.2	0.1 ± 0.5
20:4n-6 (ARA)	0.9 ± 0.3	0.7 ± 0.2 †	0.5 ± 0.1 ‡	0.9 ± 0.2	0.7 ± 0.2	0.5 ± 0.2	1.1 ± 0.4	0.8 ± 0.2	0.5 ± 0.1	0.9 ± 0.2	0.7 ± 0.2	0.6 ± 0.1
24:0	0.2 ± 0.1	0.1 ± 0.1 †	0.1 ± 0.1	0.2 ± 0.1	0.1 ± 0.1	0.1 ± 0.1	0.3 ± 0.2	0.1 ± 0.1	0.1 ± 0.1	0.2 ± 0.1	0.1 ± 0.1	0.1 ± 0.1
24:1n-9	0.4 ± 0.3	0.1 ± 0.1 †	0.1 ± 0.1 ‡	0.4 ± 0.2	0.1 ± 0.1	0.1 ± 0.1	0.4 ± 0.3	0.1 ± 0.1	0.1 ± 0.1	0.4 ± 0.3	0.1 ± 0.1	0.1 ± 0.1
22:6n-3 (DHA)	0.5 ± 0.3	0.5 ± 0.2 †	0.3 ± 0.2 ‡	0.7 ± 0.3	0.4 ± 0.4	0.3 ± 0.2	0.5 ± 0.2	0.5 ± 0.1	0.2 ± 0.1	0.5 ± 0.2	0.4 ± 0.2	0.3 ± 0.2
Total SFA	35.7 ± 3.9	38.9 ± 4.1 †	36.2 ± 4.7 ‡	36.1 ± 4.0	39.2 ± 3.8	36.9 ± 4.8	35.4 ± 3.9	41.0 ± 3.0	36.4 ± 3.9	35.0 ± 3.7	37.2 ± 4.8	34.5 ± 4.9
Total MUFA	40.7 ± 3.8	37.7 ± 4.3 †	36.9 ± 4.1	43.1 ± 3.3	39.3 ± 3.0	38.3 ± 3.6	38.4 ± 4.1	34.7 ± 3.5	34.3 ± 4.5	39.8 ± 2.6	36.2 ± 4.8	36.4 ± 4.4
MCFA	6.8 ± 2.4	13.1 ± 3.3	11.0 ± 2.6	6.3 ± 2.3	12.1 ± 3.5	10.6 ± 2.8	7.0 ± 2.2	13.8 ± 2.2	11.2 ± 2.3	7.2 ± 2.4	13.1 ± 3.8	10.9 ± 2.6
Total PUFA n-6	21.7 ± 3.6	21.6 ± 3.8	24.1 ± 5.0	18.3 ± 2.8	19.7 ± 3.4	21.1 ± 4.3	23.3 ± 3.6	22.5 ± 3.6	26.6 ± 3.9	22.8 ± 3.0	22.9 ± 3.9	25.3 ± 5.2
Total PUFA n-3	1.4 ± 0.5	1.9 ± 0.7	1.9 ± 0.9	1.4 ± 0.4	1.5 ± 0.6	1.3 ± 0.6	1.4 ± 0.4	1.6 ± 0.7	1.9 ± 1.1	1.8 ± 0.4	2.1 ± 0.6	2.4 ± 0.8
n-6 to n-3 ratio	14.4 ± 3.7	11.8 ± 3.7 †	12.5 ± 5.5	13.1 ± 3.7	13.1 ± 3.9	16.5 ± 5.6	16.6 ± 3.0	14.1 ± 3.9	13.8 ± 5.6	12.7 ± 3.8	10.9 ± 2.9	10.5 ± 4.0
ARA to DHA ratio	1.8 ± 0.7	1.6 ± 0.5	2.2 ± 0.9 †	1.3 ± 0.5	1.8 ± 0.6	1.9 ± 1.0	2.2 ± 0.7	1.6 ± 0.5	2.3 ± 0.8	1.8 ± 0.4	1.8 ± 0.5	1.9 ± 0.8

FA, Fatty acids; ARA, arachidonic; DHA, docosahexaenoic; SFA, Saturated FA; MUFA, mono-unsaturated FA; MCFA, medium-chain FA; PUFA, polyunsaturated FA. * Values are presented as median ± standard deviation (SD). Values within a row with a symbol indicate statistically significant differences. † $p < 0.05$ versus colostrum. ‡ $p < 0.05$ versus transitional milk.

3.3. Phospholipids

PL classes were determined by LC-ELSD, as previously described by Giuffrida et al. [28] and the results are listed in Table 3.

We did not measure minor constituents, such as lysophosphatidylcholine, which may contribute only to small amounts of the infant's diet.

From the total population, total PL content in HM decreased along the lactation period from 33.0 in colostrum to 24.2 mg/100 mL in mature milk, being significant lower ($p < 0.05$) in mature milk (Table 3). PtdCho was the most abundant PL in HM (from 12.0 mg/100 mL in colostrum to 8.2 mg/100 mL in mature milk) followed by CerPCho (from 9.1 mg/100 mL in colostrum to 7.2 mg/100 mL in mature milk), PtdEtn (from 8.5 mg/100 mL in colostrum to 6.4 mg/100 mL in mature milk), PtdIns (from 1.8 mg/100 mL in colostrum to 1.5 mg/100 mL in mature milk), and PtdSer (from 1.5 mg/100 mL to 1.0 mg/100 mL in mature milk). The PL class distribution was similar in colostrum, transitional, and mature milk (Figure 2).

Among the cities, PtdCho content did not show significant difference ($p > 0.05$) (Table 3); however, when considering the mature milk data at different lactation stages (Figure 3), PtdCho content was significant higher at 2–4 months in Suzhou (9.0 mg/100 mL) when compared to Beijing (7.1 mg/100 mL) and Guangzhou (6.4 mg/100 mL). CerPCho content was significant higher ($p < 0.05$) in colostrum (10.9 mg/100 mL) of lactating mothers from Beijing and in transitional milk (8.5 mg/100 mL) of lactating mothers from Suzhou (Table 3); when considering the different lactation stages of mature milk (Figure 3), Beijing showed significantly higher content (12.9 mg/100 mL) at 12–30 days and Suzhou at 1–2 months (10.9 mg/100 mL). PtdEtn content was significant lower ($p < 0.05$) in colostrum (7.6 mg/100 mL) and mature milk (5.3 mg/100 mL) of lactating mother from Beijing and significant higher ($p < 0.05$) in colostrum (12.6 mg/100 mL) and transitional milk (10.8 mg/100 mL) of lactating mothers from Suzhou (Table 3); when considering the mature of the milk data at different lactation stages (Figure 3) Suzhou showed the highest contents of PtdEtn at 1–2 months (8.6 mg/100 mL). PtdIns content was significant low ($p < 0.05$) in mature milk (1.2 mg/100 mL) of lactating mothers from Beijing and significant higher ($p < 0.05$) in colostrum (2.3 mg/100 mL), transitional (2.4 mg/100 mL), and mature milk (1.7 mg/100 mL) of lactating mothers from Suzhou (Table 3); within mature milk (Figure 3) Suzhou showed the highest content of PtdIns (2.0 mg/100 mL) at 1–2 months. PtdSer content was significant higher ($p < 0.05$) in colostrum (1.8 mg/100 mL) of lactating mothers from Beijing and significantly different ($p < 0.05$) in transitional (1.3 mg/100mL) and mature milk (1.2 mg/100 mL) of lactating mothers from Suzhou (Table 3). Within mature milk (Figure 3) Beijing showed the highest PtdSer content (1.7 mg/100 mL) at 12–30 days and Suzhou at 1–2 months (1.5 mg/100 mL, respectively). Finally, Suzhou showed significant higher ($p < 0.05$) PL content in colostrum (38.9 mg/100 mL), transitional milk (34.9 mg/100 mL), and mature milk (26.0 mg/100 mL), and Beijing showed the lowest content in mature milk (22.3 mg/100 mL) (Table 3).

3.4. Gangliosides

Gangliosides were determined by LC-MS/MS as described by Giuffrida et al. [29] and the results are listed in Table 4.

From the total population, the amount of GD changed during the lactation period (Table 4), with GM3 significantly increasing ($p < 0.05$) from 3.8 mg/mL in colostrum to 10.1 mg/L in mature milk and GD3 significantly decreasing ($p < 0.05$) from 4.1 mg/mL in colostrum to 1.0 mg/mL in mature milk. Total gangliosides increased significantly ($p < 0.05$) from 8.0 mg/L in colostrum to 11.0 mg/L in mature milk (Table 4). However, variability was high and total ganglioside content ranged from 1.66–28.44 mg/L in colostrum, 2.77–22.04 mg/L in transitional milk, and between 0.90–36.88 mg/L in mature milk; GM3 contents ranged between 0.63–13.03 mg/L in colostrum, 1.01–17.71 mg/L in transitional milk, 3.45–25.97 mg/L at 1–2 months, 3.45–25.97 mg/L at 2–4 months, and between 5.17–34.41 mg/L at 4–8 months; GD3 contents ranged between 0.55–18.04 mg/L in colostrum, 0.06–15.52 mg/L in transitional milk, 0.15–4.93 mg/L at 1–2 months, 0.06–5.0 mg/L at 2–4 months, and between 0.05 and 6.77 mg/L at 4–8 months. The GM3/GD3 ratio also increased over the lactation period, to 0.9 in colostrum and 10.1 in mature milk, consistent with the variation of GM3 and GD3 described above.

Table 3. Median phospholipids composition of HM expressed as mg/100 mL.

mg/100 mL	Total Population			Guangzhou			Beijing			Suzhou		
	Colostrum (0–5 Days) $n = 113$	Transitional (6–15 Days) $n = 81$	Mature (16 Days–8 Months) $n = 345$	Colostrum (0–5 Days) $n = 38$	Transitional (6–15 Days) $n = 22$	Mature (16 Days–8 Months) $n = 120$	Colostrum (0–5 Days) $n = 45$	Transitional (6–15 Days) $n = 21$	Mature (16 Days–8 Months) $n = 113$	Colostrum (0–5 Days) $n = 30$	Transitional (6–15 Days) $n = 38$	Mature (16 Days–8 Months) $n = 112$
PtdCho	12.0 ± 5.8	10.1 ± 5.5 [†]	8.2 ± 5.0 [†‡]	12.5 ± 4.6 [a]	11.3 ± 5.6 [b]	8.6 ± 5.1 [c]	10.9 ± 4.8 [a]	8.3 ± 3.7 [b]	7.6 ± 4.5 [c]	12.6 ± 7.7 [a]	11.9 ± 6.1 [b]	8.5 ± 5.3 [c]
CerPCho	9.1 ± 4.0	7.3 ± 4.1 [†]	7.2 ± 4.0 [†]	7.7 ± 1.6 [a]	6.8 ± 2.7 [b]	7.1 ± 4.0 [c]	10.9 ± 4.9 [d]	6.2 ± 3.8 [b]	7.3 ± 3.9 [c]	9.7 ± 3.1 [a]	8.5 ± 4.7 [e]	7.4 ± 4.2 [c]
PtdEtn	8.5 ± 5.2	8.2 ± 5.3	6.4 ± 3.4 [†‡]	9.9 ± 2.6 [a]	5.6 ± 3.7 [b]	7.1 ± 3.9 [c]	7.6 ± 3.1 [d]	7.3 ± 2.4 [b]	5.3 ± 2.6 [e]	12.6 ± 7.4 [f]	10.8 ± 5.8 [g]	7.3 ± 3.2 [c]
PtdIns	1.8 ± 0.7	1.8 ± 1.0	1.5 ± 0.7 [†‡]	1.8 ± 0.5 [a]	0.8 ± 0.5 [b]	1.5 ± 0.8 [c]	1.6 ± 0.5 [a]	1.5 ± 0.4 [b]	1.2 ± 0.5 [d]	2.3 ± 1.0 [e]	2.4 ± 1.1 [f]	1.7 ± 0.8 [g]
PtdSer	1.5 ± 1.6	1.1 ± 0.8 [†]	1.0 ± 1.0 [†]	1.3 ± 0.4 [a]	0.8 ± 0.4 [b]	1.0 ± 0.6 [c]	1.8 ± 2.3 [d]	1.0 ± 1.4 [b]	0.9 ± 1.2 [c]	1.7 ± 0.5 [a]	1.3 ± 0.5 [e]	1.2 ± 1.4 [f]
Total PL (mg/100 mL)	33.0 ± 13.2	28.5 ± 14.4 [†]	24.2 ± 11.4 [†‡]	33.2 ± 8.1 [a]	25.6 ± 11.1 [b]	25.3 ± 12.5 [c]	33.0 ± 11.2 [a]	24.4 ± 8.1 [b]	22.3 ± 9.9 [d]	38.9 ± 18.8 [e]	34.9 ± 16.6 [f]	26.02 ± 11.3 [c]

PL, phospholipids. * Values are presented as median ± standard deviation. Values within a row with a symbol indicate statistically significant differences. [†] $p < 0.05$ versus colostrum. [‡] $p < 0.05$ versus transitional milk. [a,b,c,d,e,f,g] $p < 0.05$ among cities.

Table 4. Average GD composition of HM expressed as mg/L.

GD mg/L	Total Population			Guangzhou			Beijing			Suzhou		
	Colostrum (0–5 Days) $n = 113$	Transitional (6–15 Days) $n = 81$	Mature (16 Days–8 Months) $n = 345$	Colostrum (0–5 Days) $n = 38$	Transitional (6–15 Days) $n = 22$	Mature (16 Days–8 Months) $n = 120$	Colostrum (0–5 Days) $n = 45$	Transitional (6–15 Days) $n = 21$	Mature (16 Days–8 Months) $n = 113$	Colostrum (0–5 Days) $n = 30$	Transitional (6–15 Days) $n = 38$	Mature (16 Days–8 Months) $n = 112$
GM3	3.8 ± 2.5	5.5 ± 3.2 [†]	10.1 ± 4.6 [†‡]	4.0 ± 2.7 [a]	7.7 ± 4.5 [b]	10.5 ± 4.6 [c]	3.7 ± 2.3 [a]	3.3 ± 1.6 [d]	9.0 ± 3.8 [c]	4.0 ± 2.6 [a]	5.4 ± 2.0 [e]	10.8 ± 5.2 [c]
GD3	4.1 ± 4.5	3.0 ± 3.4 [†]	1.0 ± 1.7 [†‡]	2.8 ± 2.5 [a]	3.0 ± 3.5 [b]	1.0 ± 2.3 [c]	2.2 ± 2.0 [a]	3.0 ± 2.8 [b]	0.7 ± 0.9 [c]	8.6 ± 5.9 [d]	2.9 ± 3.7 [b]	1.1 ± 1.5 [c]
GM3 + GD3	8.0 ± 5.3	8.5 ± 4.5 [†]	11.0 ± 5.0 [†‡]	6.6 ± 3.2 [a]	10.7 ± 4.7 [b]	11.5 ± 5.1 [c]	5.9 ± 2.7 [a]	6.3 ± 3.4 [d]	9.7 ± 4.0 [c]	12.6 ± 7.0 [e]	8.3 ± 4.3 [f]	11.9 ± 5.6 [c]
GM3/GD3	0.9	1.8 [†]	10.1 [†‡]	1.4	2.6	10.4	1.7	1.1	12.5	0.5	1.8	9.4

* Values are presented as average ± standard deviation. Values within a row with a symbol indicate statistically significant differences. [†] $p < 0.05$ versus colostrum. [‡] $p < 0.05$ versus transitional milk. [a,b,c,d,e,f] $p < 0.05$ among cities.

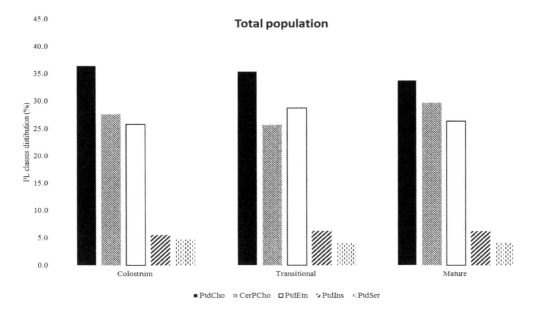

Figure 2. Change in phospholipid (PL) classes distribution in colostrum, transitional and mature milk.

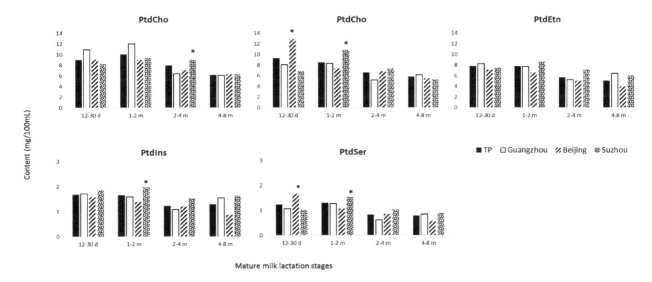

Figure 3. PL contents at different lactation stages, i.e., 12–30 days, 1–2 months, 2–4 months, and 4–8 months postpartum are shown in the total population and cities. TP stands for total population. * indicates significant difference ($p < 0.05$) among cities within the lactation stage.

Among the different cities, GM3 content was comparable ($p > 0.05$) in colostrum; GM3 highest content ($p < 0.05$) in transitional milk (7.7 mg/L) was observed in HM of lactating mothers from Guangzhou and in mature milk in lactating mothers from Guangzhou and Suzhou, at 10.5 and 10.8 mg/L, respectively (Table 4). Within mature milk (Figure 4) Beijing, Guangzhou, and Suzhou showed the highest GM3 content at 4–8 months (11.0 ± 3.9, 12.3 ± 5.5, and 15.6 ± 6.1 mg/L, respectively). The highest content ($p < 0.05$) of GD3 was observed in colostrum of lactating mothers from Suzhou (8.6 mg/L); GD3 content was comparable ($p > 0.05$) in transitional milk among the different cities and between Guangzhou and Suzhou in mature HM (Table 4). However, when considering mature milk at different lactation stages (Figure 4), Beijing, Guangzhou, and Suzhou showed the highest GD3 content at 12–30 days (0.9 ± 1.3, 1.1 ± 1.1, and 1.5 ± 2.2 mg/L, respectively). Suzhou showed the highest content ($p < 0.05$) of total GD in colostrum and mature milk (12.6 and 11.9 mg/L, respectively), the highest content ($p < 0.05$) of total GD in transitional milk was observed in Guangzhou (10.7 mg/L) (Table 4).

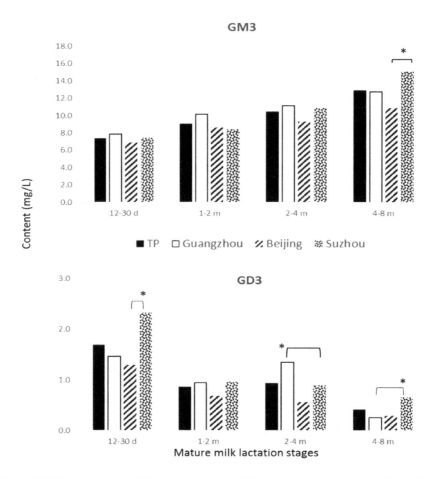

Figure 4. GM3 and GD3 contents at different mature milk lactation stages, i.e., 12–30 days, 1–2 months, 2–4 months, and 4–8 months postpartum are shown in total population (TP) and cities. * stands for significant difference (*p* < 0.05) at 4–8 months between Beijing and Suzhou for GM3, at 12–30 days between Beijing and Suzhou, and at 2–4 months and at 4–8 months between Guangzhou and Suzhou for GD3.

4. Discussion

This study measured the FA, PL, and GD content and the profile of 539 HM samples from Beijing, Guangzhou, and Suzhou.

4.1. FA

Results from the total population (Table 2) showed a total SFA content of 35.7% ± 3.9% in colostrum, of 38.9% ± 4.1% in transitional milk, and of 36.2% ± 4.7% in mature milk. Chinese studies have reported SFA level in colostrum ranging from 36.8% to 41.3% [30,31], in transitional milk from 35.2% to 42.6% [31,32] and in mature milk from 35.1% to 41.1% [30–34], in agreement with our results. When considering other populations (e.g., Caucasian, American) the SFA level in colostrum was 42.3%–43.7% [35–37], in transitional milk it ranged from 43.1% to 45.2% [36,37] and, in mature milk, from 37.4% to 57.1% [34–38], therefore, Chinese populations seem to show lower amount of total SFA in colostrum, transitional and mature milk when compared to other populations.

In this study, main SFA, lauric (12:0), myristic (14:0), palmitic (16:0), and stearic (18:0) acid contents were 2.6% ± 1.6%, 3.8% ± 1.7%, 23.2% ± 1.9%, and 5.2% ± 1.0% of total FA, respectively, in colostrum (Table 2); 6.1% ± 2.3%, 5.5% ± 2.2%, 20.5% ± 2.3%, and 5.0% ± 0.8% of total FA in transitional milk (Table 2); and 5.2% ± 1.9%, 4.2% ± 1.7%, 19.8% ± 2.6%, and 5.1% ± 1.1% of total FA, respectively, in mature milk (Table 2). Among the Chinese population, lauric, myristic, palmitic, and stearic acids ranged between 3.0%–4.9%, 5.2%–5.3%, 20.1%–23.3%, and 6.0%–7.0% of total

FA, respectively, in colostrum [30,31]; between 4.2%–6.5%, 3.8%–6.4%, 19.7%–23.3%, and 5.4%–8.1% of total FA, respectively, in transitional milk [31,32]; and finally between 3.8%–6.3%, 3.4%–6.5%, 17.3%–22.3%, and 5.0%–8.0% of total FA, respectively, in mature milk [30–34]. When considering other populations, lauric, myristic, palmitic, and stearic acids ranged between 1.2%–4.5%, 4.8%–7.3%, 24.0%–27.3%, and 5.5%–7.1% of total FA, respectively, in colostrum [35–37]; between 5.2%–6.5%, 6.5%–7.7%, 22.2%–22.6%, and 5.7%–7.4% of total FA, respectively, in transitional milk [36,37]; and finally between 3.7%–6.1%, 4.9%–7.0%, 18.7%–23.0%, and 4.8%–7.6% of total FA, respectively, in mature milk [34–38]. Philippian population showed high lauric (13.82%) and myristic (12.12%) FA contents [34] and it was reported [20,21] that 10:0, 12:0, and 14:0 FA content increases when lactating women consumed high-carbohydrate diets, whereas the secretion of the 18-carbon chain unsaturated FA, which are derived from the diet, decreased. High contents of lauric (10.2%) and myristic FA (9.1%) have been also reported in the milk of women from Nigeria [4] as a typical response to a high-carbohydrate diet.

Results from the total population (Table 2) showed total MUFA content of 40.7% ± 3.8% in colostrum, of 37.7% ± 4.3% in transitional milk, and of 36.9% ± 4.1% in mature milk. Chinese studies have reported MUFA levels in colostrum ranging from 34.7% [30] to 43.1% [31], in transitional milk from 30.8% to 42.9% [31,32], and in mature milk from 28.5% to 45.6% [30–34], in agreement with our results.

When considering other population, MUFA levels in colostrum ranged between 32.1%–44.4% of total FA [35–37], in transitional milk it was 35.1% of total FA [37], and in mature milk ranged from 30.3%–44.4% of total FA [34,35,37,38], therefore, Chinese populations seem to show comparable MUFA content in colostrum, transitional and mature milk to other populations.

Among MUFA, oleic acid was the most abundant FA and its content ranged from 34.4% in colostrum to 31.9% in transitional and mature milk. In the Chinese population oleic acid ranged from 28.4%–36.3% of total FA in colostrum [30,31]; from 25.9%–36.5% of total FA in transitional milk [31,32], and from 24.9%–38.1% in mature milk [30–34], and in other populations from 28.4%–40.1%, from 27.7%–32.1%, and from 21.9%–40.5% of total FA in colostrum [35–37], transitional [36,37], and mature milk [34–38], respectively.

Results from the total population (Table 2) showed total n-6 and n-3 PUFA content of 21.7 ± 3.6 and 1.4% ± 0.5% in colostrum, respectively, of 21.6 ± 3.8 and 1.9% ± 0.7% in transitional milk, and of 24.1 ± 5.0 and 1.9% ± 0.9% of total FA in mature milk. Chinese studies have reported PUFA levels in colostrum ranging from 14.8%–22.5% for n-6PUFA and from 2.9%–3.9% for n-3PUFA [30,31], in transitional milk from 13.7%–27.6% for n-6PUFA and from 2.5%–5.1% for n-3PUFA [31,32], and in mature milk from 14.1%–27.8% for n-6PUFA and from 2.6%–6.8% for n-3PUFA [30–34], therefore, the values are in agreement with the n-6PUFA results of this study, but higher for n-3PUFA.

When considering other populations, PUFA levels in colostrum ranged between 11.2%–14.0% for n-6PUFA and from 1.9%–3.5% of total FA for n-3PUFA [35–37], in transitional milk from 12.3%–14.1% for n-6PUFA and from 1.5%–3.3% of total FA for n-3PUFA [36,37], and in mature milk from 9.5%–20.3% for n-6PUFA and from 1.3%–3.2% of total FA for n-3PUFA [34–38]. Therefore, the Chinese populations seem to show higher contents of total n-6 PUFA when compared to other populations.

Among PUFA, LA (18:2n-6), and ALA (18:3n-3), considered essential FA because humans lack the enzymes required for their biosynthesis, were the most abundant FA we observed in colostrum, mature and transitional milk (18.9% ± 3.6%, 19.7% ± 3.8%, and 22.8% ± 4.9% of total FA for LA, respectively and for 0.9% ± 0.4%, 1.4% ± 0.6%, and 1.5% ± 0.9% of total FA for ALA, respectively).

In the Chinese population, LA and ALA ranged from 10.3%–19.2% and from 0.9%–1.3% of total FA, respectively, in colostrum [30–32]; from 9.8%–23.3% and from 0.9%–2.2% of total FA, respectively, in transitional milk [31,32]; and from 10.9%–23.7% and from 0.9%–3.0% of total FA, respectively, in mature milk [30–34], in agreement with our findings.

In other populations, LA and ALA ranged from 8.6%–11.9% and from 0.7%–1.1% of total FA, respectively, in colostrum [35–37]; from 10.3%–12.5% and from 0.8%–1.3% of total FA, respectively, in transitional milk [36,37]; and from 7.9%–17.8% and from 0.4%–1.4% of total FA, respectively, in mature milk [34–38].

Finally, in our study, DHA contents for the total population ranged from 0.3%, in mature milk, to 0.5% in colostrum and transitional milk, therefore, lower than the DHA content reported for Chinese marine populations in colostrum (1.5%) [30], transitional (0.6%) [31], and mature milk (0.5%–2.8%) [30,33]. The ratio ARA/DHA (1.8–2.2) was comparable to average worldwide ratio of about 1.5 [22].

Among different cities, over lactation time, HM from Beijing showed slightly higher SFA content (Table 2), Guangzhou the highest MUFA content (Table 2), and Suzhou the highest n-3PUFA content (Table 2).

It is known that the type of fat/oil in the maternal diet influences the FA composition of breast milk. Francois et al. [22] showed that the consumption of six different dietary fats, each providing a specific FA, caused an acute response in HM FA composition, especially within 24 h, and that the response remained significantly elevated for 1–3 days after consumption of dietary fat. Therefore, difference observed in HM FA composition may reflect variation in maternal diet [33].

However, a careful analyses of dietary habits of Guangzhou, Beijing, and Suzhou needs to be performed for correlating to HM composition.

4.2. Phospholipids

Several studies have recognized the importance of PL for infant growth [39–41]. At the same time, PL are involved in immunity and inflammatory responses [42], and in neuronal signaling [43].

PL content in HM significantly ($p < 0.005$) decreased along the lactation period from 33.0 in colostrum to 24.2 mg/100 mL in mature milk, in agreement with previous studies performed elsewhere [12,44]. The PL class distribution was similar in colostrum, transitional and mature milk (Figure 2).

PL as emulsifiers are essential for the solubilization of dietary fats and as a consequence for their digestion and absorption. In this regard, the higher content of PL in colostrum and transitional HM compared to mature milk might explain the good fat absorption from HM by the newborn, despite poor pancreatic secretion, as suggested by Harzer et al. [11]. A decrease in PL content in HM along the lactation stage might occur because the diameter of the milk fat globule membrane increases [11,45], decreasing the PL/TAG ratio [7,8].

Our study showed that PtdCho was the most abundant PL in HM (Figure 2), followed by CerPCho and PtdEtn, and PtdIns and PtdSer, in agreement with previous studies [3,11,12,44,46]. PtdCho and CerPCho are important sources of choline considered as an essential nutrient for infants. Choline is a precursory amino alcohol of the neurotransmitter acetylcholine, it acts by regulating the transduction signal, and serves as a source of methyl groups in intermediate metabolism, being considered essential for optimum development of the brain [7,8]. In addition, CerPCho can reduce cholesterol absorption between 20.4%–85.5%, depending on the ingested dose (0.1% and 5.0%, respectively) [47], being possibly involved in cholesterol regulation programming.

The amount of total PL in colostrum (33.0 ± 13.2 mg/100 mL), transitional (28.5 ± 14.4 mg/100 mL), and mature milk (24.2 ± 11.4 mg/100 mL), was comparable to the values reported by Bitman et al. [44] (35, 31, and 27 mg/100 mL, respectively), Thakkar et al. [48] (20.8–24.2 mg/100 mL in mature milk), and Garcia et al. [49] (15.3–47.4 mg/100 mL in mature milk); higher than the values reported by Sala-Vila et al. [12] (13.5, 14.0, and 9.8 mg/100 mL, respectively), Lopez et al. [50] (13.5 mg/100 mL in mature milk) and Zou et al. [51] (16.8, 22.3, and 19.2 mg/100 mL, respectively).

In the total population PtdCho contents in colostrum, transitional, and mature milk were 12.0 ± 5.8, 10.1 ± 5.5, and 8.2 ± 5.0 mg/100 mL, respectively, comparable to values reported in literature, 4.3–11.2, 5.7–9.4, and 2.0–11.2 mg/100 mL, respectively [44,48–56].

CerPCho contents in colostrum, transitional, and mature milk were 9.1 ± 4.0, 7.3 ± 4.1, and 7.2 ± 4.0 mg/100 mL, respectively, comparable to values reported in the literature of 5.3–11.0, 9.0–11.6, and 3.1–13.5 mg/100 mL, respectively [44,48–57].

PtdEtn contents in colostrum, transitional, and mature milk were 8.5 ± 5.2, 8.2 ± 5.3, and 6.4 ± 3.4 mg/100 mL, respectively, higher than values reported in the literature for colostrum and transitional milk 1.4–6.4 and 1.5–5.6 mg/100 mL, respectively [44,51], and comparable to values reported for mature milk of 0.2–8.1 mg/100 mL [3,11,12,44,48,49,51,52].

PtdIns and PtdSer contents in colostrum (1.8 ± 0.7 and 1.5 ± 1.6 mg/100 mL, respectively), transitional (1.8 ± 1.0 and 1.1 ± 0.8 mg/100mL, respectively), and mature milk (1.5 ± 0.7 and 1.0 ± 1.1 mg/100 mL, respectively) were comparable to values reported in previous studies for PtdIns, 1.4–3.3, 1.5–2.2, and 0.2–2.2 mg/100 mL, respectively, and for PtdSer, 2.1–3.6, 1.5–2.2, and 0.8–4.5 mg/100 mL [44,48–51,53].

Among the different cities, Suzhou showed the highest total PL and PtdEtn levels in colostrum, transitional, and mature milk (Table 3). Dietary sources of PtdEtn may be lecithin from rapeseed oil, whose consumption may explain also the higher content of ALA in HM from Suzhou. However, a careful analyses of dietary habits of this region needs to be performed for correlating to HM composition.

It is well known [58] that lipid and liposoluble nutrients content increases towards the latter part of a feeding session, a phenomenon that has been corroborated by biochemical analyses of total milk fat in fore-milk, and hind-milk [59,60]. Therefore, in order to assure sample homogeneity in our study all efforts have been made to collect fully-expressed milk. Among the cited studies, only Bitman et al., Thakkar et al., Holmes et al., and Fischer et al. [44,48,54,56] refer to full breast milk samples, Sala-Vila et al. [12] to fore-milk, and no detailed sampling procedure is described in the other studies. Analysis performed in fore-milk and hind-milk rather than fully-expressed milk could explain the discrepancy among results.

4.3. Gangliosides

GD are widely distributed in almost all human tissues, with the highest amount found in neural tissue and extra-neural organs, such the lung, spleen, and gut. It has been reported that during the first stages of life, dietary GD may have an important role in preventing infections [61] and in cognitive development functions [10,62].

Our data confirmed, as previously reported [14,16,17,29,63,64], that the amount of GD changes during the lactation period, with GD3 decreasing and GM3 increasing over the lactation period. Rueda et al. [15] postulated that a high concentration of GD3 in early milk may reflect its biological role in the development of organs, such as the intestine, as was observed in our study in all cities. The increase in GM3 in mature milk has been associated with signal transduction, cell adhesion, and growth factor receptors, leading to the development of the immune and central nervous systems [14,17,61]. In the studied population, the sum of GM3 and GD3 increased from 8.0 mg/L in colostrum to 11.0 mg/L in mature milk, as previously published [29]. It has been reported [64] that the sum of GM3 and GD3 can range from as low as 2 mg/L to as high as 25 mg/L, depending on breast milk sampling, population demographics, diet, and analytical methodologies. In this study, total ganglioside content ranged from 1.66–28.44 mg/L in colostrum, 2.77–22.04 mg/L in transitional milk, and between 0.90–36.88 mg/L in mature milk, covering total GD contents previous reported, i.e., 2.8–59.7 mg/L in colostrum [14,15,17,18,29,63,65], 0.9–30.7 mg/L in transitional [14,15,17,18,63,65], and 1.6–68.6 mg/L in mature milk [14,15,17,18,29,48,63,65,66]. When considering average values, in colostrum and transitional milk, GM3 content (3.8 and 5.5 mg/L, respectively) was lower than the one reported by Ma et al. [63] (6.5–7.1 and 8.3–9.6 mg/L, respectively). Within mature milk, at 1–2 months GM3 content (9.08 mg/L) was comparable to the one reported by Ma et al. [63,64] (8.3–11.3 mg/L) and higher than the content reported by Thakkar et al. [48] (2.3–2.9 mg/L); after 3–8 months GM3 content (10.46–12.92 mg/L) was lower than what reported by Ma et al. [63,64] (17.4–21.4 mg/L) and higher than the content reported by Thakkar et al. [48] (3.9 mg/L). However, when considering minimum and maximum values, GM3 contents (0.63–13.03, 1.01–17.71, and 0.8–34.41 mg/L, in colostrum, transitional, and mature milk, respectively) were comparable with GM3 contents previously reported [48,63,64].

As for GM3, when considering average values, in colostrum and transitional milk, GD3 content (4.1 and 3.0 mg/L, respectively) was lower than the one reported by Ma et al. [63] (20 and 10 mg/L, respectively). Within mature milk, at 1–2 months GD3 content (0.87 mg/L) was lower than the one reported by Ma et al. [63,64] (4.6–7.0 mg/L) and by Thakkar et al. [48] (1.9–2.3 mg/L); after 3–8 months GD3 content (0.25–0.50 mg/L) was lower than that reported by Ma et al. [63,64] (1.5–2.7 mg/L) and by Thakkar et al. [48] (1.7 mg/L). However, when considering minimum and maximum values, GD3 contents (0.6–18.0, 0.1–15.5, and 0.1–9.3 mg/L, in colostrum, transitional, and mature milk, respectively) were comparable with GD3 contents previously reported [48,63,64]. Among the cities Suzhou showed the highest GM3 and GD3 contents (Table 4) in colostrum and mature milk.

Ma et al. [64] suggested that the ganglioside concentrations in HM at any time point may be influenced by the mother's dietary intake of gangliosides or their precursors. It was demonstrated [67] that GD3 and GM3 are transferred across the human placenta using an ex vivo model of dually-perfused isolated human placental lobules, suggesting that they are available to the developing fetus. Therefore, a careful analysis of dietary habits in this region needs to be performed for correlating to HM GD composition.

5. Conclusions

In this study, FA, PL, and GD contents and compositions of HM from lactating women living in Suzhou, Guangzhou, and Beijing were evaluated.

HM was collected over a period of eight months, allowing the observation of lipid compositional changes during lactation.

SFA, MUFA, and PL content decreased during lactation, PUFA and GD content increased. Among different cities, over lactation time, HM from Beijing showed the highest SFA content, HM from Guangzhou showed the highest MUFA content, and HM from Suzhou showed the highest n-3PUFA content. The highest total PL and GD contents were observed in HM from Suzhou. In order to investigate the influence of the diet on maternal milk composition, a careful analysis of dietary habits of these population needs to be performed in future work.

Acknowledgments: The authors would like to thank the participants who volunteered for this study, Lawrence Li for project support and guidance, Celia Ning for project management, Qiaoji Li for clinical project management, Emilie Ba for data management and local project staff at Peking University School of Public Health, Guangzhou University School of Public Health and Soochow University School of Public Health for recruitment and data collection.

Author Contributions: S.K.T., G.V.-P., Y.Z. and P.W. conceived and designed the experiments; F.G., C.C.-H., E.B., P.F., I.M.E., I.T., C.M., B.S.-B. developed, validated and performed the experiments; F.G., C.C.-H., S.K.T. and C.A.D.-C. analyzed the data; F.G. wrote the paper.

Abbreviations

FA (FA), phospholipids (PL), gangliosides (GD), gas chromatography (GC), evaporative light scattering detector (ELSD), with time of flight (TOF), triacylglycerols (TAG), saturated FA (SFA), mono-unsaturated (MUFA), polyunsaturated (PUFA), long chain polyunsaturated FA (LCPUFA), linoleic (LA), linolenic acids (ALA), arachidonic (ARA), docosahexaenoic (DHA), phosphatydylinositol (PtdIns), phosphatydylethanolamine (PtdEtn), phosphatydylserine (PtdSer), phosphatidylcholine (PtdCho), sphingomyelin (CerPCho), methyl esters of FA (FAMEs).

References

1. Kramer, M.; Ritsuko, S.K. *The Optimal Duration of Exclusive Breastfeeding: A Systematic Review*; World Health Organization: Geneva, Switzerland, 2002.

2. Giovannini, M.; Riva, E.; Agostoni, C. FA in pediatric nutrition (Review). *Pediatr. Clin. North. Am.* **1995**, *42*, 861. [CrossRef]
3. Bitman, J.; Wood, L.; Metha, N.R.; Hamosh, P.; Hamosh, M. Comparison of phospholipid composition of breast milk from mothers of term and preterm infants during lactation. *Am. J. Clin. Nutr.* **1984**, *40*, 1103–1119. [PubMed]
4. Jensen, R.G. Lipids in HM. *Lipids* **1999**, *12*, 1243–1271. [CrossRef]
5. Innis, S.M. Essential FA in growth and development. *Prog. Lipid Res.* **1991**, *30*, 39–103. [CrossRef]
6. Pruett, S.T.; Bushnev, A.; Hagedorn, K.; Adiga, M.; Haynes, C.A.; Sullards, M.C.; Liotta, D.C.; Merrill, A.H., Jr. Biodiversity of sphingoid bases ("sphingosines") and related amino alcohols. *J. Lipid Res.* **2008**, *49*, 1621–1639. [CrossRef] [PubMed]
7. Zeisel, S.H.; Blusztajn, J.K. Choline and human nutrition. *Ann. Rev. Nutr.* **1994**, *14*, 269–296. [CrossRef] [PubMed]
8. Zeisel, S.H. The fetal origins of memory: The role of dietary choline in optimal brain development. *J. Pediatr.* **2006**, *149*, 131s–136s. [CrossRef] [PubMed]
9. Schauer, R. Achievements and challenges of sialic acid research. *Glycoconj. J.* **2000**, *17*, 485–499. [CrossRef] [PubMed]
10. Gurnida, D.A.; Rowan, A.M.; Idjradinata, P.; Muchtadi, D.; Sekarwana, N. Association of complex lipids containing gangliosides with cognitive development of 6-month-old infants. *Early Hum. Dev.* **2012**, *88*, 595–601. [CrossRef] [PubMed]
11. Harzer, G.; Haug, M.; Bindels, J.G. Biochemistry of human milk in early lactation. *Z. Ernahrungswissenschaft* **1986**, *25*, 77–90. [CrossRef]
12. Sala Vila, A.; Castellote, A.I.; Rodriguez-Palmero-Seuma, M.; Campoy, C.; Lopez-Sabater, M.C. Lipid composition in human breast milk from Granada (Spain): Changes during lactation. *Nutrition* **2005**, *21*, 467–473. [CrossRef] [PubMed]
13. Cilla, A.; Diego-Quintaes, K.; Barbera, R.; Alegria, A. Phospholipids in HM and infant formula: Benefits and needs for correct infant nutrition. *Crit. Rev. Food Sc. Nutr.* **2016**, *56*, 1880–1892. [CrossRef] [PubMed]
14. Takamizawa, K.; Iwamori, K.; Mutai, M.; Nagai, Y. Selective changes in gangliosides of HM during lactation: A molecular indicator for the period of lactation. *Biochim. Biophys. Acta* **1986**, *879*, 73–77. [PubMed]
15. Rueda, R.; Puente, R.; Hueso, P.; Maldonado, J.; Gil, A. New data on content and distribution of gangliosides in HM. *Biol. Chem. Hoppe-Seyler* **1995**, *376*, 723–727. [CrossRef] [PubMed]
16. Rueda, R.; Maldonado, J.; Gil, A. Comparison of content and distribution of HM gangliosides from Spanish and Panamanian mothers. *Ann. Nutr. Metab.* **1996**, *40*, 194–201. [CrossRef] [PubMed]
17. Pan, X.L.; Izumi, T. Variation of the ganglioside compositions of HM, cow's milk and infant formulas. *Early Hum. Dev.* **2000**, *57*, 25–31. [CrossRef]
18. Martin-Sosa, S.; Martin, M.-J.; Garcia-Pardo, L.A.; Hueso, P. Distribution of sialic acids in the milk of Spanish mothers of full term infants during lactation. *J. Pediatr. Gastr. Nutr.* **2004**, *39*, 111–116.
19. Uchiyama, S.-I.; Sekiguchi, K.; Akaishi, M.; Anan, A.; Maeda, T.; Izumi, T. Characterization and chronological changes of preterm HM gangliosides. *Nutrition* **2011**, *27*, 998–1001. [CrossRef] [PubMed]
20. Read, W.W.C.; Lutz, P.G.; Tashjian, A. HM lipids. II the influence of dietary carbohydrates and fat on the FA of mature milk. A study in four ethnic groups. *Am. J. Clin. Nutr.* **1965**, *17*, 180–183. [PubMed]
21. Van Beusekom, C.M.; Martini, I.A.; Rutgers, H.M.; Boersma, E.R.; Muskiet, F.A. A carbohydrate-rich diets not only leads to incorporation of medium-chain FA (6:0–14:0) in triglycerides but also in each milk-phospholipid subclass. *Am. J. Clin. Nut.* **1990**, *52*, 326–334.
22. Francois, C.A.; Connor, S.L.; Wander, R.C.; Connor, W.E. Acute effects of dietary FA on the FA of HM. *Am. J. Clin. Nutr.* **1998**, *67*, 301–308. [PubMed]
23. Samur, G.; Topcu, A.; Turan, S. Trans FA and fatty acid composition of mature breast milk in Turkish women and their association with maternal diets. *Lipids* **2009**, *44*, 405. [CrossRef] [PubMed]
24. Lauritzen, L.; Jørgensen, M.H.; Hansen, H.S.; Michaelsen, K.F. Fluctuations in HM long-chain PUFA levels in relation to dietary fish intake. *Lipids* **2002**, *37*, 237. [CrossRef] [PubMed]
25. Ryan, J.M.; Rice, E.G.; Mitchell, M.D. The role of gangliosides in brain development and the potential benefits of perinatal supplementation. *Nutr. Res.* **2013**, *33*, 877–887. [CrossRef] [PubMed]
26. Yang, T.; Zhang, Y.; Ning, Y.; You, L.; Ma, D.; Zheng, Y.; Yang, X.; Li, W.; Wang, J.; Wang, P. Breast milk macronutrient composition and the associated factors in urban Chinese mothers. *Chin. Med. J. Assoc.* **2014**, *9*, 127.

27. Cruz-Hernandez, C.; Goeuriot, S.; Giuffrida, F.; Thakkar, S.K.; Destaillats, F. Direct quantification of FA in HM by gas chromatography. *J. Chrom. A* **2013**, *9*, 174. [CrossRef] [PubMed]

28. Giuffrida, F.; Cruz-Hernandez, C.; Fluck, B.; Tavazzi, I.; Thakkar, K.S.; Destaillats, F.; Braun, M. Quantification of Phospholipids Classes in HM. *Lipids* **2013**, *48*, 1051–1058. [CrossRef] [PubMed]

29. Giuffrida, F.; Masserey-Elmelegy, I.; Thakkar, S.K.; Marmet, C.; Destaillats, F. Longitudinal Evolution of the Concentration of Gangliosides GM3 and GD3 in HM. *Lipids* **2014**, *49*, 997–1004. [CrossRef] [PubMed]

30. Wu, T.-C.; Lau, B.-H.; Chen, P.-H.; Wu, L.-T.; Tang, R.-B. Fatty acid composition of Taiwanese HM. *J. Chin. Med. Assoc.* **2012**, *73*, 581–588. [CrossRef]

31. Chen, Z.Y.; Kwan, K.Y.; Tong, K.K.; Ratnayake, W.M.N.; Li, H.Q.; Leung, S.S.F. Breast milk fatty acid composition: A comparative study between Hong Kong and Chongqing Chinese. *Lipids* **1997**, *32*, 1061–1067. [CrossRef] [PubMed]

32. Li, J.; Fan, Y.; Zhang, Z.; Yu, H.; An, Y.; Kramer, J.K.G.; Deng, Z. Evaluating the trans fatty acid, CLA, PUFA and erucic acid diversity in HM from five region in China. *Lipids* **2009**, *44*, 257–271. [CrossRef] [PubMed]

33. Ruan, C.-L.; Liu, X.-F.; Man, H.-S.; Ma, X.-L.; Lu, G.-Z.; Duan, G.-H.; DeFrancesco, C.A.; Connor, W.E. Milk composition in women from five different regions of China: The great diversity of milk FA. *Hum. Clin. Nutr.* **1995**, 2993–2998.

34. Yuhas, R.; Pramuk, K.; Lien, E.L. HM fatty acid composition from nine countries varies most in DHA. *Lipids* **2006**, *41*, 851–858. [CrossRef] [PubMed]

35. Xiang, M.; Alfvén, G.; Blennow, M.; Trygg, M.; Zetterstrom, R. Long-Chain polyunsaturated FA in HM and brain growth during early infancy. *Acta Pediatr.* **2000**, *89*, 142–147. [CrossRef]

36. Genzel-Boroviczény, O.; Wahle, J.; Koletzko, B. Fatty acid composition of HM during the 1st month after term and preterm delivery. *Eur. J. Pediatr.* **1997**, *156*, 142–147. [CrossRef] [PubMed]

37. Idota, T.; Sakurai, M.; Sugawara, Y.; Ishiyama, Y.; Murakami, Y.; Moriguchi, H.; Takeuchi, M.; Shimoda, K.; Asai, Y. The latest survey for the composition of milk obtained from Japanese mothers. Part II. Changes of fatty acid composition, phospholipids and cholesterol contents during lactation. *Jpn. J. Pediatr. Gastroenterol. Nutr.* **1991**, *5*, 159–173.

38. Chardigny, J.-M.; Wolff, R.L.; Sébédio, J.-L.; Martine, L.; Juaneda, P. Trans mono- and polyunsaturated FA in HM. *Eur. J. Clin. Nutr.* **1995**, *49*, 523–531. [PubMed]

39. Tanaka, K.; Hosozawa, M.; Kudo, N.; Yoshikawa, N.; Hisata, K.; Shoji, H.; Shinohara, K.; Shimizu, T. The pilot study: Sphingomyelin-Fortified milk has a positive association with the neurobehavioural development of very low birth weight infants during infancy, randomized control trial. *Brain Dev.* **2013**, *35*, 45–52. [CrossRef] [PubMed]

40. Küllenberg, D.; Taylor, L.A.; Schneider, M.; Massing, U. Health effects of dietary phospholipids. *Lipids Health Dis.* **2012**, *11*, 1–16. [CrossRef] [PubMed]

41. German, J.B. Dietary lipids from an evolutionary perspective: Sources, structures and functions. *Mater. Child. Nutr.* **2011**, *7*, 2–16. [CrossRef] [PubMed]

42. Nixon, G.F. Sphingolipids in inflammation: Pathological implications and potential therapeutic targets. *Br. J. Pharmacol.* **2009**, *158*, 982–993. [CrossRef] [PubMed]

43. McDaniel, M.A.; Maier, S.F.; Einstein, G.O. "Brain-specific" nutrients: A memory cure? *Nutrition* **2003**, *19*, 957–975. [CrossRef]

44. Bitman, J.; Freed, L.M.; Neville, M.C.; Wood, D.L.; Hamosh, P.; Hamosh, M. Lipid composition of prepartum human mammary secretion and postpartum milk. *J. Ped. Gastr. Nutr.* **1986**, *5*, 608–615. [CrossRef]

45. Harzer, G.; Haug, M.; Dieterich, I.; Gentner, P.G. Changing patterns of HM lipids in the course of the lactation and during the day. *Am. J. Clin. Nutr.* **1983**, *37*, 612–621. [PubMed]

46. Morrison, W.R.; Smith, L.M. Fatty Acid Composition of Milk Phospholipids. II. Sheep, Indian Buffalo and HMs. *Lipids* **1967**, *2*, 178–182. [CrossRef] [PubMed]

47. Rombaut, R.; Dewettinck, K. Properties, analysis and purification of milk polar lipids. *Int. Dairy J.* **2006**, *16*, 1362–1373. [CrossRef]

48. Thakkar, S.K.; Giuffrida, F.; Cruz-Hernandez, C.; De Castro, A.C.; Mukherjee, R.; Tran, L.-A.; Steenhout, P.; Lee, L.Y.; Destaillats, F. Dynamic composition of HM nutrient composition of women from Singapore with special focus on lipids. *Am. J. Nutr. Biol.* **2013**, *25*, 770–779.

49. Garcia, C.; Millet, V.; Coste, T.C.; Mimoun, M.; Ridet, A.; Antona, C.; Simeoni, U.; Armand, M. French Mothers' Milk Deficient in DHA Contains Phospholipid Species of Potential Interest for Infant Development. *J. Pediatr. Gastroenterol. Nutr.* **2011**, *53*, 206–212. [CrossRef] [PubMed]

50. Lopez, C.; Briard-Bion, V.; Menard, O.; Rousseau, F.; Pradel, P.; Besle, J.-M. Phospholipid, sphingolipid, and fatty acid compositions of the milk fat globule membrane are modified by diet. *J. Agric. Food Chem.* **2008**, *56*, 5226–5236. [CrossRef] [PubMed]

51. Zou, X.-Q.; Guo, Z.; Huang, J.-H.; Jin, Q.-Z.; Cheong, L.-Z.; Wang, X.-G.; Xu, X.-B. HM fat globules from different stages of lactation: A lipid composition analysis and microstructure characterization. *J. Agric. Food Chem.* **2012**, *60*, 7158–7167. [CrossRef] [PubMed]

52. Zeisel, S.H.; Char, D.; Sheard, N.F. Choline, phosphatidylcholine and sphingomyelin in human and bovine milk and infant formulas. *J. Nutr.* **1986**, *116*, 50–58. [PubMed]

53. Kynast, G.; Schmitz, C. Determination of the phospholipid content of HM, cow's milk and various infant formulas. *Z. Ernährungswiss* **1988**, *27*, 252–265. [CrossRef] [PubMed]

54. Holmes-McNary, M.Q.; Cheng, W.-L.; Mar, M.-H.; Fussell, S.; Zeisel, S.H. Choline and choline esters in human and rat milk and in infant formulas. *Am. J. Clin. Nutr.* **1996**, *64*, 572–576. [PubMed]

55. Ilcol, Y.O.; Ozbek, R.; Hamurtkin, E.; Ulus, I.H. Choline status in newborns, infants, children, breast-feeding women, breast-fed infants and human breast milk. *J. Nutr. Biochem.* **2005**, *16*, 489–499. [CrossRef] [PubMed]

56. Fischer, L.M.; Costa, K.A.; Galanko, J.; Sha, W.; Stephenson, B.; Vick, J.; Zeisel, S.H. Choline intake and genetic polymorphisms influence choline metabolite concentrations in human breast milk and plasma. *Am. J. Clin. Nutr.* **2010**, *92*, 336–346. [CrossRef] [PubMed]

57. Blaas, N.; Schüürmann, C.; Bartke, N.; Stahl, B.; Humpf, H.-U. Structural profiling and quantification of sphingomyelin in human breast milk by HPLC-MS/MS. *J. Agric. Food Chem.* **2011**, *59*, 6018–6024. [CrossRef] [PubMed]

58. Neville, M.C.; Picciano, M.F. Regulation of milk lipid secretion and composition. *Ann. Rev. Nutr.* **1997**, *17*, 159–184. [CrossRef] [PubMed]

59. Hytten, F.E. Clinical and chemical studies in human lactation. *Br. Med. J.* **1954**, *1*, 249–255. [CrossRef] [PubMed]

60. Saarela, T.; Kokkonen, J.; Koivisto, M. Macronutrient and energy contents of HM fractions during the first six months of lactation. *Acta Paediatr.* **2005**, *94*, 1176–1181. [CrossRef] [PubMed]

61. Rueda, R. The role of dietary gangliosides on immunity and the prevention of infection. *Brit. J. Nutr.* **2007**, *98*, 68–73. [CrossRef] [PubMed]

62. Wang, B.; McVeagh, P.; Petocz, P.; Brand-Miller, J. Brain gangliosides and glycoprotein sialic acid in breastfed compared with formula-fed infants. *Am. J. Clin. Nutr.* **2003**, *78*, 1024–1029. [PubMed]

63. Ma, L.; MacGibbon, A.K.H.; Mohamed, H.J.B.J.; Loy, S.L.; Rowan, A.; McJarrow, P.; Fong, B.Y. Determination of ganglioside concentrations in breast milk and serum from Malaysian mothers using a high performance liquid chromatography-mass spectrometry-multiple reaction monitoring method. *Intern. Dairy J.* **2015**, *49*, 62–71. [CrossRef]

64. Ma, L.; Liu, X.; MacGibbon, A.K.H.; Loy, S.L.; Rowan, A.; McJarrow, P.; Fong, B.Y. Lactational changes in concentration and distribution of ganglioside molecular species in human breast milk from Chinese mothers. *Lipids* **2015**, *50*, 1145–1154. [CrossRef] [PubMed]

65. Nakano, T.; Sugawara, M.; Kawakami, H. Sialic acid in HM: Composition and functions. *Acta Paediatr. Taiwan* **2001**, *42*, 11–17. [PubMed]

66. Laegreid, A.; Otnaess, A.B.K.; Fuglesang, J. Human and bovine-milk: Comparison of ganglioside composition and enterotoxin-inhibitory activity. *Pediatr. Res.* **1986**, *20*, 416–421. [CrossRef] [PubMed]

67. Mitchell, M.D.; Henare, K.; Balakrishnan, B.; Lowe, E. Transfer of gangliosides across the human placenta. *Placenta* **2012**, *33*, 312–316. [CrossRef] [PubMed]

10

Does Human Milk Modulate Body Composition in Late Preterm Infants at Term-Corrected Age?

Maria Lorella Giannì [1,*], **Dario Consonni** [2], **Nadia Liotto** [1], **Paola Roggero** [1], **Laura Morlacchi** [1], **Pasqua Piemontese** [1], **Camilla Menis** [1] and **Fabio Mosca** [1]

[1] Fondazione I.R.C.C.S. Ca Granda Ospedale Maggiore Policlinico, Neonatal Intensive Care Unit, Department of Clinical Science and Community Health, University of Milan, Via Commenda 12, 20122 Milano, Italy; nadia.liotto@unimi.it (N.L.); paola.roggero@unimi.it (P.R.); lally.morly@hotmail.it (L.M.); pasquina.piemontese@mangiagalli.it (P.P.); camilla.menis@studenti.unimi.it (C.M.); fabio.mosca@unimi.it (F.M.)

[2] Fondazione IRCCS Ca' Granda Ospedale Maggiore Policlinico, Epidemiology Unit, Via San Barnaba 8, 20122 Milan, Italy; dario.consonni@unimi.it

* Correspondence: maria.gianni@unimi.it

Abstract: (1) Background: Late preterm infants account for the majority of preterm births and are at risk of altered body composition. Because body composition modulates later health outcomes and human milk is recommended as the normal method for infant feeding, we sought to investigate whether human milk feeding in early life can modulate body composition development in late preterm infants; (2) Methods: Neonatal, anthropometric and feeding data of 284 late preterm infants were collected. Body composition was evaluated at term-corrected age by air displacement plethysmography. The effect of human milk feeding on fat-free mass and fat mass content was evaluated using multiple linear regression analysis; (3) Results: Human milk was fed to 68% of the infants. According to multiple regression analysis, being fed any human milk at discharge and at term-corrected and being fed exclusively human milk at term-corrected age were positively associated with fat-free mass content($\beta = -47.9$, 95% confidence interval (CI) $= -95.7$; -0.18; $p = 0.049$; $\beta = -89.6$, 95% CI $= -131.5$; -47.7; $p < 0.0001$; $\beta = -104.1$, 95% CI $= -151.4$; -56.7, $p < 0.0001$); (4) Conclusion: Human milk feeding appears to be associated with fat-free mass deposition in late preterm infants. Healthcare professionals should direct efforts toward promoting and supporting breastfeeding in these vulnerable infants.

Keywords: human milk; late preterm infants; body composition

1. Introduction

Late preterm birth, defined as a birth that occurs between 34 0/7 and 36 6/7 weeks of gestation, accounts for the majority of all preterm births [1]. Late preterm infants show increased mortality and morbidity compared with full-term newborn infants [2]. It has been reported that the first months of the postnatal life of late preterm infants are characterized by rapid postnatal catch-up growth, and as a result, at term-corrected age, late preterm infants achieve a weight either comparable to or higher than full-term newborns [3,4]. Evidence indicates that early body composition development in these infants is accompanied by a major deposition of fat mass so that, at term-corrected age, increased adiposity irrespective of the percentile at birth has been found. Unlike very preterm infants, however, late preterm infants appear not to develop a fat-free mass deficit [4].

It has long been recognized that early life represents a critical time window in terms of metabolic programming [5]. Indeed, increased adiposity early on may contribute to negative health outcomes later [6], whereas fat-free mass accretion has been positively associated with faster brain processing [7].

Considering the key role played by body composition development in modulating later health outcomes [6], identification of the determinants of body composition may help in tailoring nutritional interventions in infancy. Mode of feeding in early life has been reported to affect body composition development [8]. Human milk is recommended as the normal and unequalled method for feeding both preterm and term infants [9].

While some authors have investigated the determinants of body composition, including human milk feeding, in very preterm infants at the time of hospital discharge [10,11], there is a paucity of data on early determinants of body composition in late preterm infants who are recognized to be undergoing a critical period of development [12]. Huang et al. [8] have conducted a systematic review and meta-analysis, including infants born before completion of the 37th week of gestational age, to investigate whether body composition at term-corrected age differs between breastfed and formula-fed infants. However, late preterm infants were relatively underrepresented in the investigation. The aim of the present study was to investigate whether human milk consumption in early life could modulate body composition development at term-corrected age in late preterm infants.

2. Materials and Methods

2.1. Design and Setting

We conducted an observational cohort study. Approval was obtained from the institutional review board of Fondazione Istituto di Ricovero e Cura a Carattere Scientifico Cà Granda Ospedale Maggiore Policlinico (code number 506_2015, date of approval: 22 May 2015) and written informed consent from the infants' parents.

2.2. Sample

All consecutive newborns admitted to the authors' institution between July 2015 and May 2016 were screened for eligibility. The inclusion criteria were gestational age from 34 0/7 to 36 6/7, Caucasian parentage and clinical stability at term-corrected age. The exclusion criteria were presence of congenital disease; chromosomal abnormalities; cardiac, brain, renal, endocrine, gastrointestinal or infectious disease; respiratory distress syndrome, defined as the need for any respiratory support for longer than seven days; and pre-pregnancy maternal body mass index >30.

2.3. Nutritional Practices

Infants were fed on demand. Mothers were encouraged either to breastfeed their infant or express their milk according to their infant's clinical condition. According to our internal nutritional procedure, human milk was not fortified [13]. When human milk was unavailable or insufficient, formula feeding was started. Infants born at 34 weeks gestational age and infants born small for gestational age (SGA) at 35–36 weeks gestational age were fed a post-discharge formula (range of protein content: 2–2.4 g/100 mL; range of energy content: 73–82 kcal/100 mL) up to the maximum corrected age of 40 weeks. Late preterm infants, born adequate for gestational age (AGA), at 35–36 weeks of gestational age, were fed a regular-term formula (range of protein content: 1.3–1.7 g/100 mL; range of energy content: 66–68 kcal/100 mL).

2.4. Data Collection

Infants were enrolled at birth. At enrolment, basic subject characteristics such as gestational age at birth, anthropometrics parameters at birth and at discharge (weight, length and head circumference), gender, being a twin, and being adequate for gestational age or small for gestational age were recorded prospectively. Gestational age was based on the last menstrual period and first trimester ultrasonogram. Term-corrected age was calculated from the chronologic age, that is the time elapsed after birth, reduced by the number of weeks the infant was born before the expected date of delivery, that is, 40 weeks of gestation [14]. Infants with birth weight in the <10th or ≥10th percentile for gestational age, based on Fenton's growth chart [15], were, respectively, classified as having weight that was SGA or AGA. The feeding status at discharge (any human milk, including exclusively human milk or exclusively formula) and length of hospital stay were also collected. Specifically, infants fed any extent of human milk, irrespective of the quantity or the exclusivity, were categorized as fed any human milk [9]. After discharge, the parents were asked to report in a diary the mode of feeding from discharge up to term-corrected age (40 weeks $\pm$ 2 days).

2.5. Growth and Body Composition Assessment

Anthropometric measurements were assessed at birth, at discharge and at term-corrected age (40 weeks $\pm$ 2 days). Body weight, length and head circumference were measured according to standard procedures [16]. The weight of each baby was measured on an electronic scale accurate to 0.1 g (PEA POD Infant Body Composition System; Cosmed, Concord, CA, USA). Body length was measured to the nearest 1 mm on a Harpenden neonatometer (Holtain, Crymych, UK). Head circumference was measured to the nearest 1 mm using non-stretch measuring tape. All measurements were assessed by trained medical staff of the author's institution. The late preterm infants' growth (weight, length and head circumference) z-scores were then calculated using the z-score calculator provided by the University of Calgary, Calgary, Alberta, Canada [17]. Body composition was assessed at term-corrected age using an air-displacement plethysmograph (PEA POD Infant Body Composition System; COSMED, Concord, CA, USA). A detailed description of the PEA POD's physical design, operating principles, validation, and measurement procedures is provided elsewhere [18,19]. Briefly, the PEA POD assesses fat mass and fat-free mass by direct measurements of body mass and volume and the application of a classic densitometric model where percentage of body fat is calculated using body density and pre-determined fat and fat-free mass density values. Body fat was defined as body weight minus fat-free mass. A constant fat mass density value of 0.9007 g/mL [20,21] is used. Fat-free mass density values are calculated as the sum of the contribution of the various components in the fat-free mass compartment. Age- and sex-specific fat-free mass density values extrapolated from data by Fomon et al. are used [22].

2.6. Statistical Analysis

All descriptive data are expressed as the mean $\pm$ SD or n (%). The associations between neonatal characteristics (anthropometric measurements at birth and at term-corrected age, feeding status at discharge and at term-corrected age), fat mass and fat-free mass content at term-corrected age were assessed using univariate linear regression analysis. Multiple linear regression models, including variables that resulted to be significant at univariate analysis, were used to identify the determinants of fat mass and fat free mass content at term-corrected age. In order to avoid collinearity, with regard to anthropometric parameters, we included only weight at term-corrected age as independent variable since it was most closely correlated with fat-free mass and fat mass content at term-corrected age in the univariate analysis. Weight was expressed as z-scores, in order to take into account gestational age. All statistical analyses were performed using SPSS (SPSS, version 12; SPSS, Chicago, IL, USA) and Stata (StataCorp. 2013, Stata Statistical Software: Release 13. StataCorp LP, College Station, TX, USA).

3. Results

A total of 284 late preterm infants were enrolled. The flow chart of the study is reported in Figure 1. The mean hospital stay was 8.9 $\pm$ 5.05 days. The mean postmenstrual age at discharge was 36.6 $\pm$ 0.8 weeks. The mean chronological age at term-corrected age was 33.1 $\pm$ 3.6 days.

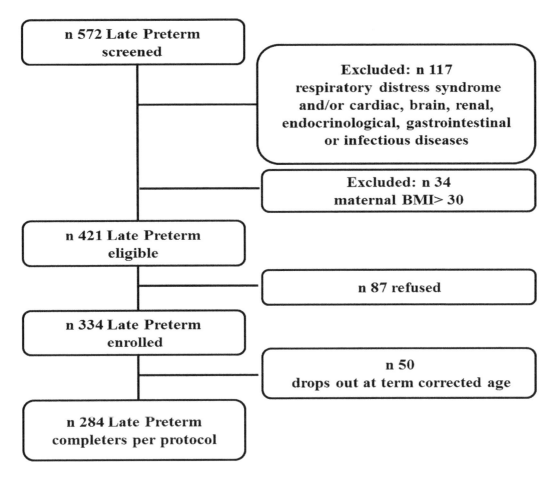

Figure 1. Flow chart of the study.

The basic characteristics of the subjects at birth are shown in Table 1.

Table 1. Basic subject characteristics at birth.

	Late Preterm Infants (*n* = 284)	Males (*n* = 147)	Females (*n* = 137)
Gestational age (weeks)	35.3 ± 0.8	35.2 ± 0.9	35.4 ± 0.7
Birth weight (g)	2413 ± 387	2427 ± 404	2397 ± 369
Length (cm)	45.3 ± 2.4	45.3 ± 2.6	45.3 ± 2.2
Head circumference (cm)	31.9 ± 1.4	31.9 ± 1.6	31.9 ± 1.2
Weight *z*-scores	−0.23 ± 0.87	−0.27 ± 0.8	−0.28 ± 0.8
Length *z*-scores	−0.33 ± 0.91	−0.31 ± 0.9	−0.28 ± 0.8
Head circumference *z*-scores	−0.09 ± 0.88	−0.06 ± 0.9	−0.01 ± 0.8
Small for gestational age *n* (%)	42 (15)	18 (12)	24 (18)
Twins *n* (%)	119 (42)	50 (34)	69 (50)

Data are presented as the mean (SD) or *n* (%).

Mode of feeding, anthropometric parameters and body composition in the enrolled late preterm infants at discharge and at term-corrected age are reported in Tables 2 and 3, respectively.

In the univariate analysis, anthropometric parameters at birth and at term-corrected age, gestational age, being male and being fed human milk at discharge and at term-corrected age were all positively associated with fat-free mass content at term-corrected age, whereas being born small for gestational age and being a twin were negatively associated. With regard to fat mass, anthropometric parameters at birth and at term-corrected age and being exclusively fed human milk at discharge were positively associated with fat mass content at term-corrected age, whereas being born small for gestational age was negatively associated (Table 4).

Table 2. Mode of feeding and anthropometric parameters of the enrolled late preterm infants at discharge.

	Late Preterm Infants (n = 284)	Males (n = 147)	Females (n = 137)
Exclusive human milk n (%)	97 (34)	53 (36)	44 (32)
Exclusive formula n (%)	91 (32)	35 (24)	56 (41)
Any human milk n (%)	193 (68)	112 (77)	81 (59)
Weight (g)	2270 ± 497	2317 ± 442	2200 ± 428
Length (cm)	45.1 ± 2.7	45.1 ± 3.4	45.1 ± 2.2
Head circumference (cm)	31.9 ± 1.4	31.9 ± 1.5	31.8 ± 1.1
Weight z-scores	−0.92 ± 0.8	−0.95 ± 0.8	−0.94 ± 0.8
Length z-scores	−0.70 ± 0.9	−0.85 ± 1.0	−0.53 ± 0.8
Head circumference z-scores	−0.38 ± 0.7	−0.51 ± 0.8	−0.30 ± 0.7

Table 3. Mode of feeding, anthropometric parameters and body composition of the enrolled late preterm infants at term-corrected age.

	Late Preterm Infants (n = 284)	Males (n = 147)	Females (n = 137)
Exclusive human milk n (%)	88 (31)	54 (37)	34 (25)
Exclusive formula n (%)	134 (47)	68 (46)	66 (48)
Any human milk n (%)	150 (53)	79 (54)	71 (52)
Weight (g)	3396 ± 504	3380 ± 526	3240 ± 521
Length (cm)	49.4 ± 2.3	49.7 ± 2.5	49.1 ± 2.2
Head circumference (cm)	35.1 ± 1.6	35.3 ± 2.0	34.7 ± 1.3
Weight z-scores	−0.31 ± 1.1	−0.38 ± 1.1	−0.23 ± 1.0
Length z-scores	−0.56 ± 1.0	−0.59 ± 1.1	−0.53 ± 0.9
Head circumference z-scores	0.14 ± 0.9	0.25 ± 0.9	−0.02 ± 0.9
Fat mass %	14.7 ± 4.7	14.2 ± 4.5	15.3 ± 4.9
Fat free mass %	85.2 ± 4.8	85.8 ± 4.6	84.7 ± 4.9
Fat mass (g)	510 ± 2.1	493.8 ± 204	527.6 ± 219
Fat free mass (g)	2878 ± 392	2934.2 ± 408	2817.1 ± 366

Table 4. Univariate linear regression analysis for associations of infant characteristics, anthropometric parameters and mode of feeding with fat-free mass and fat mass at term-corrected age.

Parameters	Fat-Free Mass at Term-Corrected Age (g)			Fat Mass at Term-Corrected Age (g)		
	β	95% Confidence Interval	p	β	95% Confidence Interval	p
Gestational age (weeks)	64.5	8.1; 120.9	0.025	−5.7	−36.5; 25.0	0.713
Being male (yes vs. no)	117.0	26.1; 207.8	0.012	−33.8	−83.2; 15.7	0.180
Being small for gestational age (no vs. yes)	−401.9	−522.3; −281.5	<0.0001	−128.5	−196.8; 60.3	<0.0001
Weight z-score at birth	280.9	238.1; 323.7	<0.0001	92.5	65.4; 119.6	<0.0001
Length z-score at birth	175.0	129; 220.9	<0.0001	60.8	34.5; 87.1	<0.0001
Head circumference z-score at birth	156.4	107.3; 205.4	<0.0001	57.5	29.9; 85.0	<0.0001
Weight z-score at term-corrected age	307.1	283.9; 330.2	<0.0001	140.3	124.1; 156.6	<0.0001
Length z-score at term-corrected age	246.4	212.4; 280.4	<0.0001	103.6	82.7; 124.4	<0.0001
Head circumference z-score at term-corrected age	232.5	191.3; 273.6	<0.0001	87.5	62.8; 112.1	<0.0001
Being twin (no vs. yes)	−187.6	−289.6; −85.6	<0.0001	−32.8	−89.8; 24.8	0.256
Being exclusively human milk fed vs. exclusively formula fed at discharge	−333	−483.6; −183.5	<0.0001	−99.1	−179.1; −19.1	0.016
Being fed any human milk vs. exclusively formula fed at discharge	−223	−337.9; −109.0	<0.0001	−43.6	−110.0; 22.9	0.197
Being exclusively human milk fed vs. exclusively formula fed at term-corrected age	−226	−344.6; 109.1	<0.0001	17.8	−48.1; 83.8	0.594
Being fed any human milk vs. exclusively formula fed at term-corrected age	−227	−327.8; −126.2	<0.0001	−7.8	−65.0; 49.4	0.788

At multiple regression analysis, when including mode of feeding at discharge, being male, weight z-score at term-corrected age and being fed any human milk at discharge were positively associated with fat-free mass content at term-corrected age (Tables 5 and 6).

Table 5. Multiple linear regression analysis for associations of gender, weight z-score at term-corrected age, being a twin and being exclusively fed human milk at discharge with fat-free mass at term-corrected age ($R^2 = 0.88$, $p < 0.0001$).

Model	Fat-Free Mass Content at Term-Corrected Age (g)		
	β	95% Confidence Interval	p
Intercept	3008.4	2898.5; 3118.3	<0.0001
Male (yes vs. no)	80.6	20.6; 140.6	0.009
Being a twin (no vs. yes)	−7.9	−73.4; 57.6	0.8
Weight z-score at term-corrected age	361.2	327.9; 394.6	<0.0001
Mode of feeding at discharge (being exclusively human milk fed vs. being exclusively formula fed)	−39.6	−102.4; 23.2	0.214

Table 6. Multiple linear regression analysis for associations of gender, weight z-score at term-corrected age, being a twin and being fed any human milk at discharge with fat-free mass at term-corrected age ($R^2 = 0.85$, $p < 0.0001$).

Model	Fat-Free Mass Content at Term-Corrected Age (g)		
	β	95% Confidence Interval	p
Intercept	3037.2	2961.2; 3113.1	<0.0001
Male (yes vs. no)	68.0	24.2; 111.7	0.002
Being a twin (no vs. yes)	−38.7	−82.3; 4.7	0.08
Weight z-score at term-corrected age	347.7	325.2; 370.2	<0.0001
Mode of feeding at discharge (being fed any human milk vs. being exclusively formula fed)	−47.9	−95.7; −0.18	0.049

With regard to fat mass content, the weight z-score at term-corrected age was positively associated with its content at term-corrected age, whereas the mode of feeding was not significantly associated (Table 7).

Table 7. Multiple linear regression analysis for associations of weight z-score at term-corrected age, and being exclusively human milk fed at discharge with fat mass at term-corrected age ($R^2 = 0.63$, $p < 0.0001$).

Model	Fat Mass Content at Term-Corrected Age (g)		
	β	95% Confidence Interval	p
Intercept	517.7	430.8; 604.5	<0.0001
Weight z-score at term-corrected age	164.9	137.8; 192.0	<0.0001
Mode of feeding at discharge (being exclusively human milk fed vs. being exclusively formula fed)	27.2	−27.0; 81.5	0.321

In the multiple regression analysis, when including the mode of feeding at term-corrected age, being male, the weight z-score at term-corrected age and being fed either exclusively or any human milk at term-corrected age were positively associated with fat-free mass content at term-corrected age (Tables 8 and 9).

Table 8. Multiple linear regression analysis for associations of gender, weight z-score at term-corrected age, being a twin and being fed exclusively human milk at term-corrected age with fat-free mass at term-corrected age ($R^2 = 0.88$, $p < 0.0001$).

Model	Fat-Free Mass Content at Term-Corrected Age (g)		
	β	95% Confidence Interval	p
Intercept	3098.2	3018.1; 3178.3	<0.0001
Male (yes vs. no)	84.3	41.1; 127.4	<0.0001
Being a twin (no vs. yes)	23.4	−23.6; 70.4	0.32
Weight z-score at term-corrected age	355.0	332.8; 377.2	<0.0001
Mode of feeding at term-corrected age (being exclusively human milk fed vs. being exclusively formula fed)	−104.1	−151.4; −56.7	<0.0001

Table 9. Multiple linear regression analysis for associations of gender, weight z-score at term-corrected age, being a twin and being fed any human milk at term-corrected age with fat-free mass at term-corrected age ($R^2 = 0.86$, $p < 0.0001$).

Model	Fat-Free Mass Content at Term-Corrected Age (g)		
	β	95% Confidence Interval	p
Intercept	3088.1	3023.3; 3152.9	<0.0001
Male (yes vs. no)	75.0	34.8; 115.2	<0.0001
Being a twin (no vs. yes)	1.5	−41.2; 44.2	0.94
Weight z-score at term-corrected age	354.5	333.7; 375.3	<0.0001
Mode of feeding at term-corrected age (being fed any human milk vs. being exclusively formula fed)	−89.6	−131.5; −47.7	<0.0001

4. Discussion

The findings of this study indicate that the consumption of human milk is associated with fat-free mass deposition in late preterm infants. It must be taken into account that the strength of this relationship appears to become stronger towards the achievement of term-corrected age, suggesting a potential cumulative effect of human milk consumption on body composition development.

Fat-free mass content has been recognized to positively modulate central nervous system development because greater fat-free mass gains during the hospital stay have been associated with improved cognitive and motor scores at one year of corrected age in very-low-birth-weight infants [23]. In addition, higher fat-free mass content in former preterm infants at four months of corrected age was found to be associated with shorter brain speed processing [7]. On the other hand, the consumption of human milk at term-corrected age was found to be negatively associated with fat mass deposition. Considering that late preterm infants are at risk for developing increased adiposity at term-corrected age [3,4], which in turn could represent a risk factor for developing metabolic syndrome later in life, it could be speculated that human milk exerts a potentially protective effect in late preterm infants against obesity risk.

The present results are consistent with previous data published in the literature. Larcade et al. [11] reported that the number of days very preterm infants were fed human milk during their hospital stay positively correlated with fat-free mass content at discharge. Accordingly, Huang et al. [8] conducted a meta-analysis investigating the effect of breastfeeding and formula feeding on the body composition of 642 preterm infants (<37 weeks of gestational age). The authors found significantly lower fat mass in breastfed infants in comparison to formula-fed infants (mean difference 0.24; 95% CI 0.17,

0.31 kg) at term-corrected age. These results differ from those reported by Gale et al. [24] who found significantly higher fat mass content in healthy, full-term, breastfed infants at three to four months of age in comparison to formula-fed infants. However, it must be taken into account that preterm infants, including those born between 34 and 36 weeks of gestation, still need to complete their organ development and present a lack of both fat-free mass and fat mass at birth because premature birth interrupts the physiologic development of body composition [25]. Furthermore, it has been demonstrated that the early postnatal growth of late preterm infants is characterized by a major deposition of fat mass so that at term-corrected age, late preterm infants show a higher fat mass content than term infants [3,4]. Hence, the promotion of fat-free mass accretion by consumption of human milk may represent a physiological compensatory mechanism aimed at recovering body composition, promoting neurodevelopment and protecting preterm infants from potential unbalanced nutritional intake provided by infant formulas.

In the present study, not surprisingly, weight z-scores at birth and at term-corrected age were positively associated with fat-free mass at term-corrected age. Indeed, the fat-free mass compartment accounts for the majority of the weight [25]. In addition, the finding that weight z-scores at term-corrected age are positively associated with fat mass content at term-corrected age can be explained by the fact that the early postnatal growth of late preterm infants is characterized by a major deposition of fat mass [4]. Consistently with previous data reported in the literature [26], being male was positively associated with fat-free mass content at term-corrected age.

While this study is of clinical interest, it presents some limitations. First of all, the data collected in the present study refer to late preterm infants not affected by comorbidities, so that their effect on body composition development has not been assessed. Furthermore, body composition was evaluated only at one time point, and as a result, the effect of human milk feeding over time has not been investigated. The main strength of the paper is represented by the fact that body composition data have been collected from a large number of late preterm infants.

5. Conclusions

The findings from this study indicate that human milk feeding appears to be associated with early fat-free mass deposition in late preterm infants. On the basis of the present results, health care professionals should direct efforts toward promoting and supporting breastfeeding in these vulnerable infants. Future research is desirable to explore the effect of comorbidities and the persistence of the effect of human milk consumption on body composition development in late preterm infants.

Author Contributions: M.L.G. conceived and designed the study and wrote the article; D.C. analyzed the data and contributed to the discussion of the results; N.L. analyzed the data and contributed to the discussion of the results; P.R. was responsible for database management; L.M., P.P. and C.M. collected the data; F.M. provided suggestions concerning the content and concept of the article.

References

1. Dong, Y.; Yu, J.L. An overview of morbidity, mortality and long-term outcome of late preterm birth. *World J. Pediatr.* **2011**, *7*, 199–204. [CrossRef] [PubMed]
2. Engle, W.A. Morbidity and mortality in late preterm and early term newborns: A continuum. *Clin. Perinatol.* **2011**, *38*, 493–516. [CrossRef] [PubMed]
3. Giannì, M.L.; Roggero, P.; Liotto, N.; Amato, O.; Piemontese, P.; Morniroli, D.; Bracco, B.; Mosca, F. Postnatal!catch-up fat after late preterm birth. *Pediatr. Res.* **2012**, *72*, 637–640. [CrossRef] [PubMed]
4. Giannì, M.L.; Roggero, P.; Liotto, N.; Taroni, F.; Polimeni, A.; Morlacchi, L.; Piemontese, P.; Consonni, D.; Mosca, F. Body composition in late preterm infants according to percentile at birth. *Pediatr. Res.* **2016**, *79*, 710–715. [CrossRef] [PubMed]

5. Koletzko, B.; Brands, B.; Chourdakis, M.; Cramer, S.; Grote, V.; Hellmuth, C.; Kirchberg, F.; Prell, C.; Rzehak, P.; Uhl, O.; et al. The Power of Programming and the EarlyNutrition project: Opportunities for health promotion by nutrition during the first thousand days of life and beyond. *Ann. Nutr. Metab.* **2014**, *64*, 187–196. [CrossRef] [PubMed]

6. Roy, S.M.; Spivack, J.G.; Faith, M.S.; Chesi, A.; Mitchell, J.A.; Kelly, A.; Grant, S.F.; McCormack, S.E.; Zemel, B.S. Infant BMI or weight-for-length and obesity risk in early childhood. *Pediatrics* **2016**, *137*. [CrossRef] [PubMed]

7. Pfister, K.M.; Gray, H.L.; Miller, N.C.; Demerath, E.W.; Georgieff, M.K.; Ramel, S.E. Exploratory study of the relationship of fat-free mass to speed of brain processing in preterm infants. *Pediatr. Res.* **2013**, *74*, 576–583. [CrossRef] [PubMed]

8. Huang, P.; Zhou, J.; Yin, Y.; Jing, W.; Luo, B.; Wang, J. Effects of breast-feeding compared with formula-feeding on preterm infant body composition: A systematic review and meta-analysis. *Br. J. Nutr.* **2016**, *116*, 132–141. [CrossRef] [PubMed]

9. American Academy of Pediatrics. Section on Breastfeeding. Breastfeeding and the use of human milk. *Pediatrics* **2012**, *129*, e827–e841.

10. Simon, L.; Frondas-Chauty, A.; Senterre, T.; Flamant, C.; Darmaun, D.; Rozé, J.C. Determinants of body composition in preterm infants at the time of hospital discharge. *Am. J. Clin. Nutr.* **2014**, *100*, 98–104. [CrossRef] [PubMed]

11. Larcade, J.; Pradat, P.; Buffin, R.; Leick-Courtois, C.; Jourdes, E.; Picaud, J.C. Estimation of fat-free mass at discharge in preterm infants fed with optimized feeding regimen. *J. Pediatr. Gastroenterol. Nutr.* **2016**. [CrossRef] [PubMed]

12. Kugelman, A.; Colin, A.A. Late preterm infants: Near term but still in a critical developmental time period. *Pediatrics* **2013**, *132*, 741–751. [CrossRef] [PubMed]

13. Giannì, M.L.; Roggero, P.; Piemontese, P.; Liotto, N.; Orsi, A.; Amato, O.; Taroni, F.; Morlacchi, L.; Consonni, D.; Mosca, F. Is nutritional support needed in late preterm infants? *BMC Pediatr.* **2015**, *15*, 194. [CrossRef] [PubMed]

14. Engle, W.A.; American Academy of Pediatrics Committee on Fetus and Newborn. Age terminology during the perinatal period. *Pediatrics* **2004**, *114*, 1362–1364. [PubMed]

15. Fenton, T.R. A new growth chart for preterm babies: Babson and Benda's chart updated with recent data and a new format. *BMC Pediatr.* **2003**, *16*, 3–13. [CrossRef] [PubMed]

16. Agostoni, C.; Grandi, F.; Scaglioni, S.; Giannì, M.L.; Torcoletti, M.; Radaelli, G.; Fiocchi, A.; Riva, E. Growth pattern of breastfed and non breastfed infants with atopic dermatitis in the first year of life. *Pediatrics* **2000**, *106*, E73. [CrossRef] [PubMed]

17. Two Apps Are Available Based on the 2013 Fenton Growth Charts. Available online: http://ucalgary.ca/fenton (accessed on 1 July 2016).

18. Roggero, P.; Giannì, M.L.; Amato, O.; Piemontese, P.; Morniroli, D.; Wong, W.W.; Mosca, F. Evaluation of air-displacement plethysmography for body composition assessment in preterm infants. *Pediatr. Res.* **2012**, *72*, 316–320. [CrossRef] [PubMed]

19. Urlando, A.; Dempster, P.; Aitkens, S. A new air displacement plethysmograph for the measurement of body composition in infants. *Pediatr. Res.* **2003**, *53*, 486–492. [CrossRef] [PubMed]

20. Going, S.B. Hydrodensitometry and air displacement plethysmography. In *Human Body Composition*, 2nd ed.; Heymsfield, S.B., Lohman, T.G., Wang, Z., Eds.; Human Kinetics: Champaign, IL, USA, 2005; pp. 17–34.

21. Brozek, J.; Grande, F.; Anderson, J.T.; Keys, A. Densitometric analysis of body composition: Revision of some quantitative assumptions. *Ann. N. Y. Acad. Sci.* **1963**, *11*, 113–340.

22. Fomon, S.J.; Haschke, F.; Ziegler, E.E.; Nelson, S.E. Body composition of reference children from birth to age 10 years. *Am. J. Clin. Nutr.* **1982**, *35*, 1169–1175. [PubMed]

23. Ramel, S.E.; Gray, H.L.; Christiansen, E.; Boys, C.; Georgieff, M.K.; Demerath, E.W. Greater early gains in fat-free mass, but not fat mass, are associated with improved neurodevelopment at 1 year corrected age for prematurity in very low birth weight preterm infants. *J. Pediatr.* **2016**, *173*, 108–115. [CrossRef] [PubMed]

24. Gale, C.; Logan, K.M.; Santhakumaran, S.; Parkinson, J.R.; Hyde, M.J.; Modi, N. Effect of breastfeeding compared with formula feeding on infant body composition: A systematic review and meta-analysis. *Am. J. Clin. Nutr.* **2012**, *95*, 656–669. [CrossRef] [PubMed]
25. Micheli, J.L.; Pfister, R.; Junod, S.; Laubscher, B.; Tolsa, J.F.; Schutz, Y.; Calame, A. Water, energy and early postnatal growth in preterm infants. *Acta Paediatr. Suppl.* **1994**, *405*, 35–42. [CrossRef] [PubMed]
26. Simon, L.; Borrego, P.; Darmaun, D.; Legrand, A.; Rozé, J.C.; Chauty-Frondas, A. Effect of sex and gestational age on neonatal body composition. *Br. J. Nutr.* **2013**, *109*, 1105–1108. [CrossRef] [PubMed]

11

Assessment of Breast Milk Iodine Concentrations in Lactating Women in Western Australia

Anita Jorgensen [1,*], Peter O'Leary [2], Ian James [3], Sheila Skeaff [4] and Jillian Sherriff [1]

[1] School of Public Health, Curtin University, Perth 6102, Australia; j.sherriff@curtin.edu.au
[2] Faculty of Health Sciences, Curtin University, Perth 6102, Australia; peter.oleary@curtin.edu.au
[3] Institute for Immunology & Infectious Diseases, Murdoch University, Murdoch 6150, Australia; i.james@murdoch.edu.au
[4] Department of Human Nutrition, University of Otago, Dunedin 9054, New Zealand; sheila.skeaff@otago.ac.nz
[*] Correspondence: a.jorgensen@curtin.edu.au

Abstract: Breast-fed infants may depend solely on an adequate supply of iodine in breast milk for the synthesis of thyroid hormones which are essential for optimal growth and cognitive development. This is the first study to measure breast milk iodine concentration (BMIC) among lactating women in Western Australian ($n = 55$). Breast milk samples were collected between 2014 and 2015 at a mean ($\pm$SD) of 38.5 ($\pm$5.5) days post-partum. The samples were analysed to determine median BMIC and the percentage of samples with a BMIC < 100 µg/L, a level considered adequate for breast-fed infants. The influence of (a) iodine-containing supplements and iodised salt use and (b) consumption of key iodine-containing foods on BMIC was also examined. The median (p25, p75) BMIC was 167 (99, 248) µg/L and 26% of samples had a BMIC < 100 µg/L. Overall, BMIC tended to be higher with iodine-containing supplement usage (ratio 1.33, 95% confidence interval (CI) (1.04, 1.70), $p = 0.030$), cow's milk consumption (ratio 1.66, 95% CI (1.23, 2.23), $p = 0.002$) and lower for Caucasians (ratio 0.61, 95% CI (0.45, 0.83), $p = 0.002$), and those with secondary school only education (ratio 0.66, 95% CI (0.46, 0.96), $p = 0.030$). For most women, BMIC was adequate to meet the iodine requirements of their breast-fed infants. However, some women may require the use of iodine-containing supplements or iodised salt to increase BMIC to adequate levels for optimal infant nutrition.

Keywords: iodine; breast milk; supplementation; iodine status

---

1. Introduction

Iodine, an essential nutrient, is required by humans for the synthesis of thyroid hormones which are vital for normal growth and development [1,2]. A regular and adequate supply of iodine is particularly important during the critical period for brain and central nervous system development, namely, from the second trimester of pregnancy to 3 years of age [1]. Iodine deficiency during this time results in a spectrum of adverse effects known as iodine deficiency disorders, with the most severe outcomes, irreversible mental impairment and cretinism, resulting from severe iodine deficiency during pregnancy. In infants, iodine deficiency leading to inadequate thyroid activity results in delayed growth and physical development, and impaired cognitive function [1,2].

During intrauterine life, iodine is transferred from the mother to the fetus [3]. This results in a pool of iodine stored in the fetal thyroid gland, with the size of the pool strongly reflecting maternal dietary iodine intake. However, even under conditions of maternal iodine sufficiency, this fetal iodine pool is small and turns over rapidly after birth to partly support the iodine demand of newborns [4]. Infants, however, rely solely on dietary sources to meet their iodine needs. Breast-fed infants are particularly vulnerable to iodine deficiency as they may be completely dependent on the iodine concentration of breast milk for their intake of iodine [5]. Consequently, maternal iodine requirements are increased during breastfeeding to provide sufficient amounts for the mother and to also meet the iodine demands of the developing infant, via breast milk. Given that 40%–45% of the iodine ingested by the mother appears in breast milk [6], a maternal iodine intake during breastfeeding of 190 μg/day (Australian Estimated Average Requirement (EAR)) would provide just under the Australian Adequate Intake (AI) of 90 μg/day for infants aged 0–6 months [7]. This is achieved by a physiological response during breastfeeding whereby iodine is strongly concentrated by the lactating mammary gland due to the increased expression of the sodium iodide symporter, the main iodine transporter in lactating breast cells [8]. This results in human milk having an iodine concentration 20–50 times higher than that of plasma [4].

Breast milk iodine concentration (BMIC) is influenced by, and may be an indicator of, maternal iodine status during breastfeeding [4,5,8–11]. BMIC is also influenced by other factors including recent maternal iodine intake [12] and duration of lactation [5]. While no reference ranges for the adequate iodine concentration of breast milk have been specified, values above 75 μg/L have been suggested to indicate sufficient maternal iodine intake [4]. An iodine balance study of full-term infants found that a positive iodine balance is only achieved when iodine intake is 15 μg/kg per day, which equates to a BMIC of 100–200 μg/L [8].

A wide range of median or mean BMIC values has been reported in several reviews conducted in areas of varying iodine sufficiency [4,8,10]. BMIC typically ranges from <50 μg/L in iodine-deficient areas [5] to 100–150 μg/L in areas of iodine sufficiency [4] and as high as 150–180 μg/L in areas of good iodine supply [8,10]. A BMIC < 100 μg/L has been identified in studies from France, Germany, Belgium, Sweden, Spain, Italy, Denmark, Thailand and Zaire while studies from Iran, China, USA and some parts of Europe have identified above this level [4]. A recent study in Nepal identified a median BMIC of 250 μg/L, and the estimated iodine intake of the infants involved (0–6 months) was 200 μg/day [13]. WHO's recommended maximum iodine intake for infants <2 years old is 180 μg/day [14], therefore some infants in this area may be consuming excessive iodine intakes through breast milk [13]. This can result in subclinical hypothyroidism and permanently affect their neurodevelopment [15].

In recent decades, Australia has been regarded as a country with mild iodine deficiency. Two initiatives introduced in response to the re-emergence of this public health issue are the mandatory fortification of all bread (except organic) with iodised salt in 2009 [16] and the 2010 National Health and Medical Research Council recommendation that all pregnant and breastfeeding women take a daily supplement containing 150 μg of iodine [17]. Despite this recommendation, only two studies have examined the iodine content of breast milk in Australia to assess either iodine provision to breastfed infants or maternal iodine status. The first was a small ($n = 50$) cross-sectional study of breastfeeding women in Sydney, conducted more than a decade ago and prior to mandatory iodine fortification. This study identified a median BMIC of 84 μg/L [18], indicating inadequate maternal iodine intake based on the adequate cut-off of 100 μg/L. The second larger and more recent study compared the BMIC of lactating women in South Australia pre- ($n = 291$) and post- ($n = 653$) mandatory fortification. The median BMIC of samples from both periods were indicative of adequate breast milk iodine levels, however, BMIC was significantly higher in the post-fortification samples compared with the pre-fortification samples (187 vs. 103 μg/L; $p < 0.05$) [19].

To date, there is no information regarding BMIC for lactating mothers in Western Australia (WA), nor for iodine status of WA breastfeeding women. WA has long been considered an iodine-sufficient area of Australia, based on measures of iodine status in studies involving school-children and adults [20,21]. However, this outcome may not reflect the iodine status in breastfeeding women, who have substantially greater requirements for iodine [1]. In the present study we examined BMIC in breastfeeding women in a local cohort to determine adequacy of iodine provision to breastfed infants. We also investigated the influence of iodine-containing supplements and iodised salt use, as well as the consumption of key iodine-containing foods, on this biomarker of iodine status.

2. Materials and Methods

2.1. Subjects and Design

Participants were recruited in 2013–2014 as part of the Perth Iodine and Pregnancy Study II (PIPS II) via advertising (flyer in private women's ultrasound practices $n = 15$ and newspaper, radio and websites $n = 7$), in-person by study coordinator (public maternity hospital antenatal clinics $n = 21$ and pathology centre $n = 3$) and word of mouth ($n = 8$). At the time of recruitment, women were aged 18 years and over and were in the first or second trimester of pregnancy (gestation range 5–22 weeks). Other inclusion criteria were no history of thyroid disease, not currently taking thyroid medication, having a singleton birth and not currently breastfeeding but with the intention to breastfeed their baby. Women were excluded from the study if English was not the main language spoken at home. The study was approved by the Curtin University (Approval No. HR 47/2013; 15 April 2013) and Women and Newborn Health Service Human Research Ethics Committees (Approval No. 2014075EW; 4 August 2014) and informed written consent was obtained from each participant.

Breast milk samples were collected between February 2014 and August 2015. Participants were mailed vials for sampling together with instructions to provide (duplicate) 5 mL nonfasted breast milk samples at home at the start of a single morning feed (preferably between 0900 and 1200 h) when their baby was aged 4–6 weeks. Women were asked to record baby's age and time of day of sampling. Participants were also asked to provide information on current medication use, daily use of dietary supplements, daily intake (yes/no) of any amount of six key iodine-containing foods (cow's milk, cheese, ice cream, yoghurt, bread/bread products, eggs), use of iodised salt (yes/no) and whether or not they smoke cigarettes. Sociodemographic characteristics of the women, namely parity, age, postcode, ethnicity, household income and education, had been collected previously.

2.2. Laboratory Procedures

Breast milk samples were stored at $-20\ ^\circ$C from time of sampling until collection and then at $-80\ ^\circ$C until analysis. After thawing, milk samples were homogenized before analysis by inductively coupled plasma mass spectrometry (ICPMS) in an accredited commercial laboratory (PathWest Laboratory Medicine WA, Nedlands, Australia). ICPMS is considered the gold standard to determine iodine concentration in complex sample matrices such as breast milk [9,22]. An optimised ICPMS method for breast milk has been published recently [22] and was adapted for this study. In brief, sonicated breast milk samples were diluted in mild alkali solution, ionized with inductively coupled plasma and the ions separated and quantified in a Perkin Elmer NexION 300 ICP-MS mass spectrometer (PerkinElmer Inc., Waltham, MA, USA).

2.3. Statistical Analysis

Distributions of BMIC were skewed and descriptive statistics reported as medians and 25th, 75th percentile. The proportion of women with BMIC $< 100\ \mu$g/L, the suggested cut-off for providing an adequate iodine supply to breast-fed infants, was also determined. Statistical analyses of BMIC were carried out on the log base 10 scale to better approximate normality. Multiple regression analyses were used to assess associations of BMIC with: (a) use of iodine supplements and iodised salt; (b) daily consumption of six key iodine-containing foods (yes/no); and (c) all studied factors simultaneously. Associations of cohort characteristics with use of iodised salt or iodine supplements were assessed via logistic regressions. Data were analysed using IBM SPSS version 20 (IBM Corporation, Tokyo, Japan) and TIBCO Spotfire S+ version 8.2 (TIBCO Software Inc., Boston, MA, USA). A 5% level of significance was chosen.

3. Results

Sociodemographic characteristics of the 55 study participants are shown in Table 1. The mean age ($\pm$standard deviation (SD)) of the study women was 31.4 ($\pm$4.7) years. This is consistent with the average age of women who gave birth in WA in 2013 of 29.8 years [23]. The majority of women were pregnant for the first time (52.7%), were tertiary educated (72.3%), had a total household income of >$AUS100K (67.3%) and were Caucasian (80.0%). Compared with available Western Australian data from the Australian Bureau of Statistics Census 2011, our cohort included an over representation of women with a higher reported education level and higher household incomes [24]. All women provided breast milk samples, however one woman was excluded as she reported being a smoker, thus leaving 54 women for breast milk analysis. Breast milk samples were collected at 28–56 days postpartum with a mean (±SD) of 38.5 (±5.5) days. All samples were provided in the morning between 0600 h and 1200 h. The median (p25, p75) BMIC was 167 (99, 248) μg/L indicating adequate maternal iodine intake for the group. However, 26% of women had BMIC less than the suggested cut-off level for adequacy of 100 μg/L (see Figure 1).

Table 1. Sociodemographic characteristics of study participants (n = 55).

	n	%
First pregnancy		
Yes	29	52.7
No	26	47.3
Highest education [1]		
Secondary school	7	12.7
Trade or technical	3	5.5
Diploma	5	9.1
Professional	2	3.6
Bachelor degree	22	40.0
Postgraduate university	16	29.1
Total household income		
<$AUS50K	8	14.5
$AUS50–100K	8	14.5
>$AUS100K	37	67.3
Don't wish to answer	2	3.6
Ethnicity		
Caucasian	44	80.0
Non-Caucasian	11	20.0

[1] Tertiary educated includes Professional, Bachelor degree and Postgraduate university.

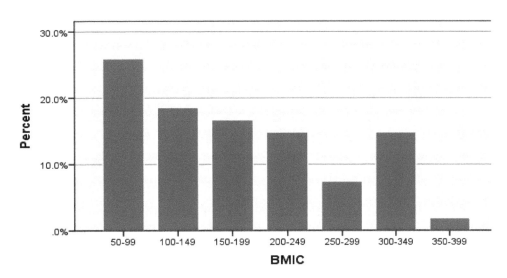

Figure 1. Percentage distribution of breast milk iodine concentration (BMIC) (μg/L).

Thirty-one women (57.4%) reported the daily use of an iodine-containing supplement, some of which contained less than the amount recommended (i.e., 150 µg). Use of iodised salt and iodine-containing supplements were independently associated with increases of similar magnitudes in BMIC (ratio 1.37, 95% CI (1.05, 1.80), $p = 0.025$ and ratio 1.37, 95% CI (1.04, 1.79), $p = 0.029$, respectively—see Table 2). There was no significant difference ($p = 0.96$) between the median BMIC values for the use of either iodised salt or iodine-containing supplements without the other. Among all cohort characteristics jointly considered only low household income (<\$AUS50K) remained significantly (negatively) associated with iodine supplement usage (1/8 vs. 30/46, $p = 0.010$ Fisher test). Exactly half of the women reported using iodised salt, with usage higher among non-Caucasians (10/11 vs. 17/43, $p = 0.005$).

Table 2. Effect of iodine supplement and iodised salt use on BMIC.

	n	Median BMIC (µg/L)
Yes supplement + Yes salt	15	272 **
Yes supplement + No salt	16	151 *
No supplement + Yes salt	12	156 *
No supplement + No salt	11	98 **

Overall $p = 0.028$; * There was no difference between the 'Yes supplement + No salt' and 'No Supplement + Yes salt' groups ($p = 0.960$); ** There was a significant difference between the 'Yes supplement + Yes salt' and 'No supplement + No salt' groups ($p = 0.003$).

For the six key iodine-containing foods, the majority of women reported daily consumption of bread/bread products (79.6%) and cow's milk (77.8%) and with just less than half of women (46.3%) reporting daily intake of cheese. Furthermore, about a third of women (37.0%) reported daily consumption of yoghurt, around a quarter (27.8%) ate eggs daily and 5.6% of women said they ate ice cream each day. However, only daily cow's milk intake was significantly associated with higher BMIC values after adjusting for the other foods or on its own (ratio 1.44, 95% CI (1.01, 2.06), $p = 0.49$ and ratio 1.44, 95% CI (1.03, 2.01), $p = 0.040$, respectively). None of the other foods were significant, jointly or marginally, in influencing BMIC values. Furthermore, cow's milk remained the only food positively associated with BMIC after adjustment for iodine-containing supplements and iodised salt use (ratio 1.50, 95% CI (1.10, 2.04), $p = 0.013$). Overall in the joint model, BMIC tended to be higher with iodine-containing supplement usage and cow's milk consumption and lower for Caucasians and those with secondary school only education (see Table 3).

Table 3. Significant joint explanatory variables for BMIC *.

Variable	Ratio ** (95% CI)	p-Value
Caucasian ethnicity	0.61 (0.45, 0.83)	0.002
School only education	0.66 (0.46, 0.96)	0.030
Iodine supplement use	1.33 (1.04, 1.70)	0.030
Cow's milk consumption	1.66 (1.23, 2.23)	0.002

* Analyses carried out on the log BMIC scale with non-significant terms (sociodemographic and dietary factors) removed by backwards elimination; ** Exponentiated coefficient from the joint model for log (BMIC) predicts the ratio of BMIC for the listed category relative to those not in the category, given fixed values of the other variables.

4. Discussion

This is the first study to report BMIC values for breastfeeding women in Western Australia. The median BMIC value of women would provide an adequate iodine supply for breastfed infants. However, BMIC levels were below the suggested adequate cut-off (100 µg/L) for 26% of women, indicating some infants may be at risk for iodine deficiency, especially if exclusively breast-fed as is recommended. These findings are consistent with results for the post-fortification cohort of the recent South Australian study. However, compared to our study, the proportion of women with BMIC below the adequate cut-off level was considerably lower in the study by Huynh et al. (26% vs. 13%) [19]. The one participant who reported being a smoker in the present study was excluded from breast milk analysis as the chemical thiocyanate found in cigarettes competitively inhibits the sodium iodide transporter in the lactating breast and impairs iodine transport into breast milk [25], thereby distorting BMIC values.

Despite the NHMRC recommendation for all breastfeeding women to use a daily 150 μg iodine supplement, only about half of the women (54%) in the present study reported behaviour consistent with this (an additional two women reported use of a daily iodine supplement containing less than the recommended iodine amount). In a recent study of breastfeeding women conducted in regional New South Wales ($n = 60$), iodine-containing supplements were being taken by 45% of women, although frequency of use and iodine content were not documented [26]. These results suggest a low level of awareness and/or compliance amongst Australian breastfeeding women regarding the national iodine supplement recommendations. In contrast, 90% of South Australian women in the post-fortification cohort reported use of supplements containing any iodine [19], although again details of frequency of use and iodine content were not documented. Furthermore, given the low use of iodine-containing supplements in low income cases compared to higher income participants (12.5% vs. 65.2%, respectively) in the present study, perhaps the availability of government subsidized iodine supplements is warranted in Australia, as is the case in New Zealand. Interestingly, in the Perth Infant Feeding Study Mark II conducted in 2002–2003 prior to the supplement recommendation, no breastfeeding women reported taking iodine supplements [27].

In addition, 50% of women in the present study reported using iodised salt. This is similar to the 45% of lactating women using iodised salt in the regional New South Wales study by Charlton et al. [26]. In the present study, use of iodised salt was significantly higher among non-Caucasians ($p = 0.013$), possibly explaining why BMIC tended to be higher in non-Caucasian mothers compared with Caucasian mothers ($p = 0.002$). This later finding is consistent with the results of the South Australian study by Huynh et al. [19].

As shown in Table 2, use of both iodine-containing supplements and iodised salt together resulted in the highest median BMIC value (272 μg/L). The use of either iodine-containing supplements or iodised salt had similar positive effects on median BMIC values, suggesting both methods are equally effective in improving the iodine content of breast milk. Our results are consistent with other recent studies that have examined the effect of supplementation and/or iodised salt use on breast milk iodine content [28,29]. The lowest median BMIC was recorded for those women using neither iodine-containing supplements nor iodised salt. This median BMIC value of 98 μg/L is borderline for inadequate BMIC using the cut-off of 100 μg/L. This suggests that for women in our study, food sources alone may not provide the amounts of iodine required during breastfeeding to meet maternal and infant needs. Furthermore, given breast milk samples in the present study were provided in the early post-partum period and BMIC of iodine-deficient lactating women has been shown to decrease in the first 6 months postpartum [5], the use of some form of iodine supplementation by these women is important.

Of the six key iodine-containing foods examined in the study, only daily cow's milk consumption was significantly associated with higher BMIC values, independent of other foods and supplement and iodised salt use. Some cow's milk was consumed daily by more than three-quarters of women in the study. Despite quantity not being examined in the present study, this suggests the importance of cow's milk consumption in terms of iodine intake for breastfeeding women. Interestingly, milk and dairy foods were the highest contributors to iodine intake in the study by Charlton et al. which used a self-administered validated iodine-specific food frequency questionnaire to assess dietary iodine intake of Australian breastfeeding women [26]. Conversely, daily consumption of bread/bread products was not associated with higher BMIC values, despite the fact that a very high proportion of women reported consumption of these foods daily and their known fortification with iodine. This finding therefore questions the impact of the bread fortification initiative for lactating women in relation to BMIC.

There are some limitations to the interpretation of our study findings. Firstly, the impact of time of supplement intake, iodised salt use and consumption of key iodine-containing foods relative to breast milk sampling were not examined. Leung et al. [12] reported a rise in BMIC following acute oral ingestion of 600 μg potassium iodide, with peak levels at 6 h post-ingestion, and concluded that recent maternal iodine intake would influence the interpretation of BMIC values. Furthermore, as BMIC values fluctuate throughout the day, single breast milk samples provide an imprecise measurement of daily iodine output or maternal iodine sufficiency [30]. In addition, actual compliance with reported supplement use, use of iodised salt or intake of foods examined in the 24-h prior to breast milk sampling could not be confirmed with participants. Finally, while the study included a cross-section of breastfeeding women from both public and private health care systems, the sample size is relatively small and all women who participated (bar one) lived in the Perth metropolitan area, so generalisability of results to the wider breastfeeding population is made with qualifications.

5. Conclusions

Despite these limitations, for the majority of women in the present study, BMIC was adequate to meet the iodine requirement of their breast-fed infants. However, the study also indicates that some breast-fed infants may be at risk of iodine deficiency, which could potentially be reduced by the maternal use of iodine-containing supplements and/or iodised salt. Further studies of women representing the social and regional diversity of the population will be needed to confirm our findings.

Acknowledgments: The authors sincerely thank the women who participated in the study, staff at recruitment sites for their cooperation and staff at PathWest Laboratory Medicine WA for their assistance with sample analysis.

Author Contributions: J.S., S.S. and P.O.L. conceived, designed and supervised the study; A.J. performed the data collection; I.J. and A.J. analysed and interpreted the data; A.J. wrote the first draft of the manuscript; J.S., S.S. and P.O.L. edited the manuscript. All authors reviewed and approved the manuscript submitted.

References

1. World Health Organisation; United Nations International Children's Emergency Fund; International Council for Control of Iodine Deficiency Disorders. *Assessment of Iodine Deficiency Disorders and Monitoring Their Elimination, a Guide for Programme Managers*; World Health Organisation Press: Geneva, Swizerland, 2007.
2. Zimmermann, M.B.; Jooste, P.L.; Pandav, C.S. Iodine-deficiency disorders. *Lancet* **2008**, *372*, 1251–1262. [CrossRef]
3. Delange, F. Optimal iodine nutrition during pregnancy, lactation and the neonatal period. *Int. J. Endocrinol. Metab.* **2004**, *2*, 1–12.
4. Azizi, F.; Smyth, P. Breastfeeding and maternal and infant iodine nutrition. *Clin. Endocrinol.* **2009**, *70*, 803–809. [CrossRef] [PubMed]
5. Mulrine, H.M.; Skeaff, S.A.; Ferguson, E.L.; Gray, A.R.; Valeix, P. Breast-milk iodine concentration declines over the first 6 mo postpartum in iodine-deficient women. *Am. J. Clin. Nutr.* **2010**, *92*, 849–856. [CrossRef] [PubMed]
6. Laurberg, P.; Andersen, S.L. Nutrition: Breast milk—A gateway to iodine-dependent brain development. *Nat. Rev. Endocrinol.* **2014**, *10*, 134–135. [CrossRef] [PubMed]
7. National Health and Medical Research Council (NHMRC); New Zealand Ministry of Health. *Nutrient Reference Values for Australia and New Zealand Including Recommended Dietary Intakes*; Commonwealth of Australia: Canberra, Australia, 2006.
8. Semba, R.D.; Delange, F. Iodine in human milk: Perspectives for infant health. *Nutr. Rev.* **2001**, *59*, 269–278. [CrossRef] [PubMed]

9. Dold, S.; Baumgartner, J.; Zeder, C.; Krzystek, A.; Osei, J.; Haldimann, M.; Zimmermann, M.B.; Andersson, M. Optimization of a new mass spectrometry method for measurement of breast milk iodine concentrations and an assessment of the effect of analytic method and timing of within-feed sample collection on breast milk iodine concentrations. *Thyroid* **2016**, *26*, 287–295. [CrossRef] [PubMed]

10. Dorea, J.G. Iodine nutrition and breast feeding. *J. Trace Elem. Med. Biol.* **2002**, *16*, 207–220. [CrossRef]

11. Zimmermann, M. Iodine deficiency. *Endocr. Rev.* **2009**, *30*, 376–408. [CrossRef] [PubMed]

12. Leung, A.M.; Braverman, L.E.; He, X.; Heeren, T.; Pearce, E.N. Breastmilk iodine concentrations following acute dietary iodine intake. *Thyroid* **2012**, *22*, 1176–1180. [CrossRef] [PubMed]

13. Henjum, S.; Kjellevold, M.; Ulak, M.; Chandyo, R.; Shrestha, P.; Frøyland, L.; Strydom, E.; Dhansay, M.; Strand, T. Iodine concentration in breastmilk and urine among lactating women of Bhaktapur, Nepal. *Nutrients* **2016**, *8*, 255. [CrossRef] [PubMed]

14. Andersson, M.; de Benoist, B.; Delange, F.; Zupan, J. Prevention and control of iodine deficiency in pregnant and lactating women and in children less than 2-years-old: Conclusions and recommendations of the technical consultation. *Public Health Nutr.* **2007**, *10*, 1606–1611. [PubMed]

15. Zimmermann, M.B. The role of iodine in human growth and development. *Semin. Cell Dev. Biol.* **2011**, *22*, 645–652. [CrossRef] [PubMed]

16. Food Standards Australia New Zealand. *Proposal p1003—Mandatory Iodine Fortification for Australia—Approval Report*; Food Standards Australia New Zealand (FSANZ): Canberra, Australia, 2008.

17. National Health and Medical Research Council. *NHMRC Public Statement: Iodine Supplementation for Pregnant and Breastfeeding Women*; National Health and Medical Research Council: Canberra, Australia, 2010.

18. Chan, S.S.Y.; Hams, G.; Wiley, V.; Wilcken, B.; McElduff, A. Postpartum maternal iodine status and the relationship to neonatal thyroid function. *Thyroid* **2003**, *13*, 873–876. [CrossRef] [PubMed]

19. Huynh, D.; Condo, D.; Gibson, R.; Makrides, M.; Muhlhausler, B.; Zhou, S.J. Comparison of breast-milk iodine concentration of lactating women in Australia pre and post mandatory iodine fortification. *Public Health Nutr.* **2016**. [CrossRef] [PubMed]

20. Li, M.; Ma, G.; Boyages, S.C.; Eastman, C.J. Re-emergence of iodine deficiency in australia. *Asia Pac. J. Clin. Nutr.* **2001**, *10*, 200–203. [CrossRef] [PubMed]

21. Australian Bureau of Statistics. *Australian Health Survey: Biomedical Results for Nutrients, 2011–2012. Feature Article: Iodine*; Australian Bureau of Statistics: Canberra, Australia, 2013.

22. Huynh, D.; Zhou, S.J.; Gibson, R.; Palmer, L.; Muhlhausler, B. Validation of an optimized method for the determination of iodine in human breast milk by inductively coupled plasma mass spectrometry (ICPMS) after tetramethylammonium hydroxide extraction. *J. Trace Elem. Med. Biol.* **2015**, *29*, 75–82. [CrossRef] [PubMed]

23. Hutchinson, M.; Joyce, A. *Western Australia's Mother's and Babies, 2013: 31st Annual Report of the Western Australian Midwives' Notification System*; Department of Health, Western Australia: Perth, Australia, 2016.

24. Australian Bureau of Statistics. *Census of Population and Housing: Community Profile Western Australia*; Australian Bureau of Statistics: Canberra, Australia, 2011.

25. Laurberg, P.; Nøhr, S.B.; Pedersen, K.M.; Fuglsang, E. Iodine nutrition in breast-fed infants is impaired by maternal smoking. *J. Clin. Endocrinol. Metab.* **2004**, *89*, 181–187. [CrossRef] [PubMed]

26. Charlton, K.; Yeatman, H.; Lucas, C.; Axford, S.; Gemming, L.; Houweling, F.; Goodfellow, A.; Ma, G. Poor knowledge and practices related to iodine nutrition during pregnancy and lactation in Australian women: Pre- and post-iodine fortification. *Nutrients* **2012**, *4*, 1317–1327. [CrossRef] [PubMed]

27. Kyung Lee, M.; Binns, C.; Zhao, Y.; Scott, J.; Oddy, W. Nutritional supplements during breastfeeding. *Curr. Pediatr. Rev.* **2012**, *8*, 292–298. [CrossRef]

28. Andersen, S.L.; Møller, M.; Laurberg, P. Iodine concentrations in milk and in urine during breastfeeding are differently affected by maternal fluid intake. *Thyroid* **2013**, *24*, 764–772. [CrossRef] [PubMed]

29. Brough, L.; Jin, Y.; Shukri, N.H.; Wharemate, Z.R.; Weber, J.L.; Coad, J. Iodine intake and status during pregnancy and lactation before and after government initiatives to improve iodine status, in Palmerston North, New Zealand: A pilot study. *Matern. Child Nutr.* **2013**, *11*, 646–655. [CrossRef] [PubMed]

30. Kirk, A.B.; Kroll, M.; Dyke, J.V.; Ohira, S.I.; Dias, R.A.; Dasgupta, P.K. Perchlorate, iodine supplements, iodized salt and breast milk iodine content. *Sci. Total Environ.* **2012**, *420*, 73–78. [CrossRef] [PubMed]

12

A Comparison of Nutritional Antioxidant Content in Breast Milk, Donor Milk and Infant Formulas

Corrine Hanson [1,*], **Elizabeth Lyden** [2], **Jeremy Furtado** [3], **Matthew Van Ormer** [4] and **Ann Anderson-Berry** [4]

[1]   College of Allied Health Professions, University of Nebraska Medical Center, Medical Nutrition Education, 984045 Nebraska Medical Center, Omaha, NE 68198-4045, USA

[2]   College of Public Health, University of Nebraska Medical Center, 984375 Nebraska Medical Center, Omaha, NE 68198-4375, USA; elyden@unmc.edu

[3]   Department of Nutrition, Harvard School of Public Health, 655 Huntington Avenue, Boston, MA 02215, USA; jfurtado@hsph.harvard.edu

[4]   Pediatrics, University of Nebraska Medical Center, 981205 Nebraska Medical Center, Omaha, NE 68198-1205, USA; Matthew.vanormer@unmc.edu (M.V.O.); alanders@unmc.edu (A.A.-B.)

*   Correspondence: ckhanson@unmc.edu

Abstract: Human milk is the optimal food for human infants, including infants born prematurely. In the event that a mother of a hospitalized infant cannot provide breast milk, donor milk is considered an acceptable alternative. It is known that the macronutrient composition of donor milk is different than human milk, with variable fat content and protein content. However, much less is known about the micronutrient content of donor milk, including nutritional antioxidants. Samples of breast milk from 12 mothers of infants hospitalized in the Newborn Intensive Care Unit until were collected and analyzed for concentrations of nutritional antioxidants, including α-carotene, β-carotene, β-cryptoxanthin, lycopene, lutein + zeaxanthin, retinol, and α-tocopherol. Additionally, a homogenized sample of donor milk available from a commercial milk bank and samples of infant formulas were also analyzed. Concentrations of nutritional antioxidants were measured using high-performance liquid chromatography. Compared to breast milk collected from mothers of hospitalized infants, commercially available donor milk had 18%–53% of the nutritional antioxidant content of maternal breast milk. As donor milk is becoming a common nutritional intervention for the high risk preterm infant, the nutritional antioxidant status of donor milk–fed premature infants and outcomes related to oxidative stress may merit further investigation.

Keywords: antioxidants; breast milk; infant feeding; infant formula; breast milk substitutes; human milk

1. Introduction

Human milk is the optimal food for infants, including infants born prematurely. In the event that a mother of a hospitalized infant cannot provide breast milk, donor milk is often considered an acceptable or even ideal alternative to the mother's own milk. It is known that the macronutrient composition of donor milk is different from human milk, with variable fat content and protein content lower than that of mature milk [1–4]. However, much less is known about the micronutrient content of donor milk, including nutritional antioxidants.

There is increasing evidence that links early exposure to oxidative stress with potentially lifelong consequences. The premature infant is especially susceptible to damage from oxidative stress for two reasons: (1) adequate concentrations of antioxidants may be absent at birth; (2) the ability to increase synthesis of antioxidants is impaired. This can lead to an increased risk for the development of oxidative stress–induced diseases such as bronchopulmonary dysplasia (BPD), retinopathy of prematurity (ROP), necrotizing enterocolitis (NEC), and periventricular leukomalacia (PVL) [5,6]. Therefore, it is critical in premature infants to ensure an adequate supply of dietary antioxidants. The objective of this analysis was to compare the nutritional antioxidant profile of different types of feedings for premature infants, including samples of maternal breast milk collected during neonatal hospitalization and pasteurized pooled donor milk.

2. Materials and Methods

A total of 12 breast milk samples from women with singleton infants who were admitted to the Neonatal Intensive Care Unit were collected for analysis. These samples were obtained as a subset of subjects ($n = 30$) who were enrolled in a study of nutritional antioxidant status of Newborn Intensive Care Unit (NICU) hospitalized infants who had excess breast milk available after clinical use. Institutional Review Board approval was obtained prior to collection of any samples. The median gestational age was 37.1 weeks, with a range 30.3–42.0 weeks. A 2.0 mL sample was collected from each participant in a sterile plastic tube, protected from heat and light, and stored at -80 °F freezers until they were analyzed. In addition, a single 2 mL aliquot of the commercially available, pooled donor milk sample was collected for analysis, and single 2 mL samples of the commercially available preterm infant formula, transitional infant formula, and term infant formula used in the study unit were collected. All formulas were from a single manufacturer (Abbott Nutrition®). Analysis of samples was performed at the Biomarker Research Institute at the Harvard School of Public Health. Measurements of lutein + zeaxanthin, β-cryptoxanthin, *trans*-lycopene, *cis*-lycopene, total lycopene, α-carotene, *trans*-β-carotene, *cis*-β-carotene, total-β-carotene, retinol, α-tocopherol and γ-tocopherol were obtained. Concentrations in plasma samples were measured as described by El-Sohemy et al [7]. Plasma samples (250 µL) were mixed with 250 mL ethanol containing 10 µg *rac*-tocopherol/mL (Tocol) as an internal standard, extracted with 4 mL hexane, evaporated to dryness under nitrogen, and reconstituted in 100 mL ethanol-dioxane (1:1, by vol) and 150 mL acetonitrile. Samples are quantitated by high-performance liquid chromatography (HPLC) on a Restek Ultra C_{18} 150 mm × 4.6 mm column with a 3 µm particle size encased in a column oven (Hitachi L-2350, Hitachi, San Jose, CA, USA) to prevent temperature fluctuations, and equipped with a trident guard cartridge system (Restek, Corp., Bellefonte, PA, USA). A mixture of acetonitrile, tetrahydrofuran, methanol, and a 1% ammonium acetate solution (68:22:7:3) was used as the mobile phase at a flow rate of 1.1 mL/min, with a Hitachi L-2130 pump in isocratic mode, a Hitachi L-2455 diode array detector (300 nm and 445 nm), and a Hitachi L-2200 auto-sampler with water-chilled tray. The Hitachi System Manager software (D-2000 Elite, Version 3.0) was used for peak integration and data acquisition. Because lutein and zeaxanthin co-elute on the chromatogram, the two are grouped and provided as lutein + zeaxanthin. Internal quality control was monitored with four control samples analyzed within each run. These samples consisted of two identical high-level plasmas and two identical low-level plasmas. Comparison of data from these samples allowed for within-run and between-run variation estimates. In addition, external quality control was monitored by participation in the standardization program for carotenoid analysis from the National Institute of Standards and Technology U.S.A. Descriptive statistics included means and standard deviations. A one sample t-test was used to compare the mean value from the 12 maternal breast milk (MBM) to the known value of the donor or infant formulas values $p < 0.05$ was considered statistically significant.

3. Results

The results for the concentrations of α-carotene, total β-carotenes, β-cryptoxanthin, total lycopenes, lutein + zeaxanthin, retinol, α-tocopherol, and γ-tocopherol for each of the feeding types are shown in Table 1.

When the concentrations of carotenoids between the 12 breast milk samples and the pooled donor milk sample were compared, the donor milk sample was descriptively lower in all carotenoids.

A statistically significant difference was found between concentrations of total lycopene ($p = 0.006$). A comparison of levels of carotenoids breast milk vs. donor milk is shown in Figure 1.

Table 1. Nutrition antioxidant content of infant feedings.

Nutritional Antioxidant (µg/L)	Premature Formula	Transitional Formula	Term Standard Formula	Breast Milk Mean (SD) N = 12	Donor Milk
α-carotene	0.51	1.40	0.5	7.7 (14.5)	3.6
β-carotene	71.1	63.9	25.0	49.1 (75.5)	13.7
β-cryptoxanthin	0.9	0.9	0.48	21.7 (40.0)	3.8
Lycopene	1.5	5.8	79.8	66.1 (55.9)	11.9
Lutein + zeaxanthin	65.5	56.9	58.4	40.1 (42.5)	21.4
Retinol	3086.2	911.8	571.2	401.6 (516.3)	185.8
α-tocopherol	20,109.1	13,360.2	8520.0	5880.8 (4971.7)	1381.9
γ-tocopherol	6787.1	6561.6	4204.0	1207.1 (668.4)	622.8

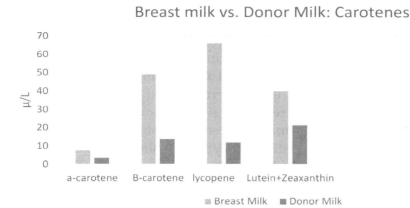

Figure 1. The concentrations of α-carotene, β-carotene, lycopene, and lutein + zeaxanthin in maternal breast milk vs. donor milk samples. Lycopene was statistically significant ($p = 0.006$).

Samples of the transitional formula and premature formula were also significantly lower in lycopene when compared to breast milk ($p = 0.003$ and 0.002, respectively) (see Table 1).

When concentrations of tocopherols between the 12 breast milk samples and the pooled donor milk sample were compared, a statistically significant difference was found between concentrations of both α- and γ-tocopherols ($p = 0.009$ and 0.01, respectively). A comparison of concentrations of tocopherols in breast milk vs. donor milk is shown in Figure 2.

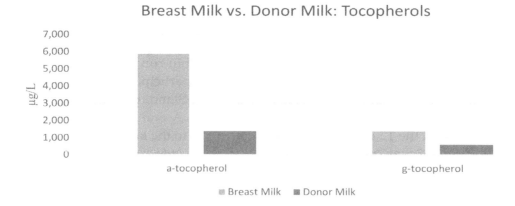

Figure 2. The concentrations of α-tocopherol and γ-tocopherol in maternal breast milk vs. donor milk samples. All values were significantly different ($p = 0.009$ and 0.01 for α-tocopherol and γ-tocopherol, respectively).

Samples of the transitional formula and premature formula were significantly higher in α-tocopherol when compared to breast milk ($p = 0.003$ and 0.002) and all infant formulas were significantly higher in γ-tocopherol when compared to breast milk ($p < 0.0001$ for term, transitional, and premature formulas) (see Table 1).

4. Discussion

Donor milk is considered to be an effective alternative source of nutrition when the mother's own milk is not available, and preterm infants are the primary recipients. Donor milk is obtained from healthy, lactating mothers who consent to donate their surplus which is collected, processed, and stored by specialized centers such as human milk banks. Donor milk is pasteurized to reduce microbial growth and ensure its safety for consumption. The most common pasteurization procedure is Holder pasteurization, in which milk is exposed to a temperature of approximately 62.5 °C (144.5 °F) for at least 30 min [8]. Pasteurization is necessary to inactivate most viral and bacterial compounds, but can affect the nutrition and immunological properties of breast milk. While it has been shown that pasteurized mother's milk retains some of the beneficial and protective effects [1,4,9] there does appear to be an impact on the antioxidant capacity of donor milk [10,11]. Significant decreases in the anti-oxidant compounds malondialdehye and glutathione have been found after pasteurization [12]. The pasteurization of human milk has also been shown to result in significant losses of vitamin D, with reductions of 10%–20% [13].

Preterm infants are born relatively deficient in antioxidant defenses, with increased oxidant stress [5]. Many events, such as infection, mechanical ventilation, intravenous nutrition, and blood transfusions result in oxidative stress. Oxidative stress is associated with serious conditions in the newborn, such as bronchopulmonary dysplasia (BPD), respiratory distress, retinopathy of prematurity (ROP), and necrotizing enterocolitis (NEC), as well as an increased risk of infection [6]. Ensuring adequate nutritional antioxidant status may provide protective benefits to infants at an increased risk of developing these conditions or may positively impact an infant's recovery from these complications.

Studies have shown that there are significant differences in the antioxidant capacity of different types of infant feeding. One study has shown that the total antioxidant capacity in the breast milk of mothers who deliver prematurely is higher than the breast milk of mothers who deliver at term [14], while another study has found them to be equal [15]. However, both have superior antioxidant capacity when compared to formula [15,16]. Breast-fed and formula-fed infants show significant differences in plasma antioxidant nutrient concentrations [17]. The mother's diet also affects the antioxidant capacity of human milk. An increased consumption of dairy products, fruits and vegetables, cereals and nuts has been shown to increase the total antioxidant capacity of the breastmilk [16].

Major nutritional antioxidants include α- and β-carotenes, lutein + zeaxanthin, lycopene, and α-tocopherol. Humans cannot synthesize these compounds and thus they must be provided exogenously through dietary intake. Carotene levels in colostrum have been shown to be five times higher than in mature breast milk [17]. Similarly, breast-fed premature infants have been shown to have higher serum carotenoids than formula-fed premature infants [18]. In one study, carotenoid supplementation was associated with a blunted increase in C-reactive protein (CRP) concentrations from one to 40 weeks post-menstrual age, whereas CRP levels rose in controls [19]. The association of a lower CRP with higher carotenoid consumption likely reflects carotenoid antioxidant and immunomodulatory properties. In populations of children with acute infections, a significant inverse correlation was shown between serum CRP and carotene concentrations [20]. Plasma β-carotene concentrations have indeed been found to be lower in infants with bronchopulmonary dysplasia [21], which may result in a reduction of their antioxidant protection. Our study does report that β-carotene concentrations in donor milk were less than one-third of those in fresh breast milk, and our p-value of 0.13, which approaches statistical significance, may be more likely due to the limited power of our study. This may indicate that further investigation into carotenoid anti-inflammatory effects in sick, preterm infants is warranted.

It is thought that lutein + zeaxanthin influence the maturation of cells in the macular region of the retina [22] and protect against stress and oxidation in the retinal pigment epithelium [23]. Vishwanathan et al. determined that the mean concentration of lutein was significantly greater than the other carotenoids in brain tissue samples of infants who died within the first 18 months of life [22]. Preterm infants also had significantly lower concentrations of lutein + zeaxanthin compared to term infants in most of the brain regions [22]. These findings, in addition to previous research, help support the role lutein + zeaxanthin plays in visual and cognitive development. Breast-fed infants have been shown to have higher serum lutein levels than formula-fed infants, possibly due to increased bioavailability of the compound in breast milk, and a dose-dependent relationship exists between lutein in the diet and lutein in the serum [24]. It was calculated that four times more lutein is needed in infant formula than in human milk to achieve similar serum lutein concentrations among breast-fed and formula-fed infants [24]. In a recent pilot randomized controlled trial in healthy newborns, lutein administration proved effective in increasing the levels of biological antioxidant potential by decreasing the total hydroperoxides as markers of oxidative stress [25]. In another study by Mazoni et al., the effect of lutein + zeaxanthin on prevention of BPD appears relevant, although not statistically significant ($p = 0.07$) [26]. Lutein supplementation also has been shown to result in greater rod photoreceptor sensitivity responses when compared to controls [19]. A pilot study showed a potential antioxidant effect of lutein in the neonatal period [25]; however, another study showed that lutein supplementation did not enhance the biological antioxidant capacity [27], although this second study did not achieve a statistically significant difference in the serum lutein concentrations between the placebo and intervention group. A positive association was seen between plasma lutein levels and total antioxidant status ($r = 0.13$, $p = 0.02$) [27]. Our study finds that concentrations of lutein + zeaxanthin were approximately half of the concentrations found in maternal breast milk. Both donor milk and maternal breast milk had lower lutein + zeaxanthin concentrations when compared to the infant formulas tested; however, given the study that demonstrated possible improved bioavailability from breast milk [24], it cannot be assumed that the formula-fed infants would have higher serum concentrations. Additionally, it is important to note that not all formula manufacturers provide supplemental lutein in preterm formula, and therefore infant intake may vary widely based on formula selection.

Vitamin E is an antioxidant that protects cell membranes against free radicals [28]. Although vitamin E deficiency is thought to be rare in healthy adults, it is much more common in premature infants [29]. Vitamin E occurs naturally in several different isoforms, including α- and γ-tocopherol. These isoforms differ by one methyl group and are not interconvertible in human metabolism [30]. As a result, increased intakes of α- or γ-tocopherol will cause a rise in serum concentrations of that specific tocopherol [31,32]. Importantly, serum and tissue levels of vitamin E isoforms correlate [33], meaning the dietary intake of tocopherols has the potential to influence biological mechanisms.

One change in infant nutrition that has occurred in the last several decades is the increase in the γ-tocopherol isoform in the diet of infants. This is primarily due to in the use of soy oils, which are extremely high in γ-tocopherol, as the primary lipid component in infant formulas [34]. While human breast milk has been shown to contain some γ-tocopherol, previous studies have shown the content of γ-tocopherol in infant formula to be up to seven times higher than that in human milk [35]. Our findings concur with this report, demonstrating γ-tocopherol levels in our formula samples to be 3.5–5.6 times higher than in maternal breast milk samples. This level of γ-tocopherol in infant formula does not appear to provide similar protection from lipid peroxidation as human milk [36]. Serum levels of γ-tocopherol in infants have been shown to increase during the first week of life [37], presumably from dietary sources [35]. Recently, our understanding of these tocopherols isoforms has expanded as new evidence indicates that vitamin E isoforms have different roles in influencing inflammation. In contrast to the anti-inflammatory properties of the α-tocopherol isoform, the γ-tocopherol isoform has been shown to increase cytokine production (i.e., IL-2) and demonstrate pro-inflammatory properties [38–42].

Importantly, serum γ-tocopherol isoforms at as little as 10% of the concentration of α-tocopherol have been shown to ablate the anti-inflammatory benefit of alpha-tocopherol [41]. With regard to α-tocopherol, long-term supplementation (six months minimum and up to 24 months) has been shown to positively impact mental development, particularly intelligence quocient (IQ), in school-age children who were extremely low-birth-weight infants (ELBW) [43], raising the possibility that α-tocopherol might be a functional molecule in a developing brain. Although some NICU infants receive donor milk for only a limited amount of time, other institutions use donor milk as a primary source of nutrition throughout NICU hospitalization; our finding that α-tocopherol levels in donor milk samples were significantly decreased when compared to breast milk may make consideration of vitamin E status important in these infants.

Donor milk still has unique advantages compared to formula and continues to represent an important alternative if maternal milk is not available, specifically with regard to necrotizing enterocolitis [44]. In a Cochrane systematic review and meta-analysis, Quigley et al. demonstrated both benefits and risks associated with the use of donor milk. Importantly, there was a higher incidence of NEC among infants with birth weights <2500 g and in those fed formula versus those fed donor milk (relative risk of 2.5 (95% CI, 1.2, 5.1) [44]. Because NEC is the most common gastrointestinal emergency among very-low-birth-weight (VLBW) infants, its prevention is a powerful argument in favor of donor milk as an alternative supplement to formula when the mother's own milk is not available. The Quigley et al. review and meta-analysis, however, concluded that infants fed donor milk experienced slower weight ($p < 0.0001$), length ($p < 0.0003$) and head circumference ($p < 0.0001$) gains than those fed formula [44]. These risks associated with donor milk are of significant concern because VLBW infants are born with impoverished nutrient reserves, and are subject to metabolic stresses that further elevate nutritional requirements [45]. Nutrient deficits and sub-optimal growth have significant long-term neurodevelopmental consequences [46,47]. Quigley et al. point out that all but one of the randomized controlled trials examined in their meta-analysis were >25 years old, when smaller VLBW infants did not survive, and these studies also may not be reflective of current practice [44]. In a more recent study conducted in 2012–2014, The Early Nutrition Study Randomized Clinical Trial found no difference in infections, necrotizing enterocolitis, or mortality during the first 60 days of life in 373 infants fed pasteurized donor milk or preterm formula for supplemental feedings [48]. Another study 2014 of 201 ELBW infants found no difference in NEC or infection rates between infants receiving human milk (including donor milk) and infants receiving formula; however, the duration of mechanical ventilation was significantly higher among formula-fed infants (24 vs. 60 h, $p = 0.016$) in the group exposed to formula [48].

Our analysis has several limitations. First, the antioxidant capacity of breast milk includes many other compounds than the ones highlighted in this study, including uric acid, enzymes, and lipids. However, the antioxidants targeted in this study are modifiable by maternal diet, which may allow for interventions targeted at increasing the antioxidant potential of human milk. Additionally, we did not have the serum levels of donor milk–fed infants to compare to infants receiving maternal breast milk to compare the impact of decreased intake. Additionally, our statistical power was limited by low numbers of analyzed breast milk, a precious commodity to a premature neonate. The median gestational age of 37 weeks in our cohort includes preterm breast milk samples, and the donor milk samples are from a commercial pooled supply. Future studies evaluating the serum nutritional antioxidant status of infants receiving the mother's own milk, donor milk, and infant formulas will expand our knowledge in this area.

5. Conclusions

As donor milk is becoming a common nutritional intervention for the high risk preterm infant, the nutritional antioxidant status of donor milk–fed premature infants and outcomes related to oxidative stress may merit further investigation.

Acknowledgments: This research and publication was supported by a grant from the Department of Pediatrics, University of Nebraska Medical Center.

Author Contributions: C.H., E.L., J.F., M.O. and A.A.B. conceived and designed the experiments, performed the experiments, analyzed the data, and wrote the paper.

References

1.   ESPGHAN Committee on Nutrition; Arslanoglu, S.; Corpeleijn, W.; Moro, G.; Braegger, C.; Campoy, C.; Colomb, V.; Decsi, T.; Domellöf, M.; Fewtrell, M.; et al. Donor human milk for preterm infants: Current evidence and research directions. *J. Pediatr. Gastroenterol. Nutr.* **2013**, *57*, 535–542. [CrossRef] [PubMed]

2.   Bertino, E.; Giuliani, F.; Baricco, M.; Di Nicola, P.; Peila, C.; Vassia, C.; Chiale, F.; Pirra, A.; Cresi, F.; Martano, C.; et al. Benefits of donor milk in the feeding of preterm infants. *Early Hum. Dev.* **2013**, *89* (Suppl. 2), S3–S6. [CrossRef] [PubMed]

3.   Vieira, A.A.; Soares, F.V.; Pimenta, H.P.; Abranches, A.D.; Moreira, M.E. Analysis of the influence of pasteurization, freezing/thawing, and offer processes on human milk's macronutrient concentrations. *Early Hum. Dev.* **2011**, *87*, 577–580. [CrossRef] [PubMed]

4.   Bertino, E.; Arslanoglu, S.; Martano, C.; Di Nicola, P.; Giuliani, F.; Peila, C.; Cester, E.; Pirra, A.; Coscia, A.; Moro, G. Biological, nutritional and clinical aspects of feeding preterm infants with human milk. *J. Biol. Regul. Homeost. Agents* **2012**, *26* (Suppl. 3), 9–13. [PubMed]

5.   Sandal, G.; Uras, N.; Gokmen, T.; Oguz, S.S.; Erdeve, O.; Dilmen, U. Assessment of oxidant/antioxidant system in newborns and their breast milks. *J. Matern. Fetal Neonatal Med.* **2013**, *26*, 540–543. [CrossRef] [PubMed]

6.   Weber, D.; Stuetz, W.; Bernhard, W.; Franz, A.; Raith, M.; Grune, T.; Breusing, N. Oxidative stress markers and micronutrients in maternal and cord blood in relation to neonatal outcome. *Eur. J. Clin. Nutr.* **2014**, *68*, 215–222. [CrossRef] [PubMed]

7.   El-Sohemy, A.; Baylin, A.; Kabagambe, E.; Ascherio, A.; Spiegelman, D.; Campos, H. Individual carotenoid concentrations in adipose tissue and plasma as biomarkers of dietary intake. *Am. J. Clin. Nutr.* **2002**, *76*, 172–179. [PubMed]

8.   O'Connor, D.L.; Ewaschuk, J.B.; Unger, S. Human milk pasteurization: Benefits and risks. *Curr. Opin. Clin. Nutr. Metab. Care* **2015**, *18*, 269–275. [CrossRef] [PubMed]

9.   Peila, C.; Coscia, A.; Bertino, E.; Cavaletto, M.; Spertino, S.; Icardi, S.; Tortone, C.; Visser, G.H.A.; Gazzolo, D. Effects of holder pasteurization on the protein profile of human milk. *Ital. J. Pediatr.* **2016**, *42*. [CrossRef] [PubMed]

10.   Ewaschuk, J.B.; Unger, S.; Harvey, S.; O'Connor, D.L.; Field, C.J. Effect of pasteurization on immune components of milk: Implications for feeding preterm infants. *Appl. Physiol. Nutr. Metab.* **2011**, *36*, 175–182. [CrossRef] [PubMed]

11.   Ewaschuk, J.B.; Unger, S.; O'Connor, D.L.; Stone, D.; Harvey, S.; Clandinin, M.T.; Field, C.J. Effect of pasteurization on selected immune components of donated human breast milk. *J. Perinatol.* **2011**, *31*, 593–598. [CrossRef] [PubMed]

12.   Silvestre, D.; Miranda, M.; Muriach, M.; Almansa, I.; Jareno, E.; Romero, F.J. Antioxidant capacity of human milk: Effect of thermal conditions for the pasteurization. *Acta Paediatr.* **2008**, *97*, 1070–1074. [CrossRef] [PubMed]

13.   Gomes, F.P.; Shaw, P.N.; Whitfield, K.; Koorts, P.; McConachy, H.; Hewavitharana, A.K. Effect of pasteurisation on the concentrations of vitamin D compounds in donor breastmilk. *Int. J. Food Sci. Nutr.* **2016**, *67*, 16–19. [CrossRef] [PubMed]

14.   Turhan, A.H.; Atici, A.; Muslu, N. Antioxidant capacity of breast milk of mothers who delivered prematurely is higher than that of mothers who delivered at term. *Int. J. Vitam. Nutr. Res.* **2011**, *81*, 368–371. [CrossRef] [PubMed]

15. Friel, J.K.; Martin, S.M.; Langdon, M.; Herzberg, G.R.; Buettner, G.R. Milk from mothers of both premature and full-term infants provides better antioxidant protection than does infant formula. *Pediatr. Res.* **2002**, *51*, 612–618. [CrossRef] [PubMed]

16. Oveisi, M.R.; Sadeghi, N.; Jannat, B.; Hajimahmoodi, M.; Behfar, A.O.; Jannat, F.; MokhtariNasab, F. Human breast milk provides better antioxidant capacity than infant formula. *Iran. J. Pharm. Res.* **2010**, *9*, 445–449. [PubMed]

17. Sommerburg, O.; Meissner, K.; Nelle, M.; Lenhartz, H.; Leichsenring, M. Carotenoid supply in breast-fed and formula-fed neonates. *Eur. J. Pediatr.* **2000**, *159*, 86–90. [CrossRef] [PubMed]

18. Chan, G.M.; Chan, M.M.; Gellermann, W.; Ermakov, I.; Ermakova, M.; Bhosale, P.; Bernstein, P.; Rau, C. Resonance Raman spectroscopy and the preterm infant carotenoid status. *J. Pediatr. Gastroenterol. Nutr.* **2013**, *56*, 556–559. [CrossRef] [PubMed]

19. Rubin, L.P.; Chan, G.M.; Barrett-Reis, B.M.; Fulton, A.B.; Hansen, R.M.; Ashmeade, T.L.; Oliver, J.S.; Mackey, A.D.; Dimmit, R.A.; Hartmann, E.E. Effect of carotenoid supplementation on plasma carotenoids, inflammation and visual development in preterm infants. *J. Perinatol.* **2012**, *32*, 418–424. [CrossRef] [PubMed]

20. Cser, M.A.; Majchrzak, D.; Rust, P.; Rust, P.; Sziklai-Laszlo, I.; Kovacs, I.; Bocskai, E.; Elmadfa, I. Serum carotenoid and retinol levels during childhood infections. *Ann. Nutr. Metab.* **2004**, *48*, 156–162. [CrossRef] [PubMed]

21. Vogelsang, A.; van Lingen, R.A.; Slootstra, J.; Dikkeschei, B.D.; Kollen, B.J.; Schaafsma, A.; van Zoeren-Grobben, D. Antioxidant role of plasma carotenoids in bronchopulmonary dysplasia in preterm infants. *Int. J. Vitam. Nutr. Res.* **2009**, *79*, 288–296. [CrossRef] [PubMed]

22. Vishwanathan, R.; Kuchan, M.J.; Sen, S.; Johnson, E.J. Lutein and preterm infants with decreased concentrations of brain carotenoids. *J. Pediatr. Gastroenterol. Nutr.* **2014**, *59*, 659–665. [CrossRef] [PubMed]

23. Lipkie, T.E.; Morrow, A.L.; Jouni, Z.E.; McMahon, R.J.; Ferruzzi, M.G. Longitudinal survey of carotenoids in human milk from urban cohorts in China, Mexico, and the USA. *PLoS ONE* **2015**, *10*, e0127729. [CrossRef] [PubMed]

24. Bettler, J.; Zimmer, J.P.; Neuringer, M.; DeRusso, P.A. Serum lutein concentrations in healthy term infants fed human milk or infant formula with lutein. *Eur. J. Nutr.* **2010**, *49*, 45–51. [CrossRef] [PubMed]

25. Perrone, S.; Longini, M.; Marzocchi, B.; Picardi, A.; Bellieni, C.V.; Proietti, F.; Rodriguez, A.; Turrisi, G.; Buonocore, G. Effects of lutein on oxidative stress in the term newborn: A pilot study. *Neonatology* **2010**, *97*, 36–40. [CrossRef] [PubMed]

26. Manzoni, P.; Guardione, R.; Bonetti, P.; Priolo, C.; Maestri, A.; Mansoldo, C.; Mostert, M.; Anselmetti, G.; Sardei, D.; Bellettato, M.; et al. Lutein and zeaxanthin supplementation in preterm very low-birth-weight neonates in neonatal intensive care units: A multicenter randomized controlled trial. *Am. J. Perinatol.* **2013**, *30*, 25–32. [CrossRef] [PubMed]

27. Costa, S.; Giannantonio, C.; Romagnoli, C.; Barone, G.; Gervasoni, J.; Perri, A.; Zecca, E. Lutein and zeaxanthin concentrations in formula and human milk samples from Italian mothers. *Eur. J. Clin. Nutr.* **2015**, *69*, 531–532. [CrossRef] [PubMed]

28. Food and Nutrition Board, Institute of Medicine. *Dietary Reference Intakes for Vitamin C, Vitamin E, Selenium, and Carotenoids*; National Academy Press: Washington, WA, USA, 2000.

29. Tanaka, H.; Mino, M.; Takeuchi, T. A nutritional evaluation of vitamin E status in very low birth weight infants with respect to changes in plasma and red blood cell tocopherol levels. *J. Nutr. Sci. Vitaminol. (Tokyo)* **1988**, *34*, 293–307. [CrossRef] [PubMed]

30. Cook-Mills, J.M. Isoforms of vitamin E differentially regulate PKC and inflammation: A review. *J. Clin. Cell Immunol.* **2013**, *4*. [CrossRef] [PubMed]

31. Wu, D.; Han, S.N.; Meydani, M.; Meydani, S.N. Effect of concomitant consumption of fish oil and vitamin E on T cell mediated function in the elderly: A randomized double-blind trial. *J. Am. Coll. Nutr.* **2006**, *25*, 300–306. [CrossRef] [PubMed]

32. Meydani, M.; Cohn, J.S.; Macauley, J.B.; McNamara, J.R.; Blumberg, J.B.; Schaefer, E.J. Postprandial changes in the plasma concentration of α- and γ-tocopherol in human subjects fed a fat-rich meal supplemented with fat-soluble vitamins. *J. Nutr.* **1989**, *119*, 1252–1258. [PubMed]

33. Redlich, C.A.; Grauer, J.N.; van Bennekum, A.M.; Clever, S.L.; Ponn, R.B.; Blaner, W.S. Characterization of carotenoid, vitamin A, and α-tocopheral levels in human lung tissue and pulmonary macrophages. *Am. J. Respir. Crit. Care Med.* **1996**, *154*, 1436–1443. [CrossRef] [PubMed]

34. Uauy, R.; Hoffman, D.R.; Birch, E.E.; Birch, D.G.; Jameson, D.M.; Tyson, J. Safety and efficacy of omega-3 fatty acids in the nutrition of very low birth weight infants: Soy oil and marine oil supplementation of formula. *J. Pediatr.* **1994**, *124*, 612–620. [CrossRef]

35. Martysiak-Zurowska, D.; Szlagatys-Sidorkiewicz, A.; Zagierski, M. Concentrations of α- and γ-tocopherols in human breast milk during the first months of lactation and in infant formulas. *Matern. Child. Nutr.* **2013**, *9*, 473–482. [CrossRef] [PubMed]

36. Elisia, I.; Kitts, D.D. Differences in vitamin E and C profile between infant formula and human milk and relative susceptibility to lipid oxidation. *Int. J. Vitam. Nutr. Res.* **2013**, *83*, 311–319. [CrossRef] [PubMed]

37. Bell, E.F.; Hansen, N.I.; Brion, L.P.; Ehrenkranz, R.A.; Kennedy, K.A.; Walsh, M.C.; Shankaran, S.; Acarregui, M.J.; Johnson, K.J.; Hale, E.C.; et al. Serum tocopherol levels in very preterm infants after a single dose of vitamin E at birth. *Pediatrics* **2013**, *132*, e1626–e1633. [CrossRef] [PubMed]

38. Cook-Mills, J.M.; Abdala-Valencia, H.; Hartert, T. Two faces of vitamin E in the lung. *Am. J. Respir. Crit. Care Med.* **2013**, *188*, 279–284. [CrossRef] [PubMed]

39. McCary, C.A.; Yoon, Y.; Panagabko, C.; Cho, W.; Atkinson, J.; Cook-Mills, J.M. Vitamin E isoforms directly bind PKCα and differentially regulate activation of PKCα. *Biochem. J.* **2012**, *441*, 189–198. [CrossRef] [PubMed]

40. McCary, C.A.; Abdala-Valencia, H.; Berdnikovs, S.; Cook-Mills, J.M. Supplemental and highly elevated tocopherol doses differentially regulate allergic inflammation: Reversibility of α-tocopherol and γ-tocopherol's effects. *J. Immunol.* **2011**, *186*, 3674–3685. [CrossRef] [PubMed]

41. Berdnikovs, S.; Abdala-Valencia, H.; McCary, C.; McCary, C.; Somand, M.; Cole, R.; Garcia, A.; Bryce, P.; Cook-Mills, J.M. Isoforms of vitamin E have opposing immunoregulatory functions during inflammation by regulating leukocyte recruitment. *J. Immunol.* **2009**, *182*, 4395–4405. [CrossRef] [PubMed]

42. Abdala-Valencia, H.; Berdnikovs, S.; Cook-Mills, J.M. Vitamin E isoforms as modulators of lung inflammation. *Nutrients.* **2013**, *5*, 4347–4363. [CrossRef] [PubMed]

43. Kitajima, H.; Kanazawa, T.; Mori, R.; Hirano, S.; Ogihara, T.; Fujimura, M. Long-term α-tocopherol supplements may improve mental development in extremely low birthweight infants. *Acta Paediatr.* **2015**, *104*, e82–e89. [CrossRef] [PubMed]

44. Quigley, M.; McGuire, W. Formula versus donor breast milk for feeding preterm or low birth weight infants. *Cochrane Database Syst. Rev.* **2014**. [CrossRef]

45. Stoll, B.J.; Hansen, N.I.; Bell, E.F.; Shankaran, S.; Laptook, A.R.; Walsh, M.C.; Hale, E.C.; Newman, N.S.; Schibler, K.; Carlo, W.A.; et al. Neonatal outcomes of extremely preterm infants from the NICHD neonatal research network. *Pediatrics* **2010**, *126*, 443–456. [CrossRef] [PubMed]

46. Ehrenkranz, R.A.; Dusick, A.M.; Vohr, B.R.; Wright, L.L.; Wrage, L.A.; Poole, W.K. Growth in the neonatal intensive care unit influences neurodevelopmental and growth outcomes of extremely low birth weight infants. *Pediatrics* **2006**, *117*, 1253–1261. [CrossRef] [PubMed]

47. Corpeleijn, W.E.; de Waard, M.; Christmann, V.; van Goudoever, J.B.; der Jansen-van Weide, M.C.; Kooi, E.M.; Koper, J.F.; Kouwenhoven, S.M.; Lafeber, H.N.; Mank, E.; et al. Effect of donor milk on severe infections and mortality in very low-birth-weight infants: The Early Nutrition Study randomized clinical trial. *JAMA Pediatr.* **2016**, *170*, 654–661. [CrossRef] [PubMed]

48. Verd, S.; Porta, R.; Botet, F.; Gutierrez, A.; Ginovart, G.; Barbero, A.H.; Ciurana, A.; Plata, I.I. Hospital outcomes of extremely low birth weight infants after introduction of donor milk to supplement mother's milk. *Breastfeed Med.* **2015**, *10*, 150–155. [CrossRef] [PubMed]

13

Usual Intake of Key Minerals among Children in the Second Year of Life, NHANES 2003–2012

Heather C. Hamner *, Cria G. Perrine and Kelley S. Scanlon

National Center for Chronic Disease Prevention and Health Promotion, Centers for Disease Control and Prevention (CDC), Atlanta, GA 30341, USA; hgk3@cdc.gov (C.G.P.); kelley.scanlon@fns.usda.gov (K.S.S.)
* Correspondence: hfc2@cdc.gov

Abstract: Iron, calcium, and zinc are important nutrients for the young, developing child. This study describes the usual intake of iron, calcium, and zinc among US children in the second year of life using two days of dietary intake data from the National Health and Nutrition Examination Survey 2003–2012. Estimates were calculated using PC-SIDE to account for within and between person variation. Mean usual iron, calcium, and zinc intakes were 9.5 mg/day, 1046 mg/day, and 7.1 mg/day, respectively. Over a quarter of children had usual iron intakes less than the Recommended Dietary Allowance (RDA) (26.1%). Eleven percent of children had usual calcium intakes below the RDA and over half of children had usual intakes of zinc that exceeded the tolerable upper intake level (UL). Two percent or less had usual intakes below the Estimated Average Requirement (EAR) for iron, calcium, and zinc. Our findings suggest that during 2003–2012, one in four children and one in ten children had usual intakes below the RDA for iron and calcium, respectively. Children who are not meeting their nutrient requirements could be at increased risk for developing deficiencies such as iron deficiency or could lead to a shortage in adequate nutrients required for growth and development. One in every two children is exceeding the UL for zinc, but the interpretation of these estimates should be done with caution given the limited data on adverse health outcomes. Continued monitoring of zinc intake and further assessment for the potential of adverse health outcomes associated with high zinc intakes may be needed.

Keywords: iron; calcium; zinc; young children; usual nutrient intake; NHANES

1. Introduction

Iron, calcium, and zinc are key minerals needed to ensure optimal cognitive development [1,2], bone health [3], and growth [1]. For young children, the American Academy of Pediatrics (AAP) has identified iron and zinc as critical nutrients—especially for children who are exclusively breastfed and are transitioning to the introduction of complementary foods [4]. Although the majority of children 12–23 months of age have transitioned to solid foods, this time period is still an important period of physical and cognitive development and adequate nutrient intakes are needed [5]. Iron, calcium, and zinc are needed throughout early childhood. Iron is important for optimal cognitive development [1]; calcium is critical in the development of bones and teeth and can be especially important during growth spurts [3], and zinc is important in growth [1]. Ensuring adequate intake of iron, calcium, and zinc can help reduce the risk of developing severe deficiencies such as iron deficiency anemia [1,2] or impaired growth, such as rickets [1,3]. Conversely, nutrient intakes exceeding cut points such as the tolerable upper intake level (UL) could lead to adverse consequences; however, limited data are available on functional outcomes for young children with regard to higher intake values [1,3].

Nationally representative data on the nutrient intake for this age group as well as the proportions who are meeting Dietary Reference Intakes, such as the Estimated Average Requirement (EAR), the Recommended Dietary Allowance (RDA), and those exceeding the UL, are lacking. Nutrition intake estimates among this age group can inform clinicians about key nutrient intakes during a critical growth period, as well as provide a basis for population level estimates that can support efforts, such as the United States Department of Agriculture (USDA)/Health and Human Services (HHS) Dietary Guidance Development Project for Birth to 24 Months and Pregnancy (B24/P) [6]. We focus this analysis on three key minerals needed for growth and development (iron, calcium, and zinc) for children 12–23 months of age and present the proportion meeting the EAR, RDA, and those exceeding the UL.

2. Materials and Methods

2.1. National Health and Nutrition Examination Survey

NHANES is an ongoing nationally representative survey of the noninstitutionalized civilian US population [7]. The survey is conducted using a stratified multistage probability design. Data from NHANES are released in 2-year cycles. This analysis includes data from 2003 to 2012. Survey respondents participate in a household interview in which participants are asked a variety of questions including information on demographics and health-related questions and a physical examination in which participants undergo a medical exam and participate in a dietary interview. Analyses reported by race/ethnicity were restricted to non-Hispanic white, non-Hispanic black, and Mexican American respondents because of the small number of individuals of other racial and ethnic groups; however, all race/ethnicities are included in analyses not stratified by race/ethnicity. We limited our analyses to children who were aged 12–23 months at the time of the physical examination. All participants in NHANES provide written informed consent or by proxy for those who are under 7 years of age. The National Center for Health Statistics Research Ethics Review Board provided the following protocol approval numbers for the presented survey years: Protocol #98-12 (NHANES 1999–2004), Protocol #2005-06 (NHANES 2005–2006), Continuation of Protocol #2005-06 (NHANES 2007–2010), and Protocol #2011-17 (NHANES 2011–2012).

2.2. Nutrient Intake

Usual nutrient intake (calories, iron, calcium, and zinc) was estimated using two 24 h dietary recall questionnaires. The first dietary recall was conducted in-person and the second dietary recall was conducted 3–10 days later via telephone. Dietary interviews for children less than 6 years of age were conducted using a proxy (i.e., a parent) who was most familiar with the child's dietary intake [8]. The USDA Food and Nutrient Database for Dietary Studies was used to determine the nutrient amount for foods that are reported in NHANES 2003–2012 [9–13]. Total nutrient intake for day one and day two of the 24 h dietary recall were used in analyses.

2.3. Analytic Sample

There were a total of 1534 children aged 12–23 months at the time of the physical examination from 2003 to 2012 and were eligible to complete a dietary recall. Children were excluded if they reported consuming any breast milk on either day one or day two of the dietary interview ($n = 94$) because nutrient intakes from breast milk were not available and therefore, total nutrient intake could not be calculated. Additionally, children who did not have a dietary intake record for day one and day two, or who had a dietary record that was coded as not reliable, were excluded ($n = 318$), leaving a final sample size of 1122 (78% of the eligible sample who did not consume any breast milk).

2.4. Covariates

Information on age, race/ethnicity, and income to poverty ratio were obtained through the household interview questionnaire. Race/ethnicity was based on respondents'/parental answers to questions on race and Hispanic origin. The income to poverty ratio, a ratio of family income to poverty guidelines, was based on the family's reported household income. The income to poverty ratio was split into three categories: (1) income to poverty ratios <1.85; (2) income to poverty ratios between 1.85 and less than 3.5; and (3) income to poverty ratios ⩾3.5. These income to poverty ratios correspond to income eligibility cut-offs used in the United States Department of Agriculture Women, Infants, and Children Program.

2.5. Statistical Analyses

Using data from the two 24-h dietary recalls, the usual intakes of total caloric intake (for reference), iron, calcium, and zinc for children 12–23 months of age were estimated using software developed by Iowa State University, PC-SIDE version 1.02 (Iowa State University, Ames, IA, USA) and within-person variation of nutrient intake were accounted for across days. In addition, the proportion of children below two specific cut-points, i.e., estimated average requirement (EAR) and recommended dietary allowance (RDA), and the proportion above the cut-points for tolerable upper intake level (UL) for each mineral were assessed. The EAR is the average daily nutrient intake estimated to meet the needs of half the healthy children of this age; whereas, the RDA is the average daily nutrient intake estimated to meet the needs of nearly all healthy children of this age [14]. The UL is the highest average daily intake likely to pose no adverse health effects [14]. Usual intakes were adjusted for the intake day of the week and interview method (in person vs. telephone). Estimates of usual intake and proportions were calculated by sex, race/ethnicity, and income to poverty ratio. Since usual intakes cannot be negative, any estimates that were negative (i.e., lower bound for 95% Confidence Interval (CIs)) were truncated at zero. Additionally, if a cut-point fell on the distribution of intakes such that no individual was included, these values did not have a standard error; thus, a zero value was given and no 95% CIs were provided.

SPSS Complex Samples Design version 23.0 (SPSS Inc., Chicago, IL, USA) was used to account for the survey design and calculate frequencies and Chi-square tests. All analyses were conducted using 10-year dietary weights calculated from day two dietary weights for the period 2003–2012, as recommended by the National Center for Health Statistics, Centers for Disease Control and Prevention [15,16]. For analyses conducted with PC-SIDE, standard errors were calculated using a set of 150 Jackknife replicate weights calculated using the 10-year dietary weights. T-tests were calculated to assess differences in mean usual intakes; statistical significance defined as $p < 0.05$.

3. Results

A total of 1122 children aged 12–23 months of age were included in the analysis. Approximately half of children were male (52%) (weighted percent). Over half (53.6%) of children were non-Hispanic white, 14.4% were non-Hispanic black, and 17.8% were Mexican American (weighted percent). Among the analytic sample, 49.3% reported an income to poverty ratio <1.85 (weighted percent).

Among children 12–23 months of age, the mean usual caloric intake was 1264 kcal/day (95% CI: 1225, 1302). Caloric intake did not differ by sex or income to poverty ratio, but non-Hispanic black children had significantly higher usual caloric intake than either non-Hispanic white children or Mexican American children (1350 kcal/day, 1267 kcal/day, and 1218 kcal/day, respectively) ($p < 0.05$). Mean usual iron intake was 9.5 mg/day (Table 1). Compared to non-Hispanic white and non-Hispanic black children, Mexican-American children had significantly lower reported mean usual iron intake (9.6 mg, 10.2 mg, and 8.5 mg, respectively) ($p < 0.05$). Mean usual calcium intake was 1046 mg/day; no differences were observed by sex, race/ethnicity, or poverty status. Mean usual zinc intake was 7.1 mg/day; girls had significantly lower zinc intake compared to boys (6.9 mg vs. 7.3 mg, respectively) ($p < 0.05$).

Less than 1% of children had usual iron intakes below the EAR (3 mg/day) [1]; however, 26.1% had usual intakes below the RDA (7 mg/day) [1]. Mexican American children had significantly higher proportions below the RDA for iron compared to non-Hispanic white and non-Hispanic black children

(36.4%, 24.3%, and 18.7%, respectively) ($p < 0.05$). No children had usual iron intakes exceeding the UL (40 mg/day) [1].

Table 1. Mean usual iron, calcium, and zinc intake for children age 12 to 23 months [1,2] by select demographic characteristics, NHANES 2003–2012.

	Mean (95% Confidence Interval)		
	Iron (mg)	Calcium (mg)	Zinc (mg)
Total ($n = 1122$)	9.5 (9.0, 10.0)	1046 (1002, 1090)	7.1 (6.9, 7.4)
Sex			
Male ($n = 574$)	9.8 (9.1, 10.5)	1050 (992, 1108)	7.3 (7.0, 7.7) [a]
Female ($n = 548$)	9.1 (8.5, 9.7)	1041 (985, 1097)	6.9 (6.7, 7.2) [b]
Race/ethnicity [3]			
Non-Hispanic white ($n = 332$)	9.6 (8.9, 10.4) [a]	1055 (981, 1128)	7.2 (6.8, 7.6)
Non-Hispanic black ($n = 261$)	10.2 (9.4, 11.1) [a]	983 (909, 1056)	7.2 (6.6, 7.7)
Mexican American ($n = 357$)	8.5 (8.0, 9.1) [b]	1047 (993, 1100)	7.2 (6.8, 7.5)
Poverty status			
Income to poverty ratio <1.85 ($n = 684$)	9.4 (8.8, 9.9)	1020 (973, 1068)	7.2 (6.9, 7.5)
Income to poverty ratio 1.85 to <3.5 ($n = 204$)	9.2 (8.3, 10.1)	1056 (962, 1149)	7.0 (6.5, 7.5)
Income to poverty ratio ≥3.5 ($n = 174$)	9.8 (8.7, 10.9)	1095 (1011, 1180)	7.1 (6.6, 7.6)

[1] Does not include any children who reported consuming breast milk on either day one or day two of the 24-h dietary recall; [2] age in months at time of exam in Medical Examination Center; [3] race/ethnicity subanalyses are limited to those individuals who report being either non-Hispanic white, non-Hispanic black, and Mexican American; values with superscript letters that differ are significantly different, p-value < 0.05; abbreviations: National Health and Nutrition Examination Survey (NHANES).

Two percent of children 12–23 months had usual calcium intake below the EAR (500 mg/day) [3] and 11.2% had usual calcium intakes below the RDA (700 mg/day) [3] (Table 2). Non-Hispanic black children and children with an income to poverty ratio <1.85 had significantly higher proportions below the RDA for calcium ($p < 0.05$). There were no children 12–23 months with usual calcium intakes that exceeded the UL (2500 mg/day) [3].

Less than 1% of children had usual zinc intakes below either the EAR (2.5 mg/day) [1] or the RDA (3 mg/day) [1]. Over 50% of children had usual zinc intakes that exceeded the UL (7 mg/day) [1]; no differences by sex, race/ethnicity, or income to poverty ratio were observed.

4. Discussion

Our analyses presented nationally representative usual mean intake for children 12–23 months of age on key minerals needed for healthy growth and development [1,3]. Our findings indicate that one in four children and one in ten children 12–23 months of age are not consuming enough iron and calcium to meet current RDA recommendations, respectively. However, one in two children 12–23 months of age are exceeding the UL for zinc.

Our findings, presented here, are similar to what was reported in the 2008 Feeding Infants and Toddler Study (FITS) [17], a cross-sectional consumer panel survey weighted to be nationally representative. For example, FITS reported usual intake of zinc 7.2 mg/day and our analysis indicated a usual intake of 7.1 mg/day. However, FITS data had slightly lower usual intakes of calories and calcium and higher usual intakes of iron as compared to our results using NHANES (FITS: 1141 kcal/day; 892 mg/day calcium; 10.3 mg/day iron; NHANES: 1264 kcal/day; 1046 mg/day calcium; 9.5 mg/day iron) [17]. The FITS 2008 findings assessed both the proportion below the EAR and the proportion exceeding the UL and found similar results as those presented here. Although FITS is considered nationally representative, it may not be truly representative if the consumer panel used as the sampling frame is not representative of the US population. Although the surveys had slightly different estimates, both came to similar conclusions in regard to nutrient intake of key minerals for children in the second year of life (12–23 months of age).

Table 2. Percent of children aged 12 to 23 months [1,2] not meeting recommendations for iron, calcium and zinc by select demographic characteristics, NHANES 2003–2012 [3].

	Iron			Calcium			Zinc		
	% below EAR (3 mg/Day)	% below RDA (7 mg/Day)	% above UL (40 mg/Day)	% below EAR (500 mg/Day)	% below RDA (700 mg/Day)	% above UL (2500 mg/Day)	% below EAR (2.5 mg/Day)	% below RDA (3 mg/Day)	% above UL (7 mg/Day)
Total (n = 1122)	0.4 (0.2, 0.6)	26.1 (21.7, 30.4)	0	2.0 (1.3, 2.7)	11.2 (8.7, 13.7)	0	0	0.1 (0, 0.2)	50.8 (45.4, 56.1)
Sex									
Male (n = 574)	0.5 (0.1, 0.8)	25.0 (18.9, 31.1)	0	2.8 (1.4, 4.2) [a]	13.1 (8.7, 17.6)	0	0	0.2 (0, 0.3)	46.8 (39.0, 54.6)
Female (n = 548)	0.4 (0.7)	26.9 (20.5, 33.3)	0	1.2 (0.6, 1.8) [b]	9.4 (6.5, 12.4)	0	0	0.1 (0, 0.2)	55.3 (48.2, 62.5)
Race/ethnicity [4]									
Non-Hispanic white (n = 332)	0.3 (0, 0.7) [a,b]	24.3 (18.1, 30.4) [a]	0	2.1 (1.0, 3.1) [a,b]	11.5 (7.0, 16.1) [a,b]	0	0	0 [a]	48.2 (37.6, 58.9)
Non-Hispanic black (n = 261)	0 (0, 0.2) [a]	18.7 (12.7, 24.8) [a]	0	3.6 (1.1, 6.1) [b]	17.4 (10.4, 24.4) [b]	0	0 (0, 0)	0.3 (0.1, 0.4) [b]	51.7 (40.7, 62.6)
Mexican American (n = 357)	0.8 (0.2, 1.4) [b]	36.4 (29.6, 43.1) [b]	0	1.3 (0.5, 2.2) [a]	9.6 (6.4, 12.8) [a]	0	0	0 (0, 0.2) [a]	50.6 (42.4, 58.9)
Poverty status									
Income to poverty ratio <1.85 (n = 684)	0.2 (0.1, 0.4)	23.1 (16.7, 29.4)	0	2.3 (1.3, 3.2)	13.8 (10.2, 17.4) [a]	0	0	0.1 (0, 0.2) [a,b]	50.0 (43.2, 56.7)
Income to poverty ratio 1.85 to <3.5 (n = 204)	0.7 (0.1, 1.4)	32.8 (22.8, 42.8)	0	2.5 (0.8, 4.1)	12.0 (6.9, 17.1) [a,b]	0 (0, 0)	0	0.2 (0, 0.4) [a]	53.3 (42.7, 63.8)
Income to poverty ratio ≥3.5 (n = 174)	0.5 (1.1)	27.8 (19.5, 36.1)	0	1.8 (0.2, 3.4)	9.0 (4.5, 13.4) [b]	0 (0, 0)	0	0 [b]	50.4 (38.0, 62.7)

[1] Does not include any children who reported consuming breast milk on either day one or day two of the 24 h dietary recall; [2] age in months at time of exam in Medical Examination Center; [3] since usual intakes cannot be negative, any estimates that were negative (i.e., lower bound for 95% Confidence Interval (CIs)) were truncated at zero and 95% CIs are provided. If a cut-point fell on the distribution of intakes such that no individual was included, these values did not have a standard error; thus, a zero value was given and no 95% CIs were provided; [4] race/ethnicity subanalyses are limited to those individuals who report being either non-Hispanic white, non-Hispanic black, and Mexican American; values with superscript letters that differ are significantly different, p-value < 0.05; abbreviations: Estimated Average Requirement (EAR), National Health and Nutrition Examination Survey (NHANES), Recommended Dietary Allowance (RDA), Tolerable Upper Intake Level (UL).

Our analysis expanded on the FITS assessment by looking at the proportion of children 12–23 months of age with usual intakes below the RDA. One in every four children, and one in every three children who was Mexican American, reported having an iron intake below the RDA and the intake value recommended by the AAP [1,2]. A recent study by Grimes et al. reported the top food sources of iron for this age group and found ready-to-eat cereals, baby foods, breads, rolls and tortillas, mixed dishes—grains, and cooked cereals were responsible for half of a child's total daily iron intake [18]. These sources are a combination of multiple foods and could represent fortified sources (i.e., ready-to-eat cereals), as well as heme-rich sources (i.e., baby foods with meat) or non-heme sources (i.e., baby foods with fruit and/or vegetables). Adequate intake of iron can help reduce the likelihood of developing iron deficiency and iron deficiency anemia [2]. According to data from NHANES 2007–2010, 13.5% of children 1–2 years of age were considered iron deficient [19]. Given the importance of iron in optimal cognitive development at this age [1,2], the reported estimates of iron deficiency [19] and iron intake suggest the need to ensure young children are consuming adequate iron and to continue monitoring iron status.

Calcium has also been identified as a key mineral to ensuring adequate growth and development of young children, especially for bone health [3]. With the development of the 2011 Institute of Medicine report on calcium and vitamin D, there are now EARs and RDAs for calcium for children 1–3 years of age; these values were not available in the previous 1997 IOM report for calcium and vitamin D [3,20]. Our data indicate that although very few children 12–23 months of age have a usual calcium intake below the EAR, one in ten, and almost one in five non-Hispanic black children (17.4%), have an intake below the RDA. Milk is the main food group that contributes to calcium intake for this age group with over 50% of daily intake of calcium coming from milk [18]. However, trends in beverage consumption indicate a significant decline in milk consumption among 1 year olds (3.8% decline) and an increase in 100% fruit juice consumption (21.9% increase) from 1988–1994 to 2001–2006 [21]. Continued support for ensuring adequate calcium intake through sources like milk is important.

Ensuring adequate zinc intake for young children, especially during the transition from breast milk to complementary foods, has been one of the cornerstones of AAP recommendations [4]. However, our data indicate that over half of children 12–23 months have usual zinc intakes that exceed the UL, which is similar to what Butte et al. reported using FITS [17]. Milk and ready-to-eat cereals were the top two food sources contributing 39.1% of total zinc intake among children 12–23 months of age [18]. Ready-to-eat cereals may be fortified with zinc and could be one of the reasons for higher zinc intakes in this age group. Data were not available on children 1–3 years of age to set a UL value for zinc for this age group[1]; however, data were available from one study among 68 infants 0–6 months of age receiving infant formula with 5.8 mg zinc/L of formula for six months found no adverse effects [22]. Using this study as a basis, the UL value for zinc among children 1–3 years of age was extrapolated and then adjusted for body weight [1]. Two case reports of children receiving ⩾16 mg of zinc for ⩾6 months developed a copper-induced anemia [23,24]; however, evidence of zinc toxicity in young children is not often reported [25,26] and may not be a concern at the population level. Additionally, the potential that the zinc UL for children is too low has been raised [27,28]. Therefore, interpreting whether the proportion of children above the UL for zinc is of concern should be done with caution since limited data are available supporting population-level indications of adverse health outcomes associated with high intake and the relevance of the current UL value has been questioned. Continued monitoring of zinc intake and the potential for adverse health outcomes could be warranted.

This analysis provides pediatricians, other health care providers, and public health practitioners with evidence on the nutritional intake of young children, specifically for key minerals needed for healthy growth and development. Compared with developing countries, children in the United States may not be considered as at risk for specific nutritional deficiencies; however, this analysis indicates that for specific minerals, such as iron, there may be a need for a renewed focus on ensuring children are consuming adequate nutrients. A further assessment of nationally representative data on the nutritional status of young children using biomarkers could help provide context to national level policies and recommendations for foods and food groups to encourage. Biomarkers, with the exception of iron, on this age group are not routinely collected through surveys, such as NHANES, but specific biomarkers may need to be considered given the assessment of current intake and the development of the B24/P Guidance.

This study is subject to several limitations. First, we combined multiple survey years. Although this provides a larger sample size and smaller standard errors, the data span a period of ten years. Sociodemographic characteristics did not differ by survey year; however, we did find that usual caloric intake was significantly higher in 2003–2004. We did not correct for this because we were not assessing trends over time and recommendations, such as the EAR, RDA and UL are set values and are not dependent on total caloric intake. Second, we did not include any nutrient intake coming from dietary supplements, which could contribute to mineral intake. This decision was based on a change in methodology for reporting supplement intake during the survey years included in our analysis. When we assessed the frequency of supplement use in a subset of the population with similar supplement intake methodology, we concluded that the inclusion of dietary supplements would not change the overall interpretation of our results. Specifically, we found that among children 12–23 months of age surveyed in 2007–2012, 13.3% reported consuming any dietary supplement on day 1 Lastly, we limited our analyses to children not reporting the consumption of breast milk during the second year of life on day one or day two of the dietary intake recall. This was done because nutrient intakes were not reported for children who reported consuming any breast milk. A total of 94 children reported some consumption of breastmilk (6% of the original sample). As a result, these findings may not be generalizable to children consuming breast milk during the second year of life. There were also several strengths of this study. First, NHANES is a nationally representative study. Second, usual dietary intake assessment was possible because two 24-h dietary recalls were collected and nutrients examined were consumed on a daily basis and were not episodic. This allowed for the estimation of the proportions of the population at specific cut-points (i.e., EAR, RDA, and UL). Lastly, because we combined survey years, we were able to have adequate sample size to stratify by different sociodemographic factors.

5. Conclusions

During 2003–2012, one in every four and one in every ten children 12–23 months of age is not meeting the recommended iron and calcium intake, respectively. Efforts to ensure children are consuming optimal amounts of both iron and calcium are important for their growth and development. One in every two children 12–23 months of age is exceeding the UL for zinc, but the interpretation of these estimates should be done with caution given the limited data on adverse health outcomes.

Acknowledgments: No funding was secured for this study.

Author Contributions: H.C.H. conceived the research question and analyzed the data; H.C.H., C.G.P. and K.S.S. reviewed and interpreted the statistical analyses and wrote the paper.

Disclaimer: The findings and conclusions in this report are those of the authors and do not necessarily represent the official position of the Centers for Disease Control and Prevention.

Abbreviations

AAP	American Academy of Pediatrics
B24/P	Birth to 24 Months and Pregnancy
CI	Confidence Interval
EAR	Estimated Average Requirement
FITS	Feeding Infants and Toddler Study

HHS   Health and Human Services
NHANES   National Health and Nutrition Examination Survey
RDA   Recommended Dietary Allowance
UL   Tolerable Upper Intake Level
USDA   United States Department of Agriculture

References

1.   Institute of Medicine. *Dietary Reference Intakes: Vitamin A, Vitamin K, Arsenic, Boron, Chromium, Copper, Iodine, Iron, Manganese, Molybedenum, Nickel, Silicon, Vanadium, and Zinc*; National Academy Press: Washington, DC, USA, 2001.

2.   Baker, R.D.; Greer, F.R. American Academy of Pediatrics Committe on Nutrition. Clinical report—Diagnosis and prevention of iron deficiency and iron-deficiency anemia in infants and young children (0–3 years of age). *Pediatrics* **2010**, *126*, 1040–1050. [CrossRef] [PubMed]

3.   Institute of Medicine. *Dietary Reference Intakes for Calcium and Vitamin D*; The National Academies Press: Washington, DC, USA, 2011.

4.   American Academy of Pediatrics Committe on Nutrition. Chapter 6: Complementary feeding. In *Pediatric Nutrition*, 7th ed.; Kleinman, R.E., Greer, F.R., Eds.; American Academy of Pediatrics: Elk Grove Village, IL, USA, 2014.

5.   Dewey, K.G.; Vitta, B.S. *Strategies for Ensuring Adequate Nutrient Intake for Infants and Young Children during the Period of Complementary Feeding*; A & T Technical Brief: Washington, DC, USA, 2013; pp. 1–14.

6.   Raiten, D.J.; Raghavan, R.; Porter, A.; Obbagy, J.E.; Spahn, J.M. Executive summary: Evaluating the evidnce base to support the inclusion of infants and children from birth to 24 months of age in the Dietary Guidelines for Americans—"The B-24 Project". *Am. J. Clin. Nutr.* **2014**, *99*, 663S–691S. [CrossRef] [PubMed]

7.   National Center for Health Statistics. About the National Health and Nutrition Examination Survey. Available online: http://www.cdc.gov/nchs/nhanes/about_nhanes.htm (accessed on 7 March 2016).

8.   National Center for Health Statistics. National Health and Nutrition Examination Survey: Dietary Data. Available online: http://wwwn.cdc.gov/Nchs/Nhanes/Search/DataPage.aspx?Component=Dietary&CycleBeginYear=2011 (accessed on 14 December 2015).

9.   US Department of Agriculture. Food and Nutrient Database for Dietary Studies, 2.0. Available online: http://www.ars.usda.gov/SP2UserFiles/Place/80400530/pdf/fndds/fndds2_doc.pdf (accessed on 28 July 2016).

10. US Department of Agriculture. Food and Nutrient Database for Dietary Studies, 3.0. Available online: http://www.ars.usda.gov/SP2UserFiles/Place/80400530/pdf/fndds/fndds3_doc.pdf (accessed on 28 July 2016).

11. US Department of Agriculture. Food and Nutrient Database for Dietary Studies, 4.0. Available online: http://www.ars.usda.gov/SP2UserFiles/Place/80400530/pdf/fndds/fndds4_doc.pdf (accessed on 28 July 2016).

12. US Department of Agriculture. Food and Nutrient Database for Dietary Studies, 5.0. Available online: http://www.ars.usda.gov/SP2UserFiles/Place/80400530/pdf/fndds/fndds5_doc.pdf (accessed on 28 July 2016).

13. US Department of Agriculture. Food and Nutrient Database for Dietary Studies 2011–2012. Available online: http://www.ars.usda.gov/SP2UserFiles/Place/80400530/pdf/fndds/fndds_2011_2012_doc.pdf (accessed on 28 July 2016).

14. Institute of Medicine. *Dietary Reference Intakes: Application in Dietary Assessment*; National Academy Press: Washington DC, USA, 2000.

15. National Center for Health Statistics. *National Health and Nutrition Examination Survey: Analytic Guidelines, 2011–2012*; Centers for Disease Control and Prevention: Hyattsville, MD, USA, 2013.

16. Johnson, C.L.; Paulose-Ram, R.; Ogden, C.L.; Carroll, M.D.; Kruszon-Moran, D.; Dohrmann, S.M.; Curtin, L.R. National health and nutrition examination survey: Analytic guidelines, 1999–2010. *Vital Health Stat.* **2013**, *2*, 1–24.

17. Butte, N.F.; Fox, M.K.; Briefel, R.R.; Siega-Riz, A.M.; Dwyer, J.T.; Deming, D.M.; Reidy, K.C. Nutrient intakes of US infants, toddlers, and preschoolers meet or exceed Dietary Reference Intakes. *J. Am. Diet. Assoc.* **2010**, *110*, S27–S37. [CrossRef] [PubMed]

18. Grimes, C.A.; Szymlek-Gay, E.A.; Campbell, K.J.; Nicklas, T.A. Food sources of total energy and nutrients among US infants and toddlers: National Health and Nutrition Examination Survey 2005–2012. *Nutrients* **2015**, *7*, 6797–6836. [CrossRef] [PubMed]

19. Gupta, P.M.; Perrine, C.G.; Mei, Z.; Scanlon, K.S. Iron, anemia, and iron deficiency anemia among young children in the United States. *Nutrients* **2016**, *8*. [CrossRef] [PubMed]

20. Institute of Medicine. *Dietary Reference Intakes for Calcium, Phosphorus, Magnesium, Vitamin D, and Fluoride*; National Academy Press: Washington, DC, USA, 1997.

21. Fulgoini, V.L.; Quann, E.E. National trends in beverage consumption in children from birth to 5 years: Analysis of NHANES across three decades. *Nutr. J.* **2012**, *11*, 1–11. [CrossRef] [PubMed]

22. Walravens, P.A.; Hambidge, M. Growth of infants fed a zinc supplemented formula. *Am. J. Clin. Nutr.* **1976**, *29*, 1114–1121. [PubMed]

23. Botash, A.S.; Nasca, J.; Dubowy, R.; Weinberger, H.L.; Oliphant, M. Zinc-induced copper deficiency in an infant. *Am. J. Dis. Child.* **1992**, *146*, 709–711. [CrossRef] [PubMed]

24. Sugiura, T.; Goto, K.; Ito, K.; Ueta, A.; Fujimoto, S.; Togari, H. Chronic zinc toxicity in an infant who received zinc theraphy for atopic dermatitis. *Acta Paediatr.* **2005**, *94*, 1333–1335. [CrossRef] [PubMed]

25. Krebs, N.F. Update on zinc deficiency and excess in clinical pediatirc practice. *Ann. Nutr. Metab.* **2013**, *62*, 19–29. [CrossRef] [PubMed]

26. Willoughby, J.L.; Bowen, C.N. Zinc deficiency and toxicity in pediatric practice. *Curr. Opin. Pediatr.* **2014**, *26*, 579–584. [CrossRef] [PubMed]

27. King, J.C.; Brown, K.H.; Gibson, R.S.; KrebS, N.F.; Lowe, N.M.; Siekmann, J.H.; Raiten, D.J. Biomarkers of nutrition for development (BOND)—Zinc review. *J. Nutr.* **2016**. [CrossRef] [PubMed]

28. Bertinato, J.; Simpson, J.R.; Sherrard, L.; Taylor, J.; Plouffe, L.J.; Van Dyke, D.; Geleynse, M.; Dam, Y.Y.; Murphy, P.; Knee, C.; et al. Zinc supplementation does not alter sensitive biomarkers of copper status in healthy boys. *J. Nutr.* **2013**, *143*, 284–289. [CrossRef] [PubMed]

14

Changes in Biochemical Parameters of the Calcium-Phosphorus Homeostasis in Relation to Nutritional Intake in Very-Low-Birth-Weight Infants

Viola Christmann [1,*], Charlotte J. W. Gradussen [1], Michelle N. Körnmann [1], Nel Roeleveld [2,3], Johannes B. van Goudoever [4,5] and Arno F. J. van Heijst [1]

[1] Department of Paediatrics, Subdivision of Neonatology, Radboudumc Amalia Children's Hospital, Radboud University Medical Center, Nijmegen 6500HB, The Netherlands; charlotte.gradussen@radboudumc.nl (C.J.W.G.); michelle.kornmann@radboudumc.nl (M.N.K.); arno.vanheijst@radboudumc.nl (A.F.J.v.H.)

[2] Department for Health Evidence, Radboud Institute for Health Science, Radboud University Medical Center, Nijmegen 6500HB, The Netherlands; nel.roeleveld@radboudumc.nl

[3] Department of Paediatrics, Radboudumc Amalia Children's Hospital, Radboud University Medical Center, Nijmegen 6500HB, The Netherlands

[4] Department of Paediatrics, VU university medical center Amsterdam, Amsterdam 1081HV, The Netherlands; h.vangoudoever@vumc.nl

[5] Department of Paediatrics, Emma Children's Hospital-AMC Amsterdam, Amsterdam 1105AZ, The Netherlands

* Correspondence: viola.christmann@radboudumc.nl

Abstract: Preterm infants are at significant risk to develop reduced bone mineralization based on inadequate supply of calcium and phosphorus (Ca-P). Biochemical parameters can be used to evaluate the nutritional intake. The direct effect of nutritional intake on changes in biochemical parameters has not been studied. Our objective was to evaluate the effect of Ca-P supplementation on biochemical markers as serum (s)/urinary (u) Ca and P; alkaline phosphatase (ALP); tubular reabsorption of P (TrP); and urinary ratios for Ca/creatinin (creat) and P/creatinin in Very-Low-Birth-Weight infants on Postnatal Days 1, 3, 5, 7, 10, and 14. This observational study compared two groups with High ($n = 30$) and Low ($n = 40$) intake of Ca-P. Birth weight: median (IRQ) 948 (772–1225) vs. 939 (776–1163) grams; and gestational age: 28.2 (26.5–29.6) vs. 27.8 (26.1–29.4) weeks. Daily median concentrations of biochemical parameter were not different between the groups but linear regression mixed model analyses showed that Ca intake increased the uCa and TrP ($p = 0.04$) and decreased ALP ($p = 0.00$). Phosphorus intake increased sP, uP and uP/creat ratio and ALP ($p \leq 0.02$) and caused decrease in TrP ($p = 0.00$). Protein intake decreased sP ($p = 0.000$), while low gestational age and male gender increased renal excretion of P ($p < 0.03$). Standardized repeated measurements showed that biochemical parameters were affected by nutritional intake, gestational age and gender.

Keywords: blood; bone mineralization; minerals; monitoring; nutrition; renal tubular reabsorption; supplementation; urine

1. Introduction

Bone development is one of the key processes of intrauterine and postnatal growth [1]. Preterm infants are at significant risk to develop reduced bone mineral content based on inadequate supply of calcium and phosphorus (Ca-P) [2,3]. During normal pregnancies in healthy mothers, there is an active, placental transfer of Ca-P to the fetus leading to a high mineral accretion during the last trimester, while after birth the infant is dependent on nutritional supply of minerals [4,5].

In clinical practice, postnatally it is difficult to meet the high fetal needs, because of limited solubility of parenteral fluids, low content of Ca-P of human milk and impaired intestinal absorption through formula feeding [6–9]. Studies tried to define nutritional requirements, but, in clinical practice, it is often uncertain whether the nutritional intake of Ca-P provided to preterm infants is sufficient and is actually used for bone mineralization [10–12].

Assuming that biochemical parameters of Ca-P homeostasis within a normal range will lead to optimal bone mineralization, evaluation of electrolyte disturbances is standard of care in many neonatal units [13–28]. However, there is currently neither a consensus on the appropriateness of either parameter or the frequency of measurements [29,30]. A recent survey among U.S. neonatologists showed a great lack of consensus and variation in practices regarding definition and screening methods for metabolic bone disease [31]. Reference values in relation to adequate nutritional intake have not been developed. Urinary excretion of minerals in spot urine samples has been shown to be an easy tool for routine evaluation. Pohlandt proposed to aim for a small "surplus of minerals" in urine samples, while Aladangady et al. developed reference values for urinary Ca-P/creatinine ratios for preterm infants [17,23]. Staub et al. compared both methods with regard to an agreement between their results and found neither method to be superior [32]. None of the studies evaluated the direct effect of nutritional intake on biochemical parameter of Ca-P homeostasis. It is not sure whether biochemical parameters are able to indicate sufficiency of nutritional intake.

The aim of this study was to evaluate changes in biochemical parameters of the Ca-P homeostasis in blood and urine in relation to different nutritional intake during the first 14 days of life in Very Low Birth Weight (VLBW) infants. Our hypothesis was that the nutritional intake of calcium and phosphorus would have an effect on biochemical parameters of the calcium–phosphorus homeostasis.

2. Materials and Methods

2.1. Study Design and Randomization

The current study (Early Supplementation Study (ESS)) was part of the Early Nutrition Study (ENS), a multi-center double-blinded randomized controlled trial. While the ENS evaluated the effects of human milk on postnatal outcome, the primary objective of the ESS was bone mineralization in relation to early and late enteral supplementation of minerals [33]. The studies were approved by the Ethical Committee of the VU university medical center (Amsterdam, The Netherlands), 13 September 2013 (CMO file number: NL37296.029.11, Dutch Trial Registry: NTR 3225). Patients were distributed into three groups through two steps of randomization. The first step randomized eligible infants either into the early supplementation group (High) or the late supplementation group (Low) being part of the ENS. The second step of the randomization was only performed if infants were assigned to late supplementation and randomized them to either "ENS A" or "ENS B" as part of the ENS. Both randomization steps were performed before the first enteral nutrition was administered resulting in basically three groups.

2.2. Study Population

Participants for the ENS/ESS were recruited at the level III neonatal intensive care unit of the Radboud university medical center (Radboudumc), Nijmegen, The Netherlands. The inclusion criteria were a birth weight below 1500 grams and written informed consent of both parents. The exclusion criteria were maternal drugs and/or alcohol use during pregnancy, birth defects, congenital infection within 72 h after birth, perinatal asphyxia with a pH < 7.0 and any intake of cow's milk based products prior to randomization. For the current study, infants who died or were discharged before the end of the study period of 14 days were excluded from analysis.

2.3. Intervention and Nutritional Protocol

Parenteral nutrition (PN) was started directly within the first hour after birth. The PN solution consisted of 2.5 mmol/dL calcium-gluconate (calcium-gluconate 10%; B. Braun, Melsungen, Germany) and 1.6 mmol/dL sodium-glycerophosphate (Glycophos; Fresenius Kabi BV, Zeist, The Netherlands) and 2.25 grams/dL amino acids (Primene; Clintec, Brussels). Additional parenteral supplementation with 10% calcium-gluconate or sodium glycero-phosphate was administrated depending on biochemical parameters. Table A1 presents the standard protocol for PN. The decision to start additional supplementation was left to the attending neonatologist based on biochemical parameter as being a standard procedure of our department.

Enteral feeding was started on the first day of life with daily increments, while PN was gradually reduced to maintain a daily fluid intake within the protocol range. Late supplementation was assumed to provide a low intake of nutrients because "Group Low", comprising of group ENS A and ENS B, received no additional enteral supplementation or fortification of human milk during the first 10 days of life. Group ENS A received donor milk if mother's own milk (MOM) was not available. Group ENS B received preterm formula (Hero Baby Prematuur Start; Hero Kindervoeding, Breda, The Netherlands) if MOM was not available, containing 2.4 mmol/dL calcium, 1.7 mmol/dL phosphorus and 2.6 grams/dL proteins. The additional nutrition in ENS A and ENS B was blinded to all caretakers and parents. After 10 days, all infants received nutrition according to the standard protocol of the Radboudumc.

Early supplementation was assumed to provide a high intake (Group High). This group received enteral nutrition from Day 1 onwards according to the local protocol. They received additional enteral supplementation and human milk fortifier (Nutrilon Neonatal BMF; Nutricia, Zoetermeer, The Netherlands; BMF) by the time the enteral intake was 50 mL per day. The human milk fortifier added 1.65 mmol/dL calcium, 1.22 mmol/dL phosphorus and 0.8 grams/dL protein to human milk. They received preterm formula if MOM was not available. The decision to start additional enteral supplementation was left to the attending neonatologist based on biochemical parameter and postnatal growth as being a standard procedure of our department. The additional enteral supplementation could comprise of either a supplement of protein (Nutrilon Nenatal Protein Fortifier; Nutricia, Zoetermeer, The Netherlands) or a potassium phosphate (KPO_4) and calcium chloride ($CaCl_2$) suspension for enteral supplementation.

Group ENS A received 100% human milk during the first 10 days and reflected a group with low intake of minerals and protein, because human milk has a very low nutrient content. Group High reflected a high intake of nutrients, because human milk was enriched with minerals and protein as soon as possible. Group ENS B could be considered as intermediate depending on the amount of MOM or preterm formula an infant received, since preterm formula contained approximately the same amount of minerals as fortified human milk.

2.4. Biochemical Parameters of Bone Mineralization

For this study, blood and urine samples were analyzed according to the local protocol of the department. Samples were taken on Days 1, 3, 5, 7, 10 and 14 after birth. Urine was collected through spot samples [25]. The following parameters were analyzed: serum calcium (sCa), serum phosphorus (sP), serum alkaline phosphatase (ALP), urine calcium (uCa), urine phosphorus (uP), urine calcium/creatinin ratio (uCa/Creat), urine phosphorus/creatinin ratio (uP/Creat), and tubular reabsorption of phosphorus (TrP).

2.5. Data Registration and Handling

Patient characteristics, clinical course, growth and intake of all nutrients were recorded daily from the patient records and abstracted for this study. Amounts of enteral, parenteral and additional supplementation (parenteral and enteral) of all nutrients were calculated separately for each patient. The total intakes were calculated per kg per day per infant. The intake through human milk was calculated based on the reference of Gidrewicz et al. [34]. The calcium/phosphorus ratio was calculated per day by dividing the daily intake of calcium in mmol/kg through the daily intake of phosphorus in mmol/kg.

After closure of patient enrollment and de-blinding of the ENS, we performed a reallocation procedure for the intermediate group ENS B. Infants who received more than 90% MOM were considered to reflect a low intake of minerals and were allocated to group Low together with the infants of group ENS A. Infants who received more than 90% of preterm formula were considered to reflect a high intake of minerals and were allocated to High. Infants in between these extremes were not included in the analyses.

2.6. Statistical Analysis

The primary objective of the ESS was bone mineralization in relation to mineral supplementation, and the original power calculation was based on bone mineral content at term corrected age. For the evaluation of changes in biochemical parameters in relation to nutritional intake the power calculation was based on sP. In a previous evaluation of our nutritional protocol performed at our department, we found a mean 1.7 mmol/L of sP during the first week [35]. A concentration of 2.0 mmol/L was defined as target for optimal bone mineralization by Hellstern et al. [20]. Assuming an expected mean of 1.7 mmol/L, we determined that 24 infants were required in each group to find a difference of 0.3 mmol/L in sP between High and Low with $\alpha = 0.05$ (two-sided) and a power of $\beta = 0.80$.

The statistical analyses were performed using IBM SPSS statistics 22.0 for Windows (IBM SPSS Inc., Chicago, IL, USA). Differences in patient characteristics, nutritional characteristics and biochemical parameters between the High and Low group were determined using the Mann-Whitney U test or the chi-square test, depending on the variable under examination. Due to non-normality of the continuous variables, the data were presented as median (with interquartile range (IQR)), unless otherwise indicated. A p-value < 0.05 was considered statistically significant.

To account for repeated outcome measurements, we used a mixed model analysis to determine the effects of daily nutritional intake of calcium and phosphorus on each biochemical parameter. We included the total intake of Ca/P and protein, the percentage of enteral amount of Ca/P intake, and a number of clinical parameter that could affect the Ca/P homeostasis such as birth weight, gestational age, gender, caesarian section, multiple births, sepsis, and days of caffeine, furosemide, steroids, and sedation during the first two weeks as co-variables in the initial models. Necrotizing enterocolitis was not included as co-variable because of small numbers. Using manual backward selection, variables were kept in the model when they contributed statistically significantly with a p-value < 0.1.

3. Results

3.1. Patient Characteristics

Enrollment of patients occurred between January 2013 and December 2014. The distribution of the infants is presented in the consort diagram (Figure 1). Finally, 109 infants were randomized, eithe to Late Supplementation (Low; $n = 72$; distributed into Group ENS A ($n = 40$) and ENS B ($n = 32$) or Early Supplementation (High; $n = 37$).

The characteristics of all infants included in the three groups of the ENS/ESS study are presented in Table A2. After de-blinding of group Low, four infants of group ENS B were reallocated to High and 13 to Low so that Low and High consisted of 53 and 41 infants, respectively. Infants who died or were discharged before postnatal Day 14 (13 in Low, 11 in High) were excluded. Finally, data of 40 infants of Low and 30 of High were analyzed. The baseline patient characteristics, morbidity, medication and nutritional characteristics for these patients are presented in Table 1. Infant characteristics were well balanced between the groups Low and High and comparable to the original groups.

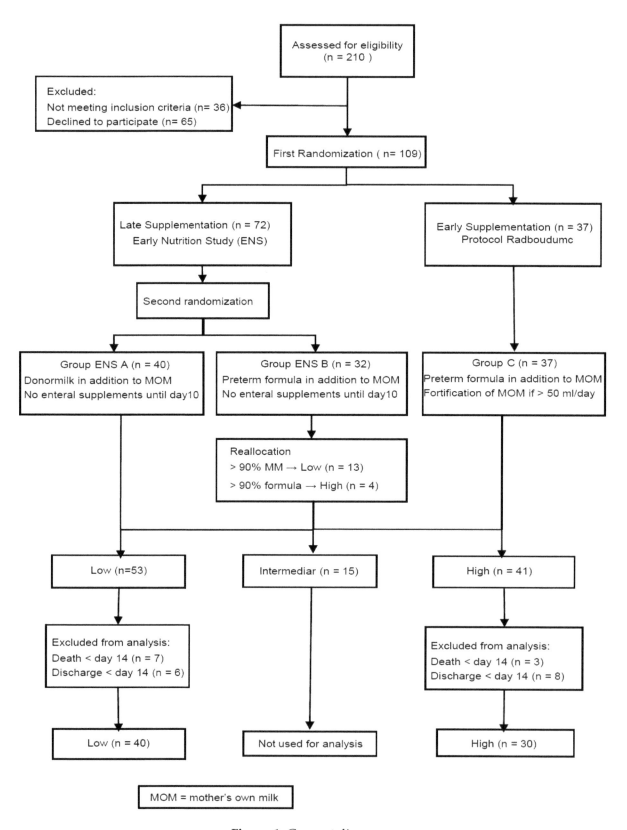

Figure 1. Consort diagram.

Table 1. Patient characteristics, morbidity, medication, and nutritional characteristics.

	Low (*n* = 40)	High (*n* = 30)	*p*-Value
Characteristics			
Birth weight, grams; median (IQR)	948 (772–1225)	939 (776–1163)	0.85
<1000 gram, *n* (%)	22 (55.0)	16 (53.3)	0.89
Gestational age, median (IQR)	28.2 (26.5–29.6)	27.8 (26.1–29.4)	0.76
SGA, *n* (%)	8 (20.0)	4 (13.3)	0.46
Male, *n* (%)	19 (47.5)	15 (50.0)	0.84
Singletons, *n* (%)	28 (70.0)	16 (53.3)	0.15
Cesarean section, *n* (%)	18 (45.0)	20 (66.7)	0.07
Apgar score (5 min), median (IQR)	7.0 (6.3–9.0)	7.5 (7.0–8.0)	0.71
Apgar score (5 min) <7, *n* (%)	10 (25.0%)	6 (20.0%)	0.62
Morbidity			
Sepsis, *n* (%)	8 (20.0%)	9 (30.0%)	0.33
NEC ≥ stage 2, *n* (%)	1 (2.5%)	2 (6.7%)	0.39
IVH Grade 3–4 *n* (%)	5 (12.5)	3 (10)	0.75
Medication			
Caffeïne; *n* (%)	39 (97.5%)	28 (93.3%)	0.39
Furosemide, *n* (%)	3 (7.5%)	4 (13.3%)	0.42
Corticosteroids	3 (7.5)	1 (3.3)	0.46
Sedation, *n* (%)	8 (20.0%)	9 (30.0%)	0.33
Nutritional characteristics			
PN, days, median (IQR)	11.0 (9.0–14.0)	12.0 (10.0–14.0)	0.10
150 mL/kg enteral, study day, median (IQR)	12.0 (9.8–17.0)	13.0 (10.5–20.0)	0.59
Start day of BMF, median (IQR)	11 (11.0–13.0)	7.9 (5.0–10.0)	0.00
Human milk in mL/kg/day *, median (IQR)	50.9 (24.0–82.2)	30.0 (8.5–54.6)	0.01
Formula in mL/kg/day *, median (IQR)	0.0 (0.0–0.2)	1.1 (0.1–7.3)	0.00
Nutritional intake			
Ca (total) W1, mmol/kg; median (IQR)	10.7 (9.9–12.0)	13.1 (11.1–14.6)	0.00
Ca (total) W2, mmol/kg; median (IQR)	16.4 (12.9–17.7)	21.7 (15.3–24.4)	0.00
P (total) W1, mmol/kg; median (IQR)	10.8 (9.3–12.4	12.3 (11.1–14.2)	0.00
P (total) W2, mmol/kg; median (IQR)	16.4 (12.9–19.6)	18.2 (16.0–22.1)	0.02
Prot (total) W1, grams/kg; median (IQR)	18.6 (15.9–21.1)	20.0 (16.9–23.4)	0.16
Prot (total) W2, grams/kg; median (IQR)	23.2 (21.0–26.6)	27.0 (24.1–30.6)	0.00

Low: no enteral supplementation of human milk before Day 11; High: standard protocol: enteral supplementation of human milk if intake was ≥50 mL/day; IQR: Interquartile range; SGA: small for gestational age: <p10; Sepsis: >72 h postnatally and positive blood culture, prevalence within the first 14 days; NEC: necrotizing enterocolitis according to Bell stage [36], prevalence within the first 14 days; IVH: Intraventricular hemorrhage (grade according to Papile) [37]; PN: parenteral nutrition; BMF: breast milk fortifier; *: during the intervention period; Ca: calcium; P: phosphorus; Prot: protein; W1: Week 1; W2: Week 2.

3.2. Nutritional Intake

The nutritional characteristics and intake of calcium, phosphorus and protein during Weeks 1 and 2 are presented in Table 1. The median and interquartile range (IQR) for the duration of PN was 12.0 (10.0–14.0) versus 11.0 (9.0–14.0) days for High versus Low, while the median day of reaching an enteral intake of 150 mL/kg was Day 13.0 (10.5–20.0) versus Day 12.0 (9.8–17.0), respectively. In accordance with the study protocol, Low received a higher amount of human milk. The median start day of BMF in groups High and Low was 7.9 (5.0–10.0) and 11.0 (11.0–13.0) respectively. As a result, High received a significant higher total intake of calcium and phosphorus during the first two weeks and of protein during Week 2 compared to Low. Table A3 presents the nutritional intake divided into four routes of administrations: parenteral, enteral and additional supplementation either par- or enteral. This shows that differences in intake were mainly based on differences in enteral intake. Further, both groups received additional parenteral supplementation of phosphorus, based on low sP concentrations.

Figure 2 presents the daily changes in nutritional intake during the first 14 days. Figure 2A,B,D demonstrate the total calcium, phosphorus and protein intake. High had a steady increase in intake during the study period, whereas Low showed a temporary decrease, and plateau at the end of the observational period, probably due to the decreasing amount of PN and increasing amount of unfortified human milk. Except for Day 1, both groups received a median total calcium, phosphorus and protein intake according to the ESPGHAN recommendations for parenteral and enteral nutrition [38,39]. The calcium/phosphorus ratios were highly variable. Both groups showed a decrease in the calcium/phosphorus ratio on Day 5 that lasted until Day 11 (Figure 2C), most likely caused by the transition from parenteral nutrition to enteral nutrition. For both groups, the ratio was below the recommendations of ESPGHAN on all days [38,39].

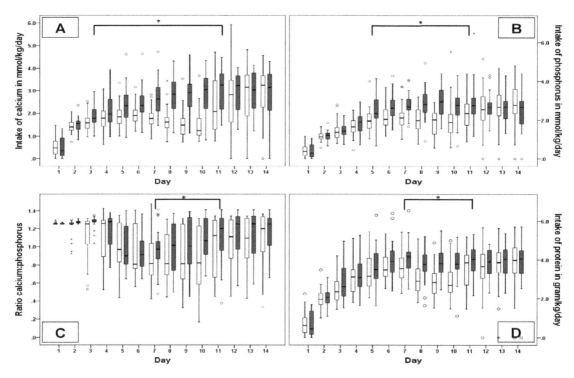

Figure 2. Nutritional intake during the first 14 days: white bars: Low; black bars: High; The horizontal black bars with * indicate the days on which the intake was statistically significant different. (**A**) Daily intake of calcium in mmol/kg/day; * = $p < 0.05$; (**B**) daily intake of phosphorus in mmol/kg/day; * = $p < 0.05$; (**C**) daily intake of protein in gram/kg/day; * = $p < 0.05$; and (**D**) ratio calcium intake to phosphorus intake; * = $p < 0.05$ Data are presented as median, interquartile range and upper and lower limits.

3.3. Biochemical Parameters

Table A4 summarizes the median daily values of both groups for all biochemical parameters. The median serum concentrations of Ca en P were within the normal range and only showed slight differences between the two groups and an overall increase during the study period [40]. Except for the first day, the median sP concentrations remained below our target of 2 mmol/L until Days 5 and 10 for High and Low, respectively. The median uCa and uP values were above the recommended surplus (uCa > 1.2 mmol/L, uP > 0.4 mmol/L) during the entire observational period [23]. The median TrP values were above the lower normal range of 85% until Day 5, and decreased thereafter, reflecting a higher loss of phosphorus. The median ALP values were within the normal range (80–330 U/L) until Day 5, but increased steadily thereafter [40]. In both groups, the uCa/Creat ratios were above the reference value (0.5 mmol/mmol) during the complete study period [32]. The uP/Creat ratios were below the reference value (4.0 mmol/mmol) until Day 5, but above the reference thereafter [32].

The results of the mixed model analyses are summarized in Table 2.

- The sCa concentration was not related to intake of Ca/P and was only marginally affected by a number of co-variables except for daily protein intake that caused an increase of 0.107 mmol/L per gram/kg protein.
- The sP concentration increased in relation to phosphorus intake (0.13 mmol/L per mmol/kg phosphorus) and birth weight (0.0004 mmol/L per gram birth weight), whereas protein intake (−0.13 mmol/L per gram/kg/day protein), gestational age (−0.05 mmol/L per week), furosemide (−0.11 mmol/L per day) and caffeine (−0.02 mmol/L per day) decreased in sP concentration.
- The urinary excretion of Ca seemed to increase in relation to Calcium intake (0.35 mmol/L per mmol/kg calcium), and increased in relation to protein (0.36 mmol/L per gram/kg protein) and being born by cesarean section (0.65 mmol/L if born by cesarean section), whereas it was not affected by the phosphorus intake.
- The urinary excretion of P increased in relation to daily phosphorus intake (3.18 mmol/L per mmol/kg phosphorus) and gender (1.88 mmol/L if infant was a boy), whereas P excretion lowered in relation to daily intake of protein (−1.18 mmol/L per mmol/kg protein), gestational age (−0.71 mmol/L per week) and caffeine (−0.29 mmol/L per day). Calcium intake did not affect the urinary P excretion.
- The TrP increased in relation the daily Calcium intake (3.10% per mmol/kg calcium) and gestational age (3.05% per week). The reabsorption of phosphorus lowered in relation to daily phosphorus intake (−6.21% per mmol/kg phosphorus), gender (−4.60% if infant was a boy), being born by cesarean section (−5.12%), and sepsis (−6.78%).
- The ALP increased in relation protein intake (30.54 U/L per mmol/kg) and daily intake of phosphorus (23.64 U/L per mmol/kg phosphorus). A decrease in ALP was related to calcium intake (−44.94 U/L per mmol/kg calcium), gestational age (−20.71 U/L per week) and the number of days of steroid use (−23.86 U/L per day).
- The uCa/creat ratio increased in relation to daily protein intake (0.54 L/L per gram/day protein) and sepsis (0.66 L/L), but it was not affected by the total calcium and phosphorus intake.
- The uP/creat ratio increased in relation to daily phosphorus intake (4.01 L/L per mmol/kg phosphorus), gender (2.31 L/L if infant was a boy), while the P/creat ratio seemed lower in relation to daily protein intake (−0.81 L/L per gram/kg protein), and decreased with gestational age (−0.94 L/L per week), and caffeine (−0.30 L/L per day).

Table 2. Mixed Model analysis: Effect of nutritional intake and clinical characteristics on biochemical parameter.

Dependant Variable	Covariates	Estimate	95% CI	p-Value
Serum Calcium	Total intake of Ca (mmol/kg/day)	0.004	−0.046–0.054	0.89
	Total intake of P (mmol/kg/day)	−0.036	−0.073–0.002	0.06
	Enteral intake of P (%)	0.001	−0.000–0.001	0.06
	Intake of protein (grams/kg /day)	0.107	0.075–0.139	0.00
	Gestational age (weeks)	0.027	0.013–0.042	0.00
	Singleton (yes)	0.081	0.021–0.140	0.01
	Sepsis (yes)	−0.092	−0.167–−0.019	0.02
	Sedation (days)	−0.007	−0.016–0.001	0.07
Serum Phosphorus	Total intake of Ca (mmol/kg/day)	0.0345	−0.0473–0.1164	0.41
	Total intake of P (mmol/kg/day)	0.1252	0.0586–0.1918	0.00
	Enteral intake of Ca (%)	0.0035	0.0023–0.0048	0.00
	Intake of protein (grams/kg/day)	−0.1274	−0.1825–−0.0723	0.00
	Birth weight (grams)	0.0004	0.0002–0.0006	0.00
	Gestational age (weeks)	−0.0479	−0.0701–−0.0258	0.00
	Gender (boy)	−0.0698	−0.1493–0.096	0.08
	Caffeine (days)	−0.0215	−0.0354–−0.0075	0.00
	Furosemide (days)	−0.1116	−0.2029–−0.0203	0.02

Table 2. *Cont.*

Dependant Variable	Covariates	Estimate	95% CI	*p*-Value
Urine Calcium	Total intake of Ca (mmol/kg/day)	0.35	0.01–0.70	0.05
	Total intake of P (mmol/kg/day)	−0.01	−0.29–0.27	0.94
	Enteral intake of Ca (%)	−0.02	−0.02−−0.01	0.00
	Intake of protein (grams/kg/day)	0.36	0.12–0.61	0.00
	Cesarean section (yes)	0.65	0.32–0.98	0.00
Urine Phosphorus	Total intake of Ca (mmol/kg/day)	−0.05	−1.56–1.45	0.94
	Total intake of P (mmol/kg/day)	3.18	2.06–4.30	0.00
	Enteral intake of P (%)	0.07	0.04–0.09	0.00
	Intake of protein (grams/kg/day)	−1.18	−2.20−−0.16	0.02
	Gestational age (weeks)	−0.71	−1.09−−0.33	0.00
	Gender (boy)	1.88	0.26–3.50	0.02
	Caffeine (days)	−0.29	−0.54−−0.01	0.04
Tubular reabsorption of P	Total intake of Ca (mmol/kg/day)	3.10	0.160–6.04	0.04
	Total intake of P (mmol/kg/day)	−6.21	−8.78−−3.65	0.00
	Enteral intake of P (%)	−0.09	−0.15−−0.03	0.01
	Gestational age (weeks)	3.05	1.92–4.17	0.00
	Gender (boy)	−4.60	−9.22–0.01	0.05
	Cesarean section (yes)	−5.12	−9.95−−0.29	0.04
	Sepsis (yes)	−6.78	−12.72−−0.85	0.03
	Furosemide (days)	4.75	−0.53–10.03	0.07
Alkaline Phosphatase	Total intake of Ca (mmol/kg/day)	−44.94	−69.51−−20.37	0.00
	Total intake of P (mmol/kg/day)	23.64	4.14–43.14	0.02
	Enteral intake of Ca (%)	2.07	1.69–2.45	0.00
	Intake of protein (grams/kg/day)	30.54	14.08–47.01	0.00
	Gestational age (weeks)	−20.71	−30.37−−11.05	0.00
	Postnatal steroids (days)	−23.86	−44.29−−3.43	0.02
Urine Ca/Crea ratio	Total intake of Ca (mmol/kg/day)	0.138	−0.292–0.568	0.53
	Total intake of P (mmol/kg/day)	0.139	−0.204–0.481	0.43
	Enteral intake of Ca (%)	−0.023	−0.029−−0.016	0.00
	Intake of protein (grams/kg/day)	0.497	0.206–0.787	0.01
	Sepsis (yes)	0.584	0.003–1.166	0.05
Urine P/Crea ratio	Total intake of Ca (mmol/kg/day)	−1.10	−2.51–0.31	0.12
	Total intake of P (mmol/kg/day)	4.01	2.97–5.05	0.00
	Enteral intake of P (%)	0.06	0.04–0.08	0.00
	Intake of protein (grams/kg/day)	−0.81	−1.76–0.14	0.10
	Gestational age (weeks)	−0.94	−1.32−−0.55	0.00
	Gender (boy)	2.31	0.72–3.89	0.01
	Sepsis (yes)	1.72	−0.24–3.68	0.09
	Caffeine (days)	−0.30	−0.56−−0.03	0.03

sCa: serum calcium (mmol/L); uCa: urine calcium (mmol/L); sP: serum phosphorus (mmol/L); uP: urine phosphorus (mmol/L); TrP: tubular reabsorption of phosphorus (%); ALP: Alkaline phosphatase (U/L); uCa/Crea ratio: urine calcium/creatinin ratio (mmol/mmol); uP/Crea ratio: urine phosphorus/creatinine ratio (mmol/mmol); 95% CI: 95% confidence interval; Co-variables initially included: daily nutritional intake of calcium, phosphorus, and protein, the enteral amount of calcium and phosphorus intake, caesarian section, multiple births, birth weight, gestational age, gender, necrotizing enterocolitis, sepsis, caffeine, furosemide, steroids and sedation.

4. Discussion

In this observational study of initially three randomized groups providing different nutritional intake to VLBW infants during the first 10 days of life, we found no differences between groups Low and High concerning the biochemical parameters of Ca-P homeostasis. However, the mixed model analysis showed that the intake of calcium was associated with increased urinary calcium excretion and tubular reabsorption of phosphorus and a decrease in the ALP, while the nutritional intake of phosphorus was associated with a decreased sCa and an increase in sP, uP and uP/creat ratio. The nutritional intake of calcium and phosphorus affected the TrP and ALP in opposite directions. Protein intake was greatly associated with a decrease in sP, uP and an increase in ALP, sCa, and uCa, while, in addition, gestational age and male gender affected especially the phosphorus metabolism.

VLBW infants belong to one of the most vulnerable patient groups for whom adequate postnatal nutritional intake has life-long consequences [41]. Therefore, intervention studies with different nutritional intakes could be seen as unethical in the light of the right of optimal treatment for every patient. On the other hand, in clinical practice a great variation in clinical guidelines has been reported, often based on rather low evidence [42]. While fortification of human milk is generally seen as necessary nowadays, there is also concern about possible risks of introducing cow-milk based products too early [43,44]. According to our local protocol, fortification is introduced early and additional mineral supplementation is provided based on laboratory results. The intention is to optimize postnatal growth and bone mineralization but the efficacy of our protocol has not been proven. The combination of the Early Nutrition Study and the Early Supplementation Study provided the opportunity to evaluate two different nutritional concepts within the range of nutritional guidelines and therefore within the ethical limits. On the other hand, all infants participating in the ESS, independent of group allocation, received the standard treatment according to the local practice, which frequently led to additional parenteral supplementation of nutrients in case of electrolyte disturbances or impaired growth. This practice may have ameliorated the differences between the groups and therefore affected the results. By reallocating infants from group ENS B to either group Low or High and excluding infants with intermediate intake from further analysis, we tried to maximize the differences in nutritional intake between the two remaining groups. The reallocation of infants did not change the baseline patient characteristics. The detailed analysis of nutritional intake showed that additional supplementation was not different between the groups and differences in intake were mainly based on enteral nutrition.

Even though the two groups had a maximum difference in nutritional intake, the comparison of daily concentrations of the biochemical parameters showed no differences between groups High and Low, probably by leveling out inter-individual differences on group level. In contrast, the linear mixed model analysis took into account both intra- and inter-individual fluctuations, and thereby enabled us to specify effects of various co-variables.

Despite an increasing intake of phosphorus, sP remained below our target concentration during the first week. Recently, a randomized trial, evaluating nutritional support according to current recommendations in VLBW infants, observed hypophosphatemia in relation to high protein intake [45]. Jamin et al. observed electrolyte disturbances, especially hypophosphatemia and hypokalemia, in low-birth weight piglets with a high protein diet [46]. Hypophosphatemia is the hallmark of the refeeding syndrome and a well-known complication in relation to parenteral nutrition of malnourished patients [47–49]. Bonsante et al. proposed the concept of Placental Incompletely Restored Feeding (PI-Refeeding) syndrome for electrolyte disturbances found in VLBW infants [50]. This syndrome is said to be caused by an imbalanced nutritional intake of amino acids and phosphorus. Amino acids and energy are needed to maintain an anabolic state of the cell, while phosphorus is necessary for a number of cellular functions, energy homeostasis as well as for bone mineralization. Phosphorus in blood will preferably be transferred to the cell regardless of bone mineral status. A higher intake of amino acids will enhance the need for phosphorus in growing cells, and in case of low concentrations of phosphorus in blood it will be released from bone. Simultaneously with the release of phosphorus, calcium will also be released from the bone because of an unfavorable Ca/P ratio and will consecutively be excreted in urine if the sP concentrations are too low. Our results are in agreement with this concept. According to the mixed model analyses, we found that an increasing amount of protein was associated with an increase in the sCa, uCa, ALP and uCa/Creat ratio, whereas it was associated with a decrease in sP, uP and the uP/Creat ratio. Remarkably, in our study, an increase in a sP concentration of 0.13 mmol/L occurred per 1 mmol/kg intake of phosphorus and a decrease of −0.13 mmol/L per 1 gram/kg protein intake, meaning that 1 gram/kg of protein intake should be accompanied by 1 mmol/kg of phosphorus in nutrition of VLBW infants to maintain adequate sP concentrations.

The role of ALP in bone mineralization is controversial, but an increase is usually associated with poor bone mineralization [30,51]. According to our results, an increasing intake of protein was associated with an increase in ALP. Again, following the above mentioned mechanisms higher protein intake enhanced the cellular need of phosphorus and thereby decreased the sP concentration and the availability of phosphorus for bone mineralization, leading to activation of ALP. We also found that an increased ALP was associated with increasing phosphorus intake, while one would expect lowering of ALP. An explanation for this phenomenon could be a relatively insufficient intake of calcium in combination with phosphorus intake, since an increasing calcium intake was associated with decrease in ALP concentrations. In this study, for both groups, the calcium/phosphorus ratio was below recommendations, meaning that relatively more phosphorus than calcium was administered.

Gestational age at birth seemed to be an important determinant for the phosphorus metabolism in our study, meaning that infants with a lower gestational age had a higher renal excretion of phosphorus, irrespective of nutritional intake. Immaturity of the kidneys at lower gestational age has been shown to cause impaired tubular reabsorption of phosphorus [15]. Renal losses of minerals may then compromise the effect of nutritional intake on bone mineralization. However, current recommendations for nutritional intake of calcium and phosphorus usually do not take into account differences in renal function based on gestational age.

Further, we found that male gender was related to low serum phosphorus concentrations, low tubular reabsorption and increased renal excretion of phosphorus and uP/creat ratio. We speculate a retardation in maturation of the renal function in male infants compared to females as is known for the development of the pulmonary function [52].

All parameters evaluated in this study are regularly used to monitor either electrolyte homeostasis or bone mineralization. Practices among units vary greatly, measurements may be performed at later age and greater intervals and not standardized or in combination, leading to inconsistent results and handling. An explanation for the inconsistency in results of other studies could be the underestimation of the effects of inter-relationships between various co-variates. In our opinion, these associations can only be discovered with standardized repeated measurements taking into account other clinical factors. To our knowledge, this is the first study evaluating changes in biochemical parameters of the calcium-phosphorus homeostasis based on standardized repeated measurements and daily changes in nutritional intake in a mixed model linear regression analysis including also clinical factors.

Our data show that standardized repeated measurements of blood and urine samples can provide useful information with regard to the Ca-P homeostasis. This does not result in a clear advice for nutritional intake. Nevertheless, this study is a first step and its importance lies in the description and quantification of changes in a more "physiological way" that will further enable us to develop new guidelines to improve bone mineral status in preterm infants. Notwithstanding, we confirmed the relationship between the intake of protein and phosphorus, and demonstrated the effect of renal immaturity and gender. Thus, a second step could be, to relate the current results to bone mineralization and provide recommendations for nutritional intake and a third step to develop a concept of target values for biochemical parameter so that these can be used to monitor nutritional intake to achieve optimal bone mineralization in daily practice.

This study had several limitations. The mixed model analysis assumes that the effects of the different variables are linear which has not been proven yet. In addition, the biochemical parameters may have been influenced by factors that were not taken into account in our analysis. Daily sampling of biochemical parameter would have been optimal, but this was judged unethical regarding the amount of blood volume needed. Nevertheless, measurements were performed in a standardized manner and therefore provided a good reflection of changes in blood and urine concentrations for the complete study period. Further, in comparison to other studies, both groups had relatively high daily intakes. This may partly explain the small variations in biochemical parameters. This study only investigated the biochemical parameters during the first 14 days of life. Maturational changes in renal function may alter the results; however, repeated measurements will indicate these changes and thereby can be used as guide for optimal supplementation of minerals.

5. Conclusions

In conclusion, standardized repeated measurements showed that biochemical parameters of Ca-P homeostasis seemed to be affected by nutritional intake of calcium and phosphorus as well as protein, while immaturity of kidneys was related to an increase in urinary excretion of minerals irrespective of nutritional intake. Further studies are needed to define target values to stabilize electrolyte balances and improve bone mineralization taking into account nutritional intake and gestational age of the patient.

Acknowledgments: This study was part of the "Early Nutrition Study" that was sponsored by Mead Johnson Nutrition, for which J.B.v.G. received a grant. The Early Supplementation Study was sponsored by Hero Kindervoeding, Breda, Netherlands, for which V.C. and A.v.H. received a grant. The sponsors had no role in the design and conduct of the study; collection, management, analysis, and interpretation of the data, the preparation of the manuscript and the decision to submit the manuscript for publication. All other authors declare that they do not have any conflict of interest and that they do not have anything to disclose. The first draft of the manuscript was written by V.C., who did not receive an honorarium or any other form of payment to produce the manuscript. All authors gratefully thank W.R.J.C. Jansen, research nurse of the Pediatric Drug Research Center Radboudumc, for the dedicated support in patient recruitment and data collection as well as T.A.J. Antonius, neonatologist at Radboudumc, for the development of the algorithm to calculate the nutritional intakes.

Author Contributions: V.C. is the primary researcher responsible for designing the study, analyzing and interpreting the data, and writing of the manuscript; C.G. and M.K. were responsible for data acquisition, analysis of the data and review of the manuscript; N.R. contributed to the analysis and interpretation of the data, and to writing and review of the manuscript; J.B.v.G. contributed in designing the study, interpretation of the data and review of the manuscript; and A.v.H. supervised the design, analyses and interpretation of the data, and writing of the manuscript. All authors listed on the manuscript have seen and approved the manuscript and take full responsibility for the manuscript.

Appendix A

Table A1. Standard parenteral nutritional intake.

	Day 1	Day 2	Day 3	Day 4
Fluid mL/kg/day	80	100	125	150
CH grams/kg/day	8	9.6	11.7	13.8
AA grams/kg/day	0.75	1.5	2.25	3
Lipids grams/kg/day	1	2	3	3
EQ Kcal/kg/day	44	62	82	94
Calcium mmol/kg/day	0.75	1.5	2.25	3.00
Phosphorus mmol/kg/day	0.48	0.96	1.44	1.92

Parenteral nutritional intake based on standardized parenteral solutions [35,53]. For infants below 1000 grams, amino acids were additionally added according to current recommendations [12]. Amino acid solution: Primene (Baxter, the Netherlands); Lipid emulsion including vitamins: Clinoleic (20%; Baxter, The Netherlands) or SMOFlipid 20% (Fresenius Kabi; The Netherlands); CH: carbohydrates, AA: amino acids, EQ: energy quotient.

Table A2. Cohort characteristics of all patients included in the Early Supplementation Study.

Characteristics	Group ENS A (n = 40)	Group ENS B (n = 32)	Group C (n = 37)
GA, weeks; med (IQR)	28.2 (25.7–30.1)	28.3 (26.5–30.7)	27.9 (26.1–29.7)
Birth weight, grams; med (IQR)	967 (753–1245)	1012 (847–1199)	1006 (771–1220)
SGA; n (%)	9 (23)	8 (25)	6 (16)
Male; n (%)	21 (53)	20 (63)	18 (49)
Singletons; n (%)	25 (63)	24 (74)	25 (68)
Antenatal Steroids compl.; n (%)	36 (90)	31 (97)	31 (86)
Cesarean section; n (%)	19 (48)	20 (63)	25 (68)
Apgar score (5 min); med (IQR)	7.5 (6.3–9.0)	8.0 (7.0–9.0)	7.0 (7.0–8.0)
Apgar score (5 min) <7; n (%)	10 (25)	5 (16)	8 (22)
Mortality; n (%)	6 (15)	3 (9)	7 (19)
Morbidity			
IRDS	24 (60)	19 (59)	23 (62)
Days of MV; med (IQR)	1.5 (0.0–4.8)	1.0 (0.0–4.0)	1.0 (0.0–7.0)
Days of N-CPAP; med (IQR)	18.0 (6.5–38.8)	28.0 (7.0–40.8)	16.0 (6.0–36.5)

Table A2. *Cont.*

Characteristics	Group ENS A (*n* = 40)	Group ENS B (*n* = 32)	Group C (*n* = 37)
CLD; *n* (%)	12 (30)	14 (44)	10 (27)
PDA; *n* (%)	20 (50)	20 (63)	21 (57)
Ductal ligation; *n* (%)	4 (10)	2 (6.3)	1 (3)
IVH grade ≤ 2; *n* (%)	15 (38)	5 (16)	5 (14)
IVH grade ≥ 3; *n* (%)	2 (5)	7 (21)	4 (11)
Sepsis; *n* (%)	13 (33)	10 (32)	14 (38)
NEC; *n* (%)	4 (10)	5 (16)	3 (8)
Bell stage 2; *n*	2	3	1
Bell stage 3; *n*	2	2	2
Laparotomy; *n*	2	1	2
ROP; *n* (%)	4 (10)	1 (3)	5 (14)
ROP grade ≥ 3	1	0	1
Medication			
Caffeine; *n* (%)	38 (95)	30 (94)	33 (90)
Furosemide; *n* (%)	11 (28)	10 (31)	7 (19)
Diuretics (maintenance); *n* (%)	3 (8)	0	3 (8)
Corticosteroids; *n* (%)	1 (3)	2 (6)	4 (11)
Sedation; *n* (%)	13 (33)	11 (34)	15 (41)
Nutritional characteristics			
Days of PN; med (IQR)	10.0 (8.0–13.0)	10.5 (9.0–14.8)	10.5 (8.3–21.0)
120 mL/kg enteral, day; med (IQR)	9.0 (7.0–12.5)	9.0 (8.0–13.0)	9.0 (7.2–14.8)
150 mL/kg enteral, day; med (IQR)	12.0 (9.0–17.0)	11.0 (10.0–17.0)	12.0 (10.0–20.0)
Start day of BMF; med (IQR)	11.0 (11.0–12.7)	12.0 (11.0–14.0)	6.0 (4.0–8.0)

ENS A: donor milk in addition to mother's own milk (MOM) and no supplements with enteral feeding until Day 10; ENS B: preterm formula in addition to MOM and no supplements with enteral feeding until Day 10; Group C: preterm formula in addition to MOM and fortifier if intake ≥50 mL/day; med: median; IQR: inter quartile range; GA: gestational age; SGA: small for gestational age according to Fenton et al. [54]; IRDS: infant respiratory distress syndrome; MV: mechanical ventilation; N-CPAP: nasal continuous positive airway pressure; CLD: chronic lung disease defined as oxygen dependency at 36 weeks gestational age; PDA: patent ductus arteriosus with need for treatment; IVH: intra-ventricular hemorrhage; Sepsis: >72 h postnatally and positive blood culture; NEC: necrotizing enterocolitis with staging according to Bell [36]; ROP: retinopathy of prematurity; sedation: morfine and/or midazolam >24 h; PN: parenteral nutrition; BMF: breast milk fortifier.

Table A3. Nutritional intake of calcium and phosphorus by route of administration.

Nutritional Intake (mmol/kg/Week)	Low (*n* = 40) Median (IQR)	High (*n* = 30) Median (IQR)	*p*-Value
Ca (total) W1	10.7 (9.9–12.0)	13.1 (11.1–14.6)	0.00
Ca (total) W2	16.4 (12.9–17.7)	21.7 (15.3–24.4)	0.00
Ca (enteral) W1	1.7 (1.1–2.2)	3.3 (1.1–5.7)	0.00
Ca (enteral) W2	10.8 (6.2–16.0)	17.5 (2.3–22.8)	0.07
Ca (enteral suppl) W1	0.0 (0.0–0.0)	0.0 (0.0–0.0)	1.0
Ca (enteral suppl) W2	0.0 (0.0–0.0)	0.0 (0.0–0.0)	0.22
Ca (PN) W1	9.4 (8.0–10.2)	9.8 (7.9–11.5)	0.34
Ca (PN) W2	3.1 (0.7–7.9)	5.1 (1.9–10.9)	0.14
Ca (PNsuppl) W1	0.0 (0.0–0.0)	0.0 (0.0–0.0)	1.0
Ca (PNsuppl) W2	0.0 (0.0–0.0)	0.0 (0.0–0.0)	0.74
P (total) W1	10.8 (9.2–12.4)	12.3 (11.1–14.2)	0.00
P (total) W2	16.4 (12.9–19.6)	18.9 (16.0–22.1)	0.02
P (enteral) W1	1.0 (0.6–1.4)	2.1 (0.7–3.9)	0.00
P (enteral) W2	8.1 (5.0–12.0)	10.4 (1.7–17.2)	0.08
P (enteral suppl) W1	0.0 (0.0–0.0)	0.0 (0.0–0.9)	0.03
P (enteral suppl) W2	0.0 (0.0–0.0)	0.0 (0.0–1.4)	0.33
P (PN) W1	7.5 (6.4–8.2)	7.8 (6.3–9.2)	0.34
P (PN) W2	2.5 (0.6–6.3)	4.1 (1.5–8.7)	0.14
P (PN suppl) W1	2.4 (0.5–3.8)	1.8 (0.0–2.7)	0.16
P (PN suppl) W2	2.3 (0.0–4.2)	0.7 (0.0–4.3)	0.30

Low: no enteral supplementation of human milk before Day 11; High: standard protocol: enteral supplementation of human milk if intake was ≥50 mL/day; IQR: inter quartile range; Ca: calcium; P: phosphorus; total: som of all nutritional intake; enteral: enteral intake including standard fortification; enteral suppl: additional enteral supplementation; PN: parenteral intake; PN suppl: additional parenteral supplementation; W1: week 1; W2: week 2.

Table A4. Daily measurements of biochemical parameter of the calcium and phosphorus homeostasis.

		Day 1	Day 3	Day 5	Day 7	Day 10	Day 14
Serum Ca (mmol/L)	Low	2.2 (2.0–2.4)	2.4 (2.2–2.5)	2.5 (2.4–2.7)	2.6 (2.4–2.7)	2.5 (2.4–2.7)	2.6 (2.4–2.8)
	High	2.2 (2.0–2.4)	2.4 (2.3–2.6)	2.5 (2.4–2.7)	2.4 (2.3–2.6)	2.5 (2.3–2.7)	2.6 (2.5–2.8)
	p-Value	*0.94*	*0.17*	*0.34*	*0.15*	*0.69*	*0.17*
Urine Ca (mmol/L)	Low	1.3 (1.0–1.9)	2.1 (1.5–3.4)	2.6 (2.0–3.9)	2.7 (1.6–3.8)	2.0 (1.6–3.3)	1.8 (1.4–3.5)
	High	1.5 (1.2–1.7)	3.3 (2.0–4.7)	3.1 (2.3–5.8)	2.5 (1.8–3.8)	2.7 (2.0–3.4)	2.3 (1.6–3.4)
	p-Value	*0.66*	*0.03*	*0.06*	*0.84*	*0.21*	*0.50*
Serum P (mmol/L)	Low	1.8 (1.7–2.2)	1.8 (1.5–2.0)	1.7 (1.5–2.0)	1.9 (1.8–2.2)	2.0 (1.8–2.2)	2.3 (2.1–2.4)
	High	2.1 (1.8–2.3)	1.8 (1.5–2.0)	1.6 (1.3–2.2)	2.1 (1.8–2.4)	2.1 (2.0–2.4)	2.2 (2.0–2.3)
	p-Value	*0.22*	*0.88*	*0.71*	*0.21*	*0.08*	*0.16*
Urine P (mmol/L)	Low	1.7 (0.3–3.8)	2.1 (0.7–5.5)	1.3 (0.7–3.5)	4.1 (0.7–6.8)	5.4 (2.2–8.2)	10.4 (6.8–18.4)
	High	2.3 (0.2–4.6)	2.6 (0.9–4.1)	3.1 (1.6–6.9)	5.4 (3.5–9.8)	7.4 (4.5–13.7)	9.5 (5.5–16.4)
	p-Value	*0.68*	*0.98*	*0.04*	*0.02*	*0.04*	*0.46*
Tubular reabsorption of P (%)	Low	94.0 (76.8–98.2)	86.5 (76.1–95.3)	92.2 (83.8–96.9)	83.1 (72.4–96.3)	80.8 (68.8–92.7)	75.9 (64.9–85.2)
	High	85.3 (76.4–98.1)	92.7 (73.3–95.7)	88.1 (80.8–95.1)	79.4 (51.9–87.6)	76.6 (59.1–83.2)	67.4 (53.9–82.4)
	p-Value	*0.59*	*0.62*	*0.21*	*0.08*	*0.23*	*0.36*
Alkaline Phosphatase (U/L)	Low	167.0 (138.0–236.0)	213.0 (182.0–291.0)	263.5 (202.3–368.5)	329 (261.3–455.0)	379 (311.0–503.0)	423.0 (301.8–506.0)
	High	203 (146.5–232.8)	244.0 (174.3–270.8)	275.5 (206.3–307.0)	304.5 (249.3–375.0)	342.0 (213.8–414.3)	380.0 (281.8–509.8)
	p-Value	*0.76*	*0.94*	*0.76*	*0.22*	*0.10*	*0.66*
uCa/Crea ratio (mmol/mmol)	Low	2.1 (1.3–3.5)	2.5 (1.8–3.1)	3.6 (2.3–5.2)	3.8 (2.3–6.2)	2.9 (1.8–4.1)	2.3 (1.6–3.7)
	High	1.7 (1.4–3.7)	2.7 (2.0–6.1)	4.0 (2.9–6.3)	3.0 (2.1–5.4)	3.8 (2.4–5.0)	3.4 (1.9–4.8)
	p-Value	*0.98*	*0.30*	*0.35*	*0.49*	*0.21*	*0.14*
uP/Crea ratio (mmol/mmol)	Low	1.6 (0.5–5.9)	2.8 (1.0–6.8)	1.9 (0.8–5.4)	5.1 (1.1–9.3)	7.2 (2.5–12.3)	11.2 (6.2–18.6)
	High	3.8 (0.5–6.7)	1.8 (1.1–5.8)	3.5 (1.6–6.1)	7.7 (5.0–10.9)	9.4 (7.0–16.5)	14.5 (9.3–18.7)
	p-Value	*0.64*	*0.72*	*0.15*	*0.14*	*0.06*	*0.73*

All data are presented as median and interquartile range; sCa: serum calcium (mmol/L); uCa: urine calcium (mmol/L); sP: serum phosphorus (mmol/L); uP: urine phosphorus (mmol/L); TrP: tubular reabsorption of phosphorus (%); ALP: Alkaline phosphatase (U/L); uCa/Crea ration: urine calcium/creatinine ration (mmol/mmol); uP/Cre ratio (mmol/mmol).

References

1. Rauch, F.; Schoenau, E. The developing bone: Slave or master of its cells and molecules? *Pediatr. Res.* **2001**, *50*, 309–314. [CrossRef] [PubMed]
2. Greer, F.R. Osteopenia of prematurity. *Annu. Rev. Nutr.* **1994**, *14*, 169–185. [CrossRef] [PubMed]
3. Harrison, C.M.; Johnson, K.; McKechnie, E. Osteopenia of prematurity: A national survey and review of practice. *Acta Paediatr.* **2008**, *97*, 407–413. [CrossRef] [PubMed]
4. Demarini, S. Calcium and phosphorus nutrition in preterm infants. *Acta Paediatr. Suppl.* **2005**, *94*, 87–92. [CrossRef] [PubMed]
5. Kovacs, C.S. Calcium, phosphorus, and bone metabolism in the fetus and newborn. *Early Hum. Dev.* **2015**, *91*, 623–628. [CrossRef] [PubMed]
6. Ribeiro Dde, O.; Lobo, B.W.; Volpato, N.M.; da Veiga, V.F.; Cabral, L.M.; de Sousa, V.P. Influence of the calcium concentration in the presence of organic phosphorus on the physicochemical compatibility and stability of all-in-one admixtures for neonatal use. *Nutr. J.* **2009**, *8*, 51. [CrossRef] [PubMed]
7. Rigo, J.; Pieltain, C.; Salle, B.; Senterre, J. Enteral calcium, phosphate and vitamin d requirements and bone mineralization in preterm infants. *Acta Paediatr.* **2007**, *96*, 969–974. [CrossRef] [PubMed]
8. Carnielli, V.P.; Luijendijk, I.H.; van Goudoever, J.B.; Sulkers, E.J.; Boerlage, A.A.; Degenhart, H.J.; Sauer, P.J. Feeding premature newborn infants palmitic acid in amounts and stereoisomeric position similar to that of human milk: Effects on fat and mineral balance. *Am. J. Clin. Nutr.* **1995**, *61*, 1037–1042. [PubMed]
9. Abrams, S.A.; Hawthorne, K.M.; Placencia, J.L.; Dinh, K.L. Micronutrient requirements of high-risk infants. *Clin. Perinatol.* **2014**, *41*, 347–361. [CrossRef] [PubMed]
10. Schanler, R.J.; Abrams, S.A.; Garza, C. Mineral balance studies in very low birth weight infants fed human milk. *J. Pediatr.* **1988**, *113*, 230–238. [CrossRef]
11. Lapillonne, A.A.; Glorieux, F.H.; Salle, B.L.; Braillon, P.M.; Chambon, M.; Rigo, J.; Putet, G.; Senterre, J. Mineral balance and whole body bone mineral content in very low-birth-weight infants. *Acta Paediatr. Suppl.* **1994**, *405*, 117–122. [CrossRef] [PubMed]
12. Rigo, J.; Senterre, J. Nutritional needs of premature infants: Current issues. *J. Pediatr.* **2006**, *149*, S80–S88. [CrossRef]
13. Bert, S.; Gouyon, J.B.; Semama, D.S. Calcium, sodium and potassium urinary excretion during the first five days of life in very preterm infants. *Biol. Neonate* **2004**, *85*, 37–41. [CrossRef] [PubMed]
14. Catache, M.; Leone, C.R. Role of plasma and urinary calcium and phosphorus measurements in early detection of phosphorus deficiency in very low birthweight infants. *Acta Paediatr.* **2003**, *92*, 76–80. [CrossRef] [PubMed]
15. De Curtis, M.; Rigo, J. Nutrition and kidney in preterm infant. *J. Matern. Fetal. Neonatal Med.* **2012**, *25*, 55–59. [CrossRef] [PubMed]
16. Boehm, G.; Wiener, M.; Schmidt, C.; Ungethum, A.; Ungethum, B.; Moro, G. Usefulness of short-term urine collection in the nutritional monitoring of low birthweight infants. *Acta Paediatr.* **1998**, *87*, 339–343. [CrossRef] [PubMed]
17. Aladangady, N.; Coen, P.G.; White, M.P.; Rae, M.D.; Beattie, T.J. Urinary excretion of calcium and phosphate in preterm infants. *Pediatr. Nephrol.* **2004**, *19*, 1225–1231. [CrossRef] [PubMed]
18. Giapros, V.I.; Papaloukas, A.L.; Andronikou, S.K. Urinary mineral excretion in preterm neonates during the first month of life. *Neonatology* **2007**, *91*, 180–185. [CrossRef] [PubMed]
19. Giles, M.M.; Fenton, M.H.; Shaw, B.; Elton, R.A.; Clarke, M.; Lang, M.; Hume, R. Sequential calcium and phosphorus balance studies in preterm infants. *J. Pediatr.* **1987**, *110*, 591–598. [CrossRef]
20. Hellstern, G.; Poschl, J.; Linderkamp, O. Renal phosphate handling of premature infants of 23–25 weeks gestational age. *Pediatr. Nephrol.* **2003**, *18*, 756–758. [CrossRef] [PubMed]
21. Hillman, L.S.; Rojanasathit, S.; Slatopolsky, E.; Haddad, J.G. Serial measurements of serum calcium, magnesium, parathyroid hormone, calcitonin, and 25-hydroxy-vitamin D in premature and term infants during the first week of life. *Pediatr. Res.* **1977**, *11*, 739–744. [CrossRef] [PubMed]
22. Mihatsch, W.A.; Muche, R.; Pohlandt, F. The renal phosphate threshold decreases with increasing postmenstrual age in very low birth weight infants. *Pediatr. Res.* **1996**, *40*, 300–303. [CrossRef] [PubMed]

23. Pohlandt, F. Prevention of postnatal bone demineralization in very low-birth-weight infants by individually monitored supplementation with calcium and phosphorus. *Pediatr. Res.* **1994**, *35*, 125–129. [CrossRef] [PubMed]

24. Senterre, J.; Salle, B. Renal aspects of calcium and phosphorus metabolism in preterm infants. *Biol. Neonate* **1988**, *53*, 220–229. [CrossRef] [PubMed]

25. Trotter, A.; Stoll, M.; Leititis, J.U.; Blatter, A.; Pohlandt, F. Circadian variations of urinary electrolyte concentrations in preterm and term infants. *J. Pediatr.* **1996**, *128*, 253–256. [CrossRef]

26. Trotter, A.; Pohlandt, F. Calcium and phosphorus retention in extremely preterm infants supplemented individually. *Acta Paediatr.* **2002**, *91*, 680–683. [CrossRef] [PubMed]

27. Abrams, S.A.; Schanler, R.J.; Garza, C. Relation of bone mineralization measures to serum biochemical measures. *Am. J. Dis. Child.* **1988**, *142*, 1276–1278. [CrossRef] [PubMed]

28. Acar, D.B.; Kavuncuoglu, S.; Cetinkaya, M.; Petmezci, E.; Dursun, M.; Korkmaz, O.; Altuncu, E.K. Assessment of the place of tubular reabsorption of phosphorus in the diagnosis of osteopenia of prematurity. *Turk Pediatri Ars.* **2015**, *50*, 45–50. [CrossRef] [PubMed]

29. Visser, F.; Sprij, A.J.; Brus, F. The validity of biochemical markers in metabolic bone disease in preterm infants: A systematic review. *Acta Paediatr.* **2012**, *101*, 562–568. [CrossRef] [PubMed]

30. Tinnion, R.J.; Embleton, N.D. How to use... alkaline phosphatase in neonatology. *Arch. Dis. Child. Educ. Pract. Ed.* **2012**, *97*, 157–163. [CrossRef] [PubMed]

31. Kelly, A.; Kovatch, K.J.; Garber, S.J. Metabolic bone disease screening practices among US Neonatologists. *Clin. Pediatr. (Phila.)* **2014**, *53*, 1077–1083. [CrossRef] [PubMed]

32. Staub, E.; Wiedmer, N.; Staub, L.P.; Nelle, M.; von Vigier, R.O. Monitoring of urinary calcium and phosphorus excretion in preterm infants: Comparison of 2 methods. *J. Pediatr. Gastroenterol. Nutr.* **2014**, *58*, 404–408. [CrossRef] [PubMed]

33. Corpeleijn, W.E.; de Waard, M.; Christmann, V.; van Goudoever, J.B.; Jansen-van der Weide, M.C.; Kooi, E.M.; Koper, J.F.; Kouwenhoven, S.M.; Lafeber, H.N.; Mank, E.; et al. Effect of Donor Milk on Severe Infections and Mortality in Very Low-Birth-Weight Infants: The Early Nutrition Study Randomized Clinical Trial. *JAMA Pediatr.* **2016**, *170*, 654–661. [CrossRef] [PubMed]

34. Gidrewicz, D.A.; Fenton, T.R. A systematic review and meta-analysis of the nutrient content of preterm and term breast milk. *BMC Pediatr.* **2014**, *14*, 216. [CrossRef] [PubMed]

35. Christmann, V.; de Grauw, A.M.; Visser, R.; Matthijsse, R.P.; van Goudoever, J.B.; van Heijst, A.F. Early postnatal calcium and phosphorus metabolism in preterm infants. *J. Pediatr. Gastroenterol. Nutr.* **2014**, *58*, 398–403. [CrossRef] [PubMed]

36. Bell, M.J.; Ternberg, J.L.; Feigin, R.D.; Keating, J.P.; Marshall, R.; Barton, L.; Brotherton, T. Neonatal necrotizing enterocolitis. Therapeutic decisions based upon clinical staging. *Ann. Surg.* **1978**, *187*, 1–7. [CrossRef] [PubMed]

37. Papile, L.A.; Burstein, J.; Burstein, R.; Koffler, H. Incidence and evolution of subependymal and intraventricular hemorrhage: A study of infants with birth weights less than 1500 gm. *J. Pediatr.* **1978**, *92*, 529–534. [CrossRef]

38. Koletzko, B.; Goulet, O.; Hunt, J.; Krohn, K.; Shamir, R.; Parenteral Nutrition Guidelines Working Group; European Society for Clinical Nutrition and Metabolism; European Society of Paediatric Gastroenterology, Hepatology and Nutrition (ESPGHAN); European Society of Paediatric Research. 1. Guidelines on paediatric parenteral nutrition of the European Society of Paediatric Gastroenterology, Hepatology and Nutrition (Espghan) and the European Society for Clinical Nutrition and Metabolism (ESPEN), Supported by the European Society of Paediatric Research (ESPR). *J. Pediatr. Gastroenterol. Nutr.* **2005**, *41*, S1–S87. [PubMed]

39. Agostoni, C.; Buonocore, G.; Carnielli, V.P.; De Curtis, M.; Darmaun, D.; Decsi, T.; Domellof, M.; Embleton, N.D.; Fusch, C.; Genzel-Boroviczeny, O.; et al. Enteral nutrient supply for preterm infants: Commentary from the European Society of Paediatric Gastroenterology, Hepatology and Nutrition Committee on Nutrition. *J. Pediatr. Gastroenterol. Nutr.* **2010**, *50*, 85–91. [CrossRef] [PubMed]

40. Fenton, T.R.; Lyon, A.W.; Rose, M.S. Cord blood calcium, phosphate, magnesium, and alkaline phosphatase gestational age-specific reference intervals for preterm infants. *BMC Pediatr.* **2011**, *11*, 76. [CrossRef] [PubMed]

41.   Ehrenkranz, R.A.; Dusick, A.M.; Vohr, B.R.; Wright, L.L.; Wrage, L.A.; Poole, W.K. Growth in the neonatal intensive care unit influences neurodevelopmental and growth outcomes of extremely low birth weight infants. *Pediatrics* **2006**, *117*, 1253–1261. [CrossRef] [PubMed]

42.   Klingenberg, C.; Embleton, N.D.; Jacobs, S.E.; O'Connell, L.A.; Kuschel, C.A. Enteral feeding practices in very preterm infants: An international survey. *Arch. Dis. Child. Fetal. Neonatal. Ed.* **2012**, *97*, F56–F61. [CrossRef] [PubMed]

43.   Sullivan, S.; Schanler, R.J.; Kim, J.H.; Patel, A.L.; Trawoger, R.; Kiechl-Kohlendorfer, U.; Chan, G.M.; Blanco, C.L.; Abrams, S.; Cotten, C.M.; et al. An exclusively human milk-based diet is associated with a lower rate of necrotizing enterocolitis than a diet of human milk and bovine milk-based products. *J. Pediatr.* **2010**, *156*, 562–567; 562.e1–567.e1. [CrossRef] [PubMed]

44.   Cristofalo, E.A.; Schanler, R.J.; Blanco, C.L.; Sullivan, S.; Trawoeger, R.; Kiechl-Kohlendorfer, U.; Dudell, G.; Rechtman, D.J.; Lee, M.L.; Lucas, A.; et al. Randomized trial of exclusive human milk versus preterm formula diets in extremely premature infants. *J. Pediatr.* **2013**, *163*, 1592.e1–1595.e1. [CrossRef] [PubMed]

45.   Moltu, S.J.; Strommen, K.; Blakstad, E.W.; Almaas, A.N.; Westerberg, A.C.; Braekke, K.; Ronnestad, A.; Nakstad, B.; Berg, J.P.; Veierod, M.B.; et al. Enhanced feeding in very-low-birth-weight infants may cause electrolyte disturbances and septicemia—A randomized, controlled trial. *Clin. Nutr.* **2013**, *32*, 207–212. [CrossRef] [PubMed]

46.   Jamin, A.; D'Inca, R.; Le Floc'h, N.; Kuster, A.; Orsonneau, J.L.; Darmaun, D.; Boudry, G.; Le Huerou-Luron, I.; Seve, B.; Gras-Le Guen, C. Fatal effects of a neonatal high-protein diet in low-birth-weight piglets used as a model of intrauterine growth restriction. *Neonatology* **2010**, *97*, 321–328. [CrossRef] [PubMed]

47.   Mehanna, H.M.; Moledina, J.; Travis, J. Refeeding syndrome: What it is, and how to prevent and treat it. *BMJ* **2008**, *336*, 1495–1498. [CrossRef] [PubMed]

48.   Walmsley, R.S. Refeeding syndrome: Screening, incidence, and treatment during parenteral nutrition. *J. Gastroenterol. Hepatol.* **2013**, *28*, 113–117. [CrossRef] [PubMed]

49.   Ross, J.R.; Finch, C.; Ebeling, M.; Taylor, S.N. Refeeding syndrome in very-low-birth-weight intrauterine growth-restricted neonates. *J. Perinatol.* **2013**, *33*, 717–720. [CrossRef] [PubMed]

50.   Bonsante, F.; Iacobelli, S.; Latorre, G.; Rigo, J.; De Felice, C.; Robillard, P.Y.; Gouyon, J.B. Initial amino acid intake influences phosphorus and calcium homeostasis in preterm infants—It is time to change the composition of the early parenteral nutrition. *PLoS ONE* **2013**, *8*, e72880. [CrossRef] [PubMed]

51.   Lucas, A.; Brooke, O.G.; Baker, B.A.; Bishop, N.; Morley, R. High alkaline phosphatase activity and growth in preterm neonates. *Arch. Dis. Child.* **1989**, *64*, 902–909. [CrossRef] [PubMed]

52.   Peacock, J.L.; Marston, L.; Marlow, N.; Calvert, S.A.; Greenough, A. Neonatal and infant outcome in boys and girls born very prematurely. *Pediatr. Res.* **2012**, *71*, 305–310. [CrossRef] [PubMed]

53.   Christmann, V.; Visser, R.; Engelkes, M.; de Grauw, A.; van Goudoever, J.; van Heijst, A. The enigma to achieve normal postnatal growth in preterm infants—Using parenteral or enteral nutrition? *Acta Paediatr.* **2013**, *102*, 471–479. [CrossRef] [PubMed]

54.   Fenton, T.R.; Kim, J.H. A systematic review and meta-analysis to revise the Fenton growth chart for preterm infants. *BMC Pediatr.* **2013**, *13*, 59. [CrossRef] [PubMed]

15

Sensory Acceptability of Infant Cereals with Whole Grain in Infants and Young Children

Juan Francisco Haro-Vicente [1], Maria Jose Bernal-Cava [1,*], Amparo Lopez-Fernandez [2], Gaspar Ros-Berruezo [2], Stefan Bodenstab [3] and Luis Manuel Sanchez-Siles [3]

[1] Department of Research and Development, Hero Group, Alcantarilla, Murcia 30820, Spain; jfrancisco.haro@hero.es

[2] Department of Food Science and Nutrition, University of Murcia, Campus de Espinardo, Espinardo, Murcia 30071, Spain; amparolf@um.es (A.L.-F.); gros@um.es (G.R.-B.)

[3] Department of Research and Development, Hero Group, Lenzburg 5600, Switzerland; stefan.bodenstab@hero.ch (S.B.); luisma.sanchez@hero.es (L.M.S.-S.)

* Correspondence: mjose.bernal@hero.es

Abstract: In many countries, infant cereals are one of the first foods introduced during the complementary feeding stage. These cereals are usually made with refined cereal flours, even though several health benefits have been linked to the intake of whole grain cereals. Prior evidence suggests that food preferences are developed at early stages of life, and may persist in later childhood and adulthood. Our aim was to test whether an infant cereal with 30% of whole grain was similarly accepted both by parents and infants in comparison to a similar cereal made from refined flour. A total of 81 infants between 4 and 24 months old were included in the study. Parent-infant pairs participated in an 8-day experimental study. Acceptance was rated on hedonic scales (4-points for infants and 7-points for parents). Other attributes like color, smell, and taste were evaluated by the parents. Acceptability for infant cereals with whole grain and refined cereals was very similar both for infants (2.30 ± 0.12 and 2.32 ± 0.11, $p = 0.606$) and parents (6.1 ± 0.8 and 6.0 ± 0.9, $p = 0.494$). Therefore, our findings show that there is an opportunity to introduce whole grain cereals to infants, including those who are already used to consuming refined infant cereals, thereby accelerating the exposure of whole grain in early life.

Keywords: acceptability; complementary feeding; infant cereals; whole grain

1. Introduction

Scholars have long established that the complementary feeding stage is very important because of the continued rapid growth and many changes that affect children's health and development [1–3]. These changes have a major influence on nutritional status during infancy and the food preferences during childhood and adulthood [4–6]. For this reason, several authors have strongly recommended the intake of healthy foods from the very beginning of the complementary feeding stage [7–9].

Weaning practices are significantly influenced by cultural beliefs [10,11]. However, in many countries, infant cereals are one of the first foods introduced at the beginning of the complementary period [11–14]. One possible reason stems from their sensorial and digestive properties [15]. For millennia, cereals have been staples for humans and are currently a large part of U.S. Dietary Guidelines [16]. Cereals are a good source of energy and macronutrients, such as carbohydrates, proteins and fats, that are needed for growth. Cereals are also an important source of vitamins, minerals and other essential bioactive compounds necessary for health [17].

Cereals can be consumed as whole grain or refined. Although the definition of whole grain is currently under discussion, the International American Association of Cereal Chemistry (AACC)

defined whole grains as "intact, ground, cracked or flaked caryopsis, whose principal anatomical components—the starchy endosperm, germ, and bran—are present in the same relative proportions as they exist in the intact caryopsis" [18]. In 2010, the Healthgrain Consortium broadened the AACC definition of whole grain to include small losses of components—that is, less than 2% of the grain/10% of the bran. Such losses may occur through processing methods required to ensure the safety and quality of whole grain and are allowed under the above definition [19].

It should be taken into account that until the 19th century, cereals were consumed as whole grain; it was only during the Industrial Revolution with the advent of new milling techniques that the bran and germ were removed from the grain kernel, obtaining refined cereal flours with improved texture and taste and ultimately leading to longer shelf life [20].

Several organizations and scholars have acknowledged the benefits associated with the intake of whole grain cereals for adults and children above two years [21–23]. Moreover, the USDA (US Department of Agriculture) recommends that, during the second semester of life, infants should be gradually introduced to fiber-containing foods, such as whole grain cereals, vegetables, and legumes [10]. Although there is no general agreement regarding daily dietary intake recommendations for whole grain (even for adults) [23,24], these recommendations are important and should be further studied in infants and young children. As eating habits can be molded during complementary feeding time, the early introduction and consumption of infant cereals elaborated with whole grain flour could be desirable [22].

In most countries, commercial infant cereals are made with refined cereal flours (www.innovadatabase.com). One of the main problems found when whole grain is introduced into the diet of an adult is the low sensorial acceptability compared to refined cereal-based foods [23,25]. However, prior research reveals that infants and young children have a higher acceptance of new foods in the complementary feeding period until the age of 18–24 months [26–28]. In this vein, several authors recommend gradually introducing whole grain products by substituting refined cereals as an effective way of incorporating whole grain into consumers' diets [23]. This can be reinforced by the development of technological processes to improve sensorial properties of whole grain products [29,30].

The present study was designed to determine if the intake of an infant cereal-based product with 30% whole grain was similarly accepted both by parents and their children, compared to the same infant cereal without whole grain (refined cereals).

2. Materials and Methods

2.1. Infant Cereal Samples

All infant cereals used in this experiment were commercially available products from HERO ESPAÑA S.A (Murcia, Spain). We selected this brand of multicereals to conduct this study because it is one of the most widely consumed infant cereals on the Spanish market. One of two infant cereals contained 30% of whole grain flour, WGC (new recipe), and the other one 100% refined cereal flours, RC (old recipe). The ingredients for WGC were: hydrolyzed cereal flour (wheat, wheat whole grain, corn, rice, oat, barley, rye, sorghum and millet), minerals, natural flavor and vitamins where the content of wheat whole grain flour was 30% of total cereals. The ingredients of RC were: hydrolyzed cereal flours (wheat, corn, rice, oat, barley, rye, sorghum and millet), minerals, natural flavor and vitamins. The nutritional composition of the two infant cereals used in this study is described in Table 1.

Table 1. Nutritional composition of the two infant cereals used in the study.

Mean Value (100 g)	WGC	RC
Energy (kcal)	380	372
Protein (g)	9.1	8.5
Carbohydrates (g)	78	81.6
Sugars (g)	21	22
Fat (g)	2.3	1.3
Fiber (g)	5.2	3

WGC: Whole Grain Cereal and RC: Refined Cereal.

2.2. Participant Characteristics

There were 81 parents with infants between the ages of 4–24 months recruited through advertisement on the website of the University of Murcia (Spain), as well as in kindergartens and parents' circles. Eligible healthy infants had a gestational age of 37–42 weeks and a birth weight greater than 2500 g and had been fed with gluten-containing cereals prior to enrolment in the experiment. Infants that had food allergies, swallowing or digestion problems, or other medical issues that could influence the ability to eat were excluded. There were an additional 20 pairs excluded because the parents did not complete the study or did not return the questionnaire (See Supplementary Materials). Once all parent-infant pairs were recruited, they were assigned to only one group where they received two packages of infant cereals (WGC and RC). The distribution of samples was counterbalanced to avoid any possible bias. The study protocol was approved by the Research Ethical Committee of the University of Murcia. Written informed consent was obtained from both parents of all participating infants before the inclusion.

2.3. Data Collection

Testing was carried out at home during a period of eight days. For the home-use test, the parents were responsible for conducting the experiment and collecting the data requested in the questionnaire (See Supplementary Materials). Prior to testing, the parents received both detailed written and oral instructions.

2.3.1. Testing

Parents received two coded packs of cereals. During days 1 and 2, infants were accustomed to the first of the two cereals. On the third day, parents evaluated the acceptance. Over days 4 and 5, infants continued eating the cereal which they used to eat before enrollment in the present study. On day 6, the same process started with the second infant cereal—familiarization on days 6 and 7 and, on day 8, evaluation of acceptance. No additional foods or beverages were introduced into the infants' diet during the study. All samples used in this study were packaged into identical foil bags. Each bag was marked with a three-digit randomization code. At the moment of feeding, the samples were counterbalanced and randomized; consequently, a child was fed with one sample on one day and the other sample on the other day. Each parent fed his/her infant in the habitual place, at a normal pace until the infant refused the spoon or bottle three consecutive times. Rejection behaviors are typically turning the head away, closing the mouth firmly, pushing the spoon away, spitting the food out or becoming upset [14,31]. Before each feeding, it was necessary to ensure that the infant was sufficiently hungry. In particular, parents were asked not to feed their infants with infant milk, other beverages, or solid foods for 1 h before the cereal intake [14,32]. Furthermore, testing occurred at approximately the same time of the day and 30 to 60 min before the infants' next scheduled feeding, so that variation of intake was not affected by different levels of hunger or satiation, but rather reflected hedonic response to the food. Regarding mode of preparation, this depended on the parents' habits (using bottle or spoon). Parents performed the sensory evaluation of the same products only after feeding their infants to ensure no interference with their infant's reactions due to non-habitual parent behavior (product testing) during the feeding (days 3 and 8) [14,32].

2.3.2. Measure of Food Acceptance

Parents were first asked to answer questions about their infants, feeding practices as well as socio-demographic information, such as gender, age and education (See Supplementary Materials). Then, parents were asked to score their degree of liking using a 7-point hedonic scale ranging from 1 "dislikes very much" to 7 "likes very much." This test allowed us to evaluate the acceptability of each parent for the sample of cereal. Parents' liking represents one important step to deciding if this type of cereal would be suitable for their infants. For the assessment of the acceptance by children, we used a 4-point hedonic scale [14,31]. This scale uses the following scores: "— " (very negative) if the infant spit out the food, frowned, pushed the spoon away or stopped eating; "−" (negative) if the infant ate a couple of spoonful, grimaced and stopped eating; "+" (positive) if the infant ate some of the food without a specific reaction; "++" (very positive) if the infant accepted the first spoonful immediately and displayed signs of content, such as a relaxed face or a smile [14,31].

2.4. Statistical Analyses

Data are expressed as means ± standard error of mean (SEM) for the following variables: age of introduction of infant cereals and parent's perception of child's degree of liking. For variables related to sensory analysis, data were expressed as mean ± standard deviation (SD). The categorical variables were expressed as percentage (%).

Descriptive analysis was employed to describe parents' and infants' characteristics as well as all variables related to consumption, mode of preparation, frequency of intake of infant cereals and sensory analysis. The evaluation of infants' acceptance, assessed by parents, was converted into scores of −3, −1, 1 and 3 so that there were equal intervals between adjacent scores throughout the scale. Taking into account that all variables are not distributed normally (Kolmogorov–Smirnov test), non-parametric analyses were performed: the Wilcoxon test for paired samples was used to detect differences in sensorial variables between the two samples of infant cereals; in the case of cereal feeding practices, variables expressed as percentages as per the Mann–Whitney test were applied in order to detect difference between both age ranges.

All results with a significance level of $p < 0.05$ were considered statistically significant. Statistical analyses of data were performed using the Statistical Package for the Social Sciences (SPSS version 19.0; Inc., Chicago, IL, USA).

3. Results

3.1. Subject Characteristics and Cereal Feeding Practices

The characteristics of the 81parent-infant pairs are presented in Table 2. The mean age of introduction of infant cereals was 5.2 (±1.3) months. The type of milk used by parents to prepare the cereals was in 55.6% of cases as follows: 21.0% "growing-up" milk; 13.5% cow's milk; 7.4% infant formula; and 2.5% breast milk (Table 3).

Parents were asked about the cereal feeding mode (bottle and/or spoon) and the number of times infants were fed per day (Table 3). The cereal feeding mode was distributed as follows: most infants (70.4%) were taking cereals from a bottle, 16.0% took cereals with a spoon and 13.6% used both bottle and spoon. There were significant differences in the mode of preparation of infant cereals depending on the age group ($p < 0.05$). Cereal bottle feeding was higher in the group of infants between 13 and 24 months of age (80%) as compared to the group of infants below one year. In general, more than 50% of infants took two servings a day, almost 40% took one serving a day, and the rest between three or more servings (7.4%) without significant differences between the two age ranges studied (below and above one year of age) (Table 3).

Table 2. Characteristics of infants and parents who participated in this study.

Characteristics	Group (*n* = 81)
Infants	
Age (by ranges)	
4–6 months	8.6
7–9 months	13.6
10–11 months	16
12–24 months	61.8
Girls	60
Parents	
Men	12
Women	88
Age	
25–30 years	5.3
31–35 years	46
36–40 years	43.4
>41 years	5.3
Number of children	
One child	48
Two children	48
Three children	4

Values expressed as percentage.

Table 3. Cereal feeding practices used for parents to prepare the infant cereals.

	Age Range		
	4–11 Months	12–24 Months	Total
Type of Milk Used			
Breast milk	6.5 (2)	-	2.5 (2)
Infant formula	9.7 (3)	6.0 (3)	7.4 (6)
Follow on formula	77.4 (24)	42 (21)	55.6 (45)
Growing up milk	3.2 (1)	32 (16)	27 (17)
Cow's milk	3.2 (1)	20 (10)	13.6 (11)
Mode of Cereal Feeding [a]			
Bottle	54.8 (17)	80 (40)	70.4 (57)
Spoon	25.8 (8)	10 (5)	16 (13)
Both	19.4 (4)	10 (5)	13.6 (11)
Frequency of Intake			
One serving	48.4 (11)	34 (17)	39.5 (32)
Two serving	41.9 (13)	60 (30)	53.1 (43)
Three or more serving	9.7 (3)	6 (3)	7.4 (6)

Values are expressed as percentage of total infant (number of infants); [a] Superscript indicates that there is significant differences between both groups of age and mode of feeding cereals ($z = -2.281; p < 0.05$).

The average amount of WGC and RC cereals consumed by age group is shown in Figure 1. In both cases, over 75% of infants consumed the entire serving of the cereals prepared, with no significant differences between the infant cereals evaluated.

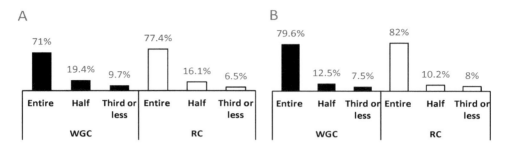

Figure 1. Infants' consumption of the serving of infant cereals prepared by parents. WGC: Whole Grain Cereal; RC: Refined Cereal. Values are expressed as percentage of total infants. (**A**) represents the consumption of cereals by infants 4–11 months of age; (**B**) consumption of cereals by infants 12–24 months of age.

3.2. Parents' Perception of Infants' Liking

As shown in Table 4, parents' rating of their infants' degree of liking was not statistically significant between the two infant cereals evaluated (WGC and RC)—neither within the two age groups ($p = 0.317$, $p = 0.666$ for group 4–11 months and group 12–24 months, respectively) nor in the total sample ($n = 81$, $p = 0.606$). Both infant cereals were highly accepted with average scores higher than 2.

Table 4. Parent's perception of child's degree of liking (mean ± SEM).

Age	WGC ($n = 81$)	RC ($n = 81$)	p-Value
4–11 months	2.35 ± 0.19	2.16 ± 0.18	0.317
12–24 months	2.29 ± 0.16	2.40 ± 0.15	0.666
Total ($n = 81$)	2.3 ± 0.12	2.32 ± 0.11	0.606

WGC: Whole Grain Cereal; RC: Refined Cereal.

3.3. Parents' Acceptability of Infant Cereals

There were no significant differences between WGC and RC in any of the attributes, as shown in Table 5. Parental rating of liking for each attribute did not differ for any infant cereal, indicating that parents reported the same liking for each sample. In general, the score for each attribute was very similar between both samples and overall acceptability was rated very high for both cereal products (6.1 for WGC and 6.0 for RC). In addition, we asked parents why they liked the infant cereals and which attributes influenced their choices. In both cases, the criteria for their choices were similar; for example, about 50% of the parents chose the taste as first choice, followed by aroma (20%), and texture (17%).

Table 5. Sensory evaluation of infant cereals by parents (mean ± SD).

Attributes	WGC	RC	p-Value
Color	6.1 ± 0.9	5.8 ± 1.1	0.090
Aroma	6.3 ± 0.9	6.3 ± 0.8	0.850
Taste	6.2 ± 0.9	6.1 ± 0.9	0.799
Texture	5.9 ± 1.1	6.2 ± 1.1	0.235
Overall acceptability	6.1 ± 0.8	6.0 ± 0.9	0.494

* Values in rows with different superscripts are significantly different ($p < 0.05$).

4. Discussion

The present study reveals that the addition of whole grain in infant cereals was similarly well accepted from the sensorial point of view by both parents and their infants as compared to refined cereals. Importantly, previous studies have observed that early exposure to foods affects infants' later taste acceptance patterns and that infants are able to communicate their acceptance by both quantity of intake and facial expression [32]. In our study, we did not observe any differences in the facial expression or in the intake, and more than 75% of the infants ate the entire cereal serving prepared by their parents. Several factors are likely to explain the high acceptability found in whole grain infant cereals such as the percentage of whole grain used in this study (30%), the milk used for the reconstitution of the cereal (already accepted by the infants) or technology advances in cereal processing which improve the sensorial characteristics of whole grain cereals.

The selected amount of whole grain tested in our study was based on the minimal amount of whole grain with possible beneficial effects. Although there is no defined adequate intake of whole grain for adults or infants, Ferruzi et al. [15] have suggested that a whole grain food should provide 8 g of whole grain per 30 g serving (27 g/100 g) in order to be defined as a whole grain food which is nutritionally meaningful.

Interestingly, it has been reported that the main factor of consumer rejection in whole grain-based products is its bitter taste and rough texture [25,33]. In our study, we did not observe any of these issues. In fact, parents were reporting similar sensory liking scores in taste and texture and high scores in both infant cereals. Our results are similar to those found in students by Magalis et al. (2016), who did not find statistical differences in bitter taste between refined and whole grain products, although sensorial preferences tended toward some refined cereal products [25]. Other sensorial studies in school children have also reported a similar degree of acceptability of whole grain versus refined cereal products, i.e., whole grain products were well accepted [34,35].

Whole grain cereals, as well as vegetables, can be bitter due to their content of polyphenolic compounds [36]. Similar to findings in our study, Lange et al. (2013) and Mennella et al. (2015) reported that when the new foods are introduced (vegetables) with other foods already accepted, the acceptability of new foods was better [14,37]. This effect was related to the reduction of the unpleasant, bitter or sour notes of the vegetables not only by dilution, but also by the sweetness of the milk. The sweetness of breast milk has been estimated as equivalent to a 2.12% solution of sucrose [38]. The sweetness of standard formula milks is similar [39]. Salty and sweet tastes have the characteristic of blocking or masking unpleasant tastes present in many foods, such as a bitter taste in vegetables [38,39]. A clinical study of school-aged children has shown that the presence of diluted solutions of a sweetener (aspartame) along with vegetables increased the liking of vegetables and decreased the perception of bitter taste [40]. For that reason, we could hypothesize that like in vegetables, our infant cereals with whole grain were highly accepted due to the fact that they were reconstituted with infant milk formulas or breast milk previously accepted by the infant. In our study, whole grain cereals were mainly prepared with milk formula and to a lesser extent with breast milk. The presence of sweet taste and its acceptance by infants could mask the bitter notes present in the whole grain cereals, leading the products to be accepted in the same way as the refined product [41,42].

Regarding infant cereal practices, our study shows that the mean age of introduction of cereals was 5.2 months. In Spain, infant cereals are usually the first food introduced at the beginning of weaning and therefore the age of introduction in our study was in line with current recommendations of first introducing products between 4 and 6 months of age [3,43].

The complementary feeding period is a "critical time window" in human development during which eating behaviors are developed [44]. For this reason, timing, type and ways the foods are introduced are important feeding practices in the development of acceptance of healthy food as part of a healthy diet. Cereals play a main role at the beginning of and during the complementary feeding period. The type of cereals consumed (whole grain or refined) may influence both health and nutritional status of infants. In adults, it has been shown that significant consumption of whole grain products is associated with a lower risk of cardiovascular diseases, diabetes, obesity, colon cancer and gastrointestinal health [36]. A previous meta-analysis concluded that there is a negative correlation between intake of whole grain and mortality, with a reduction of 7% in risk associated with each single serving/day increase in whole grain intake [45]. Due to increasing evidence of health benefits associated with whole grains, several authors have strongly recommended implementing strategies for educating consumers to gradually incorporate whole grains into their diets through the substitution of refined cereals [23]. Although the beneficial effects of whole grains have not been demonstrated in infants or young children due to the lack of clinical trials in this age range, the development of healthy dietary habits during early stages of infancy including a diet with whole grain products could be desirable [22].

Two potential risks of the use of whole grain in infant cereals should be taken in account. Firstly, as compared to refined rice, whole grain rice has a higher content of inorganic arsenic, which is concentrated in the bran layers [46,47]. Secondly, in unbalanced diets, excessive fiber content is likely to have negative effects on mineral bioavailability [48]. In order to avoid these issues, we have used whole grain wheat in compliance with European infant legislation (Directive 2006/125/CE) [48]. Also, the fiber content of the cereals used in our study was within commercial standard values.

5. Conclusions

This research was conducted as a preliminary study toward a clinical trial designed to evaluate whole grain effects in infants with ages ranging from 5 to 9 months. Interestingly, we found that infant cereals with 30% whole grain were very well accepted from a sensory point of view by infants between 4 to 24 months as well as by their parents. Moreover, there is a lack of studies showing that refined cereal flours in infants and young children are better from a nutritional point of view than whole grain infant cereals. Throughout most of human development, whole grain cereals—not refined cereals—were naturally consumed. Therefore, there might be an opportunity to (re)introduce whole grain cereals to infants who are accustomed to consuming refined infant cereals, thereby accelerating the exposure of whole grain in early life. This research represents a first step in our understanding of sensory acceptability of whole grain infant cereals in infants aged 4 to 24 months. We encourage future studies to analyze both the acceptability of higher percentages of whole grain in infant cereal-based products as well as possible imprinting of health effects on infants during the complementary feeding period.

Acknowledgments: The present study was funded by Hero Group. We are grateful to all parents who participated in this preliminary study and especially to the kindergartens as well as the university community.

Author Contributions: All authors participated in the conception, design and writing of the manuscript. All authors read and approved the final manuscript.

1.   World Health Organization. *Guiding Principles for Complementary Feeding of the Breastfed Child*; Pan American Health Organization: Washington, DC, USA, 2003.
2.   Butte, N.; Cobb, K.; Dwyer, J.; Graney, L.; Heird, W.; Rickard, K. The Start Healthy Feeding Guidelines for infants and toddlers. *J. Am. Diet. Assoc.* **2004**, *104*, 442–454. [CrossRef] [PubMed]
3.   Agostoni, C.; Decsi, T.; Fewtrell, M.; Goulet, O.; Kolacek, S.; Koletzko, B.; Michaelsen, K.F.; Moreno, L.; Puntis, J.; Rigo, J.; et al. ESPGHAN Committee on Nutrition. Complementary Feeding: A Commentary by the ESPGHAN Committee on Nutrition. *J. Pediatr. Gastroenterol. Nutr.* **2008**, *46*, 99–110. [CrossRef] [PubMed]
4.   Mennella, J.A.; Trabulsi, J.C. Complementary foods and flavor experiences: Setting the foundation. *Ann. Nutr. Metab.* **2012**, *60*, 40–50. [CrossRef] [PubMed]
5.   Schwartz, C.; Scholtens, P.; Lalanne, A.; Weenen, H.; Nicklaus, S. Development of healthy eating habits early in life: Review of recent evidence and selected guidelines. *Appetite* **2011**, *57*, 796–807. [CrossRef] [PubMed]

6. Nicklaus, S. The role of food experiences during early childhood in food pleasure learning. *Appetite* **2016**, *104*, 3–9. [CrossRef] [PubMed]
7. Nicklaus, S.; Boggio, V.; Chabanet, C.; Issanchou, S. A prospective study of food variety seeking in childhood, adolescence and early adult life. *Appetite* **2005**, *44*, 289–297. [CrossRef] [PubMed]
8. Ventura, A.K.; Worobey, J. Early influences on the development of food preferences. *Curr. Biol.* **2003**, *23*, R401–R408. [CrossRef] [PubMed]
9. Nicklaus, S.; Boggio, V.; Chabanet, C.; Issanchou, S. A prospective study of food preferences in childhood. *Food Qual. Prefer.* **2004**, *15*, 805–818. [CrossRef]
10. United States Department of Agriculture. *Infant Nutrition and Feeding. A Guide for Use in the WIC and CSF Programs*; United States Department of Agriculture: Washington, DC, USA, 2009; pp. 101–129.
11. Caroli, M.; Mele, R.M.; Tomaselli, M.A.; Cammisa, M.; Longo, F.; Attolini, E. Complementary feeding patterns in Europe with a special focus on Italy. *Nutr. Metab. Cardiovasc.* **2012**, *22*, 813–818. [CrossRef] [PubMed]
12. Siega-Riz, A.M.; Deming, D.M.; Reidy, K.C.; Fox, M.K.; Condon, E.; Briefel, R.R. Food consumption patterns of infants and toddlers: where are we now? *J. Am. Diet. Assoc.* **2010**, *110*, S38–S51. [CrossRef] [PubMed]
13. Butte, N.F.; Fox, M.K.; Briefel, R.R.; Siega-Riz, A.M.; Dwyer, J.T.; Deming, D.M.; Reidy, K.C. Nutrient intakes of US infants, toddlers, and preschoolers meet or exceed dietary reference intakes. *J. Am. Diet. Assoc.* **2010**, *110*, S27–S37. [CrossRef] [PubMed]
14. Lange, C.; Visalli, M.; Jacob, S.; Chabanet, C.; Schlich, P.; Nicklaus, S. Maternal feeding practices during the first year and their impact on infants' acceptance of complementary food. *Food Qual. Prefer.* **2013**, *29*, 89–98. [CrossRef]
15. Bernal, M.J.; Periago, M.J.; Martínez, R.; Ortuño, I.; Sánchez-Solís, M.; Ros, G.; Romero, F.; Abellán, P. Effects of infant cereals with different carbohydrate profiles on colonic function-randomized and double-blind clinical trial in infants aged between 6 and 12 months—Pilot study. *Eur. J. Pediatr.* **2013**, *172*, 1535–1542. [CrossRef] [PubMed]
16. U.S. Department of Health and Human Services and U.S. Department of Agriculture. Dietary Guidelines for Americans 2015–2020. Available online: http://health.gov/dietaryguidelines/2015/guidelines/ (accessed on 28 November 2016).
17. Topping, D. Cereal complex carbohydrates and their contribution to human health. *J. Cereal Sci.* **2007**, *46*, 220–229. [CrossRef]
18. American Association of Cereal Chemists. Definition of Whole Grain in 1999. Available online: http://www.aaccnet.org/initiatives/definitions/pages/wholegrain.aspx (accessed on 30 September 2016).
19. Van der Kamp, J.; Poutanen, K.; Seal, C.; Richardson, D. The HEALTHGRAIN definition of 'whole grain'. *Food Nutr. Res.* **2014**, *58*. [CrossRef] [PubMed]
20. Cordain, L.; Eaton, S.B.; Sebastian, A.; Mann, N.; Lindeberg, S.; Watkins, B.A.; O'Keefe, J.H.; Brand-Miller, J. Origins and evolution of the Western diet: Health implications for the 21st century. *Am. J. Clin. Nutr.* **2005**, *81*, 341–354. [PubMed]
21. World Health Organization. *Global Strategy on Diet, Physical Activity and Health Worldwide Strategy about "Feeding Regimen, Physical Activity and Health"*; World Health Organization: Washington, DC, USA, 2004.
22. Alexy, U.; Zorn, C.; Kersting, M. Whole grain in children's diet: Intake, food sources and trends. *Eur. J. Clin. Nutr.* **2010**, *64*, 745–751. [CrossRef] [PubMed]
23. Ferruzzi, M.G.; Jonnalagadda, S.S.; Liu, S.; Marquart, L.; McKeown, N.; Reicks, M.; Riccardi, G.; Seal, C.; Slavin, J.; Thielecke, F.; et al. Developing a standard definition of whole-grain foods for dietary recommendations: Summary report of a multidisciplinary expert roundtable discussion. *Adv. Nutr.* **2014**, *5*, 164–176. [CrossRef] [PubMed]
24. Slavin, J.; Tucker, M.; Harriman, C.; Jonnalagadda, S.S. Whole grains: Definition, dietary recommendations, and health benefits. *Cereal Chem.* **2016**, *93*, 209–216. [CrossRef]
25. Magalis, R.M.; Giovanni, M.; Silliman, K. Whole grain foods: is sensory liking related to knowledge, attitude, or intake? *Nut. Food Sci.* **2016**, *46*, 488–503. [CrossRef]
26. Wright, P. Development of food choice during infancy. *Proc. Nutr. Soc.* **1991**, *50*, 107–113. [CrossRef] [PubMed]
27. Cashdan, E. A sensitive period for learning about food. *Hum. Nat.* **1994**, *5*, 279–291. [CrossRef] [PubMed]
28. Olsen, A.; Møller, P.; Hausner, H. Early origins of overeating: Early habit formation and implications for obesity in later life. *Curr. Obes. Rep.* **2013**, *2*, 157–164. [CrossRef]

29. Poutanen, K. Past and future of cereal grains as food for health. *Trends Food Sci. Technol.* **2012**, *25*, 58–62. [CrossRef]

30. Poutanen, K.; Sozer, N.; Della Valle, G. How can technology help to deliver more of grain in cereal foods for a healthy diet? *J. Cereal Sci.* **2014**, *59*, 327–336. [CrossRef]

31. Schwartz, C.; Chabanet, C.; Lange, C.; Issanchou, S.; Nicklaus, S. The role of taste in food acceptance at the beginning of complementary feeding. *Physiol. Behav.* **2013**, *2011*, 646–652. [CrossRef] [PubMed]

32. Forestell, C.A.; Mennella, J.A. Early determinants of fruit and vegetable acceptance. *Pediatrics* **2007**, *120*, 1247–1254. [CrossRef] [PubMed]

33. Bakke, A.; Vickers, Z. Consumer liking of refined and whole wheat breads. *J. Food Sci.* **2007**, *72*, S473–S480. [CrossRef] [PubMed]

34. Burgess-Champoux, T.; Marquart, L.; Vickers, Z.; Reicks, M. Perceptions of Children, Parents, and Teachers Regarding Whole-Grain Foods, and Implications for a School-Based Intervention. *J. Nutr. Educ. Behav.* **2006**, *38*, 230–237. [CrossRef] [PubMed]

35. Chan, H.W.; Burgess-Champoux, T.; Reicks, M.; Vickers, Z.; Marquart, L. White whole-wheat flour can be partially substituted for refined-wheat flour in pizza crust in school meals without affecting consumption. *J. Child Nutr. Manag.* **2008**, *32*.

36. Fardet, A. New hypotheses for the health-protective mechanisms of whole-grain cereals: What is beyond fibre? *Nutr. Res. Rev.* **2010**, *23*, 65–134. [CrossRef] [PubMed]

37. Hetherington, M.M.; Schwartz, C.; Madrelle, J.; Crode, F.; Nekitsing, C.; Vereijken, C.M.J.L.; Weenen, H. A step-by-step introduction to vegetables at the beginning of complementary feeding. The effects of early and repeated exposure. *Appetite* **2015**, *84*, 280–290. [CrossRef] [PubMed]

38. McDaniel, M.R.; Barker, E.; Lederer, C.L. Sensory characterization of human milk. *J. Dairy Sci.* **1989**, *72*, 1149–1158. [CrossRef]

39. Schwartz, C.; Chabanet, C.; Boggio, V.; Lange, C.; Issanchou, S.; Nicklaus, S. À quelles saveurs les nourrissons sont-ils exposés dans la premiére année de vie? To which tastes are infants exposed during the first year of life? *Arch. Pediatr.* **2010**, *17*, 1026–1034. (In French) [CrossRef] [PubMed]

40. Mennella, J.A.; Reed, D.R.; Roberts, K.M.; Mathew, P.S.; Mansfield, C.J. Age-related differences in bitter taste and efficacy of bitter blockers. *PLoS ONE* **2014**, *9*, e103107. [CrossRef] [PubMed]

41. Mennella, J.A.; Reed, D.R.; Mathew, P.S.; Roberts, K.M.; Mansfield, C.J. "A spoonful of sugar helps the medicine go down": Bitter masking by sucrose among children and adults. *Chem. Senses* **2015**, *40*, 17–25. [CrossRef] [PubMed]

42. Capaldi, E.D.; Privitera, G.J. Decreasing dislike for sour and bitter in children and adults. *Appetite* **2008**, *50*, 139–145. [CrossRef] [PubMed]

43. EFSA Panel on Dietetic Products. Nutrition and Allergies. Scientific Opinion on the appropriate age for introduction of complementary feeding of infant. *EFSA J.* **2009**, *7*, 1423–1461.

44. Birch, L.L.; Doub, L.E. Learning to eat: Birth to age 2 years. *Am. J. Clin. Nutr.* **2014**, *99*, 723S–728S. [CrossRef] [PubMed]

45. Ma, X.; Tang, W.G.; Yang, Y.; Zhang, Q.L.; Zheng, J.L.; Xiang, Y.B. Association between whole grain intake and all-cause mortality: a meta-analysis of cohort studies. *Oncotarget* **2016**, *7*, 61996–62005. [CrossRef] [PubMed]

46. Sun, G.X.; Williams, P.N.; Carey, A.M.; Zhu, Y.G.; Deacon, C.; Raab, A.; Feldmann, J.; Islam, R.M.; Meharg, A.A. Inorganic arsenic in rice bran and its products are an order of magnitude higher than in bulk grain. *Environ. Sci. Technol.* **2008**, *42*, 7542–7546. [CrossRef] [PubMed]

47. Signes-Pastor, A.; Carey, M.; Meharg, A.A. Inorganic arsenic in rice-based products for infants and young children. *Food Chem.* **2016**, *191*, 128–134. [CrossRef] [PubMed]

48. Directive 2006/125/CE. Commission Directive 2006/125/EC of 5 December 2006 on Processed Cereal-Based Foods and Baby Foods for Infants and Young Children. Available online: http://eur-lex.europa.eu/legal-content/EN/TXT/PDF/?uri=CELEX:32006L0125&from=EN (accessed on 30 September 2016).

16

Early Taste Experiences and Later Food Choices

Valentina De Cosmi [1], Silvia Scaglioni [2] and Carlo Agostoni [3],*

[1] Valentina De Cosmi Pediatric Intensive Care Unit, Fondazione IRCCS Cà Granda Ospedale Maggiore Policlinico, Branch of Medical Statistics, Biometry, and Epidemiology "G. A. Maccacaro", Department of Clinical Sciences and Community Health, University of Milan, 20122 Milan, Italy; valentina.decosmi@gmail.com

[2] Silvia Scaglioni Fondazione De Marchi Department of Pediatrics, Fondazione IRCCS Cà Granda Ospedale Maggiore Policlinico, 20122 Milan, Italy; silviascaglioni50@gmail.com

[3] Carlo Agostoni Pediatric Intermediate Care Unit, Fondazione IRCCS Cà Granda Ospedale Maggiore Policlinico, Department of Clinical Sciences and Community Health, University of Milan, 20122 Milan, Italy

* Correspondence: carlo.agostoni@unimi.it

Abstract: Background. Nutrition in early life is increasingly considered to be an important factor influencing later health. Food preferences are formed in infancy, are tracked into childhood and beyond, and complementary feeding practices are crucial to prevent obesity later in life. Methods. Through a literature search strategy, we have investigated the role of breastfeeding, of complementary feeding, and the parental and sociocultural factors which contribute to set food preferences early in life. Results. Children are predisposed to prefer high-energy, -sugar, and -salt foods, and in pre-school age to reject new foods (food neophobia). While genetically determined individual differences exist, repeated offering of foods can modify innate preferences. Conclusions. Starting in the prenatal period, a varied exposure through amniotic fluid and repeated experiences with novel flavors during breastfeeding and complementary feeding increase children's willingness to try new foods within a positive social environment.

Keywords: early taste; food preferences; breastfeeding; complementary feeding; feeding strategy; children obesity; food choices

1. Introduction

Childhood is a period of very rapid growth and development. In this critical phase, food preferences are formed, are tracked into childhood and beyond, and foundations are laid for a healthy adult life [1]. The characterization of feeding practices is important for the determination of which factors of the early environment can be modified and thus are amenable to intervention. Since early life exposures may contribute to the risk of obesity [2], the topic is highly recognized to be of social and public health interest [3,4].

Infants' and children's eating and activity behaviors are influenced by both intrinsic (genetics, age, gender) and environmental (family, peers, community, and society) factors [5]. These factors are fully displayed in Figure 1.

Firstly, prenatal exposure, and then breastfeeding, have been associated with flavor stimulation and moderately lower childhood obesity risk in many studies [2,6,7]. Later on, the period of complementary feeding is also crucial, both for obesity prevention and for setting taste preferences and infant attitude towards food. Parents act by teaching children in different ways how, what, when, and how much to eat and by transmitting cultural and familial beliefs and practices surrounding food and eating [8]. Parents' influence is significant: it is reflected both by what is on the plate and the context in which it is offered [9].

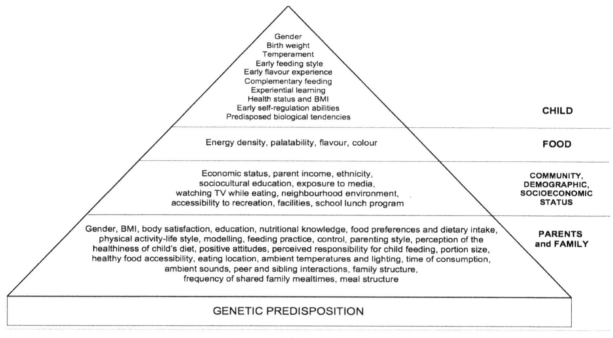

BMI: Body Mass Index

Figure 1. Environmental factors that influence child eating behavior.

Obesity is a burden social disease, linked to lifestyle and food choices changes, characterized by low level of physical activity, high energy density, and free sugar-rich food. As nutritional habits are tracked from infancy to adulthood, we investigated factors inside the child milieu, possibly connected to flavor learning and feeding practices. In particular, we focused on strictly child-related factors. Parental influence is only described in terms of food offering feeding style, while parental modeling is not a topic of our review. We reviewed (1) the biological and social early-life exposures; (2) the prenatal influence of the amniotic fluid; (3) how breast milk and formula may influence taste development; (4) the role of complementary feeding; (5) the parental and sociocultural factors associated with trajectories of health in adulthood.

2. Methods—Literature Search Strategy

Electronic databases (Pubmed, Medline, Embase, Google Scholar) were searched to locate and appraise relevant studies. We carried out the search to identify articles published in English on the relation between children's early taste experiences and their food choices during childhood. Relevant articles published after 2005 and up to August 2016 were identified using the following search words in various combinations. The literature search was not aimed to conduct a systematic review or meta-analysis of all of the available literature on this topic, but to explore the pertinent observations in a period of 10 years. Our work is a narrative review, and search terms were inserted individually and using the booleans AND and OR. The following terms were included in the search strategy: ("early taste experiences" OR "early food preferences") & ("food choices in childhood") OR ("parental feeding practices" OR "parent's feeding strategies" OR "parental modeling") & ("family environmental factors" OR "family eating environments") & ("early exposure" AND "obesity risk" AND "childhood obesity risk factors") & ("amniotic fluid" OR "breast milk" AND "taste AND flavor development") & ("early diet experiences" OR "development of eating habits") & ("Food choices"). More than 5000 references matched the terms of the search, and around 1500 had been published in the past 10 years. The authors selected the articles and assessed the potentially relevant ones.

2.1. Effects of Early Taste Experiences

According to a working hypothesis, the first thousand days of life represent a sensitive period for the development of healthy eating habits, and for this reason, interventions are likely to have a strong impact on health outcomes later during childhood and adulthood. This critical period starts with feeding through the cord during gestation, passes toward oral feeding with milk, and then the complementary feeding begins and the infant discovers a variety of foods and flavors. Humans generally have inborn positive responses to sugar and salt, and negative responses to bitter taste [10]. Genetically determined individual differences also exist, and interact with experience to ensure that children are not genetically restricted to a narrow range of foodstuffs [11]. Children are also predisposed to prefer high-energy foods, to reject new foods, and to learn associations between food flavors and the post-ingestive consequences of eating [12]. This genetic predisposition appears to have evolved over thousands of years when foods—especially those high in energy density—were scarce. Few children—PROP (6-n-propylthiouracil) tasters—are sensitive to bitter taste and have higher liking and consumption of bitter foods, such as cruciferous vegetables. Additionally, those children who are unable to taste PROP (nontasters) like and consume more dietary fat and are prone to obesity; thus, genetic variation in the ability to taste bitter compounds may have important implications as a marker for dietary patterns and chronic health in children. The available literature suggests that some children may require additional strategies to accept and consume bitter-tasting fruits and vegetables and that genetic predisposition may be modified by repeated exposures [13,14].

2.2. Amniotic Fluid and Breast Milk

The ability to recognize a variety of flavors involves multiple chemosensory sensations, primarily the sense of taste and smell. Food experiences begin prenatally, since chemosensory systems have an adaptive and evolutionary role and are functional before birth [10]. The exposure to an in utero environment may cause permanent effects on the developing tissue. These effects are referred to as "programming", and are important risk factors for chronic diseases in later adulthood [15].

Children usually prefer foods that are high in sugar and salt over those which are sour and bitter tasting, such as some vegetables. Preferences for salt and the refusal of bitter can be modified early through repeated exposure to flavors in amniotic fluid, mother's milk, and solid foods during complementary feeding. Flavor senses are well developed at birth, and continue to change throughout childhood and adolescence, serving as gatekeepers throughout the life span, controlling whether to accept or reject a foreign substance. Since amniotic fluid and breast milk both reflect to a variable degree the food composition of the maternal diet, a repeated exposure to their flavors increases infants' acceptance of foods [16]. While the knowledge of the influence of the maternal diet on breast milk is mostly indirect [17], the sensory experiences with food flavors in mothers who ate a varied diet may explain why their breastfed children tend to be less picky [18] and more willing to try new foods during childhood [11,19,20]. A cohort study [21] on 1160 mother–infant pairs showed that preponderance of breastfeeding in the first 6 months of life and breastfeeding duration were associated with less maternal restrictive behavior and less pressure to eat. Accordingly, compared with bottle-feeding, breastfeeding may promote maternal feeding styles that are less controlling and more responsive to infant cues of hunger and satiety, thereby allowing infants to develop a greater self-regulation of energy intake [21].

2.3. Formula-Fed Infants

The early flavor experience of formula-fed infants is markedly different from that of breast-fed infants. Exclusively formula-fed children do not benefit from the ever-changing flavor profile of breast milk. Their flavor experience is more monotone and lacks the flavors of the foods of the mother's diet. There are striking differences in flavors among the different types of formulas and brands of formulas, and formula-fed infants learn to prefer the flavors of the formula they are fed and foods containing these flavors [11]. There is a plethora of infant formulas on the market that differ in macronutrient composition. When evaluating the effect of diet composition on growth and health outcomes, it may no longer be appropriate to consider all formula-fed infants as a homogeneous group, because infant formulas may also differ in both fat and carbohydrate composition/structure as well as protein composition, and these differences may in turn affect growth and flavor development [22]. Consequently, it is important to understand the composition of the diet to which breastfeeding is being compared before drawing conclusions. European and US populations reveal an association between breastfeeding and a reduced prevalence of obesity in a meta-analysis; however, in a large randomized controlled trial, there was no effect of breastfeeding on body mass index in later childhood [23]. When infants are fed with a formula that is more similar in protein content to breast milk (lower vs. higher protein), their weight-for-length at 24 months of age does not differ from breastfed infants [24]. Another difference is found in infants consuming protein hydrolysate formula when compared with cow's milk formula: they are satiated sooner and have a less excessive rates of weight gain [25]. The mechanism of this effect is currently unknown, but is hypothesized to be related to differences in free glutamate (which is abundant in human breast milk) [26,27].

2.4. Complementary Feeding and Future Consumption of Fruits and Vegetables during Childhood

Early learning about flavours continues during the complementary feeding period, through the introduction of solids and changing exposures to a variety of new foods. In this peculiar time of the child's life, there is the transition from breast/formula feeding to a complementary solid diet, and infants discover the sensory (texture, taste, and flavour) and nutritional properties (energy density) of the foods that will ultimately compose their adult diet [28]. Being exposed to a variety of foods during the complementary feeding period helps modulate the acceptance of new foods in the first year, whereas exposure in the second year may have a more limited impact [29].

Young children (especially 2–5 years old) exhibit heightened levels of food neophobia during this time. This means that they are unwilling to eat novel foods; it is interpreted as an adaptive behaviour, ensuring children consume foods that are familiar and safe [30].

Distaste—dislike of the sensory characteristics of a food—appears to be the strongest driver of neophobia in young children [31]. Indeed, the two strongest predictors of young children's food preferences are familiarity and sweetness, reflecting unlearned preferences. However, these innate tendencies are paired with a predisposition to learn from early experiences through associative learning and repeated exposure, allowing the child to learn how to accept and prefer the foods that are available within his particular environment [30]. Repeated exposures to a food increase their familiarity, and it is one of the primary determinants of its acceptance. Several studies have shown that a food is consumed more and is judged as more liked by the infant after several offers. For instance, an increase in acceptance of a new green vegetable was observed after at least eight exposures to this food [31]. The effect of repeated exposure is potent enough to increase the acceptance of foods which had been previously identified by the mother as being refused by her infant during the beginning of the complementary feeding, which were most often green vegetables, but also pumpkin [32]. However, despite the efficacy of this mechanism, foods are most often only presented a limited number of times (often less than five times) before the parents decide that the infant dislikes this food [33–35].

Reactions towards new foods differ according to food groups [28]. Lange et al. (2013) asked mothers to report their infant's reactions to new foods at the beginning of complementary feeding, and they found that fruits and vegetables, which are firstly offered to infants, are less accepted than other food groups [36].

A study of de Launzon et al. investigated the long-term effects of early parental feeding practices on fruit and vegetable intake. The study used data from four European cohorts, in which data on fruits and vegetables consumption were assessed with a questionnaire. These cohorts reported different findings. Fruit and vegetable intake in early childhood varied with an average intake of <1 vegetable/day in the Greek EuroPrevall study and >3 vegetables/day in the Generation XXI Birth Cohort. Moreover, longer breastfeeding duration was found in Generation XXI than in the others.

The timing of complementary feeding varied too: complementary foods were introduced mainly between 3 and 4 months of age in ALSPAC (British Avon Longitudinal Study of Parents and Children), at ≈4 months in Generation XXI, and at ≈5 months in Greek Euro-Prevall. In EDEN (French Etude des De'terminants pre et postnatals de la sante' et du de'veloppement de l'Enfant), there was no peak age for introduction to complementary foods.

A concordant positive association between breastfeeding duration and fruit and vegetable intake was found in different cultural contexts, with a longer breastfeeding duration consistently related to higher fruit and vegetable intake in young children, whereas the associations with age of introduction to fruit and vegetable intake were weaker and less consistent [37].

Similarly, 2- to 8-year old children who were breastfed for three or more months were more likely to eat vegetables, as compared to children who were breastfed for a shorter time [28,38]. Taste may impact the acceptance of new foods, since vegetables added with salt or a salty ingredient are more easily accepted [39]. However, this observation should not encourage parents to use salt or salty ingredients, because sodium is not recommended for infants [2,35]. Furthermore, acceptance of green beans appears more difficult than that of carrot, in part due to the difference in the tastes of the two vegetables, since carrots are sweeter than beans [35].

Therefore, the attraction towards new foods in the absence of imprinting and/or learning seems to depend on their tastes and on the sensory properties of foods. At the same time, some individuals may be more sensitive to taste features. In particular, for the sour, sweet, and umami tastes, the individual sensitivity to taste in water solutions at the age of 6 months was predictive of the positive reaction towards foods bearing these tastes [39].

Nicklaus and coworkers in 2014 studied the effect of repeated exposure and of flavor-flavor learning on toddlers' (2–4 years) acceptance of a non-familiar vegetable, and concluded that repeated exposure is the simplest choice to increase vegetable intake in the short and long term [29,35]. The NOURISH is a randomized controlled trial which evaluated an intervention commencing in infancy to provide anticipatory guidance to first-time mothers on a "protective" pattern of complementary feeding practices that were hypothesized to reduce childhood obesity risk. In agreement with the results, investing in early advice on training mothers about responsive complementary feeding can improve maternal feeding practices, and suggests that complementary feeding practices promoting the self-regulation of intake and preference for healthy foods may have positive effects on obesity risk up to 5 years of age [15,40].

Early experiences with nutritious foods and flavour variety may maximize the likelihood that children will choose a healthier diet as they grow, because they like the tastes and the variety of the foods it contains. A recent investigation demonstrated that early exposure to a rotation of vegetable flavours first added to milk and then to cereals increased the intake and liking of these vegetables. Infants assigned to the intervention ate more of the target vegetables in the laboratory and at home than those assigned to the control group [12].

During childhood, the strongest predictors of what foods young children eat are (1) whether they like how the foods taste; (2) how long they were breastfed and whether their mothers ate these foods; and (3) whether they had been eating these foods from an early age [20,41]. During early childhood, infants are more likely to accept new foods, and parents should promote a varied diet and the child's curiosity towards food to reduce neophobia in toddlers [41,42]. After the age of 3–4 years, reported dietary patterns/food habits remained quite stable, further highlighting the importance of getting children on the right track from the initial stages of learning to eat [43].

2.5. Sociocultural and Family Environment

Social support plays a key role starting from birth. Accordingly, the initiation and continuation of breastfeeding and cultural beliefs—shared through kin, friend, and neighbors networks—may serve to promote or limit breastfeeding [2]. Parents create food environments for children's early experiences with food and eating, and also influence their children's eating by modeling their own eating behaviors, taste preferences, and food choices. As children grow and become more independent, familial influences on eating behavior may diminish, and other factors such as those of peers may become more influential [44]. Parents and caregivers play a role in structuring early feeding, which in turn is embedded in the larger micro- and macro-environments that shape parental beliefs, decisions, and practices [45]. It has been shown that forcing a child to eat a particular food will decrease the liking for that food, and that restricting access to particular foods increases rather than decreases preferences [14].

Social influences become increasingly important for the development of food preferences throughout infancy, and may either support or contrast the preferences learned during the prenatal and early postnatal periods [30]. Beauchamp and Moran [46] examined the preference for sweet solutions versus water in approximately 200 infants. At birth, all of the infants preferred sweet solutions to water, but by 6 months of age, the preference for sweetened water was linked to the infants' dietary experience. Infants who were routinely fed sweetened water by their mothers showed a greater preference for it than did infants who were not. Therefore, offering complementary foods without added sugars and salt may be advisable not only for short-term health but also to set the infant's threshold for sweet and salty tastes at lower levels later in life [14]. Neophobic tendencies can be reduced and preferences can be increased by exposing infants and young children repeatedly to novel foods. Children need to be exposed to a novel food between 6 and 15 times before increases in intake and preferences are seen. A recent study found that repeatedly exposing children to a novel food within a positive social environment was especially effective in increasing children's willingness to try it. These findings suggest the importance of both the act of repeatedly exposing children to new foods and the context within which this exposure occurs [30].

3. Discussion

The prevalence of childhood obesity is rising, and multiple studies indicate that most of the risk factors develop during the early phases of life. These factors may range from the prenatal to postnatal period.

Within this context, strategies to successfully promote better acceptance of vegetables should be identified. In spite of a huge body of literature, practical aspects and the results of their application are still poorly understood. This is due to the high complexity related to physiological mechanisms underlying early sensory experiences and the development of sensory preferences.

Breast-fed infants more easily accept a new vegetable, and have higher acceptance of new foods as they are introduced into the infant's diet. There are many factors which influence infants' feeding behaviours; they interact and contribute to the creation of future eating habits. Mothers who consume an array of healthy foods themselves throughout pregnancy and lactation—and subsequently feed their children these foods at the complementary feeding period—can promote healthful eating habits in their children and families. Although a large part of food-preference development occurs during early childhood, food preferences continue to change during adolescence up to adulthood, and the factors that influence these changes become more complex through the years [30]. While it is emphasized that an excessive intake of foods high in salt and refined sugars early in life may be associated with later non-communicable disorders, the individual genetic background and sensitivity to specific nutrients makes it difficult to substantiate a precise cause and effect dose-dependent relationship.

On the other side, food likes and dislikes are learned, and the learning process begins early and depends on biological and sociocultural attitudes.

4. Conclusions

Attention should be paid to the different socio-cultural contexts of eating in future studies, and cohort studies are needed to quantify the effect of early stimulation of taste and preferences. Randomized controlled trials on early diet, focusing on both caregivers and children's behaviours and adjusted for food-related genotype are also essential for understanding how preferences can be modified to promote healthful diets across the life course [30].

Acknowledgments: The authors thank all the members of the Pediatric Unit for their kindly support.

Author Contributions: Valentina De Cosmi, Silvia Scaglioni, Carlo Agostoni contributed equally in the writing and revising of the manuscript.

References

1. Alles, M.S.; Eussen, S.R.; Van Der Beek, E.M. Nutritional challenges and opportunities during the weaning period and in young childhood. *Ann. Nutr. Metab.* **2014**, *64*, 284–293. [CrossRef] [PubMed]
2. Amanda, L.T.; Margaret, E. The critical period of infant feeding for the development of early disparities in obesity. *Soc. Sci. Med.* **2013**. [CrossRef]
3. Benyshek, D.C. The developmental origins of obesity and related health disorders–prenatal and perinatal factors. *Coll. Antropol.* **2007**, *31*, 11–17. [PubMed]
4. Gillman, M.W. Developmental origins of health and disease. *N. Engl. J. Med.* **2005**, *353*, 1848–1850. [CrossRef] [PubMed]
5. Bellows, L.L.; Johnson, S.L.; Davies, P.L.; Anderson, J.; Gavin, W.J.; Boles, R.E. The Colorado LEAP study: Rationale and design of a study to assess the short term longitudinal effectiveness of a preschool nutrition and physical activity program. *BMC Public Health* **2013**. [CrossRef] [PubMed]
6. Arenz, S.; Rückerl, R.; Koletzko, B.; von Kries, R. Breast-feeding and childhood obesity—A systematic review. *Int. J. Obes.* **2004**, *28*, 1247–1256. [CrossRef] [PubMed]
7. Owen, C.G.; Martin, R.M.; Whincup, P.H.; Smith, G.D.; Cook, D.G. Effect of infant feeding on the risk of obesity across the life course: A quantitative review of published evidence. *Pediatrics* **2005**, *115*, 1367–1377. [CrossRef] [PubMed]
8. Birch, L.L.; Fisher, J.O. Development of eating behaviours among children and adolescents. *Pediatrics* **1998**, *101*, 539–549. [PubMed]
9. Mitchell, G.L.; Farrow, C.; Haycraft, E.; Meyer, C. Parental influences on children's eating behaviour and characteristics of successful parent-focussed interventions. *Appetite* **2013**, *60*, 85–94. [CrossRef] [PubMed]
10. Robinson, S.; Fall, C. Infant nutrition and later health: A review of current evidence. *Nutrients* **2012**, *4*, 859–874. [CrossRef] [PubMed]
11. Mennella, J.A. Ontogeny of taste preferences: Basic biology and implications for health. *Am. J. Clin. Nutr.* **2014**, *99*, 704S–711S. [CrossRef] [PubMed]
12. Hetherington, M.M.; Schwartz, C.; Madrelle, J.; Croden, F.; Nekitsing, C.; Vereijken, C.M.J.L.; Weenen, H. A step-by-step introduction to vegetables at the beginning of complementary feeding. The effects of early and repeated exposure. *Appetite* **2015**, *84*, 280–290. [CrossRef] [PubMed]
13. Keller, K.L.; Adise, S. Variation in the Ability to Taste Bitter Thiourea Compounds: Implications for Food Acceptance, Dietary Intake, and Obesity Risk in Children. *Annu. Rev. Nutr.* **2016**, *36*, 157–182. [CrossRef] [PubMed]
14. Agostoni, C.; Decsi, T.; Fewtrell, M.; Goulet, O.; Kolacek, S.; Koletzko, B.; Shamir, R. Complementary feeding: A commentary by the ESPGHAN Committee on Nutrition. *J. Pediatr. Gastroenterol. Nutr.* **2008**, *46*, 99–110. [CrossRef] [PubMed]
15. Muniandy, N.D.; Allotey, P.A.; Soyiri, I.N.; Reidpath, D.D. Complementary feeding and the early origins of obesity risk: A study protocol. *BMJ Open* **2016**. [CrossRef] [PubMed]
16. Forestell, C.A. The Development of Flavor Perception and Acceptance: The Roles of Nature and Nurture. *Nestle Nutr. Inst. Workshop Ser.* **2016**, *85*, 135–143. [PubMed]
17. Bravi, F.; Wiens, F.; Decarli, A.; Dal Pont, A.; Agostoni, C.; Ferraroni, M. Impact of maternal nutrition on breast-milk composition: A systematic review. *Am. J. Clin. Nutr.* **2016**, *104*, 646–662. [CrossRef] [PubMed]
18. Galloway, A.T.; Lee, Y.; Birch, L.L. Predictors and consequences of food neophobia and pickiness in young girls. *J. Am. Diet. Assoc.* **2003**, *103*, 692–698. [CrossRef] [PubMed]
19. Skinner, J.D.; Carruth, B.R.; Bounds, W.; Ziegler, P.; Reidy, K. Do food-related experiences in the first 2 years of life predict dietary variety in school-aged children? *J. Nutr. Educ. Behav.* **2002**, *34*, 310–315. [CrossRef]

20. Cooke, L.J.; Wardle, J.; Gibson, E.L.; Sapochnik, M.; Sheiham, A.; Lawson, M. Demographic, familial and trait predictors of fruit and vegetable consumption by pre-school children. *Public Health Nutr.* **2004**, *7*, 295–302. [CrossRef] [PubMed]

21. Taveras, E.M.; Scanlon, K.S.; Birch, L.; Rifas-Shiman, S.L.; Rich-Edwards, J.W.; Gillman, M.W. Association of breastfeeding with maternal control of infant feeding at age 1 year. *Pediatrics* **2004**, *114*, e577–e583. [CrossRef] [PubMed]

22. Trabulsi, J.C.; Mennella, J.A. Diet, sensitive periods in flavour learning, and growth. *Int. Rev. Psychiatry* **2012**, *24*, 219–230. [CrossRef] [PubMed]

23. Martin, R.M.; Patel, R.; Kramer, M.S.; Guthrie, L.; Vilchuck, K.; Bogdanovich, N.; Rifas-Shiman, S.L. Effects of promoting longer-term and exclusive breastfeeding on adiposity and insulin-like growth factor-I at age 11.5 years: A randomized trial. *JAMA* **2013**, *309*, 1005–1013. [CrossRef] [PubMed]

24. Koletzko, B.; von Kries, R.; Closa, R.; Escribano, J.; Scaglioni, S.; Giovannini, M.; Sengier, A. Lower protein in infant formula is associated with lower weight up to age 2 y: A randomized clinical trial. *Am. J. Clin. Nutr.* **2009**, *89*, 1836–1845. [CrossRef] [PubMed]

25. Mennella, J.A.; Ventura, A.K.; Beauchamp, G.K. Differential growth patterns among healthy infants fed protein hydrolysate or cow-milk formulas. *Pediatrics* **2011**, *127*, 110–118. [CrossRef] [PubMed]

26. Ventura, A.K.; Beauchamp, G.K.; Mennella, J.A. Infant regulation of intake: The effect of free glutamate content in infant formulas. *Am. J. Clin. Nutr.* **2012**, *95*, 875–881. [CrossRef] [PubMed]

27. Larnkjær, A.; Bruun, S.; Pedersen, D.; Zachariassen, G.; Barkholt, V.; Agostoni, C.; Michaelsen, K.F. Free Amino Acids in Human Milk and Associations with Maternal Anthropometry and Infant Growth. *J. Pediatr. Gastroenterol. Nutr.* **2016**, *63*, 374–378. [CrossRef] [PubMed]

28. Nicklaus, S. The role of food experiences during early childhood in food pleasure learning. *Appetite* **2016**, *104*, 3–9. [CrossRef] [PubMed]

29. Bouhlal, S.; Issanchou, S.; Chabanet, C.; Nicklaus, S. 'Just a pinch of salt'. An experimental comparison of the effect of repeated exposure and flavor-flavor learning with salt or spice on vegetable acceptance in toddlers. *Appetite* **2014**, *83*, 209–217. [CrossRef] [PubMed]

30. Ventura, A.K.; Worobey, J. Early influences on the development of food preferences. *Curr. Biol.* **2013**, *23*, R401–R408. [CrossRef] [PubMed]

31. Sullivan, S.A.; Birch, L.L. Infant dietary experience and acceptance of solid foods. *Pediatrics* **1994**, *93*, 271–277. [PubMed]

32. Maier, A.; Chabanet, C.; Schaal, B.; Issanchou, S.; Leathwood, P. Effects of repeated exposure on acceptance of initially disliked vegetables in 7-month old infants. *Food Qual. Preference* **2007**, *18*, 1023–1032. [CrossRef]

33. Carruth, B.R.; Ziegler, P.J.; Gordon, A.; Barr, S.I. Prevalence of picky eaters among infants and toddlers and their caregivers' decisions about offering a new food. *J. Am. Diet. Assoc.* **2004**, *104*, S57–S64. [CrossRef] [PubMed]

34. Maier, A.; Chabanet, C.; Schaal, B.; Leathwood, P.; Issanchou, S. Food-related sensory experience from birth through weaning: Contrasted patterns in two nearby European regions. *Appetite* **2007**, *49*, 429–444. [CrossRef] [PubMed]

35. Nicklaus, S. Complementary Feeding Strategies to Facilitate Acceptance of Fruits and Vegetables: A Narrative Review of the Literature. *Int. J. Environ. Res. Public Health* **2016**. [CrossRef] [PubMed]

36. Lange, C.; Visalli, M.; Jacob, S.; Chabanet, C.; Schlich, P.; Nicklaus, S. Maternal feeding practices during the first year and their impact on infants' acceptance of complementary food. *Food Qual. Preference* **2013**, *29*, 89–98. [CrossRef]

37. De Lauzon-Guillain, B.; Jones, L.; Oliveira, A.; Moschonis, G.; Betoko, A.; Lopes, C.; Charles, M.A. The influence of early feeding practices on fruit and vegetable intake among preschool children in 4 European birth cohorts. *Am. J. Clin. Nutr.* **2013**, *98*, 804–812. [CrossRef] [PubMed]

38. Wadhera, D.; Phillips, E.D.C.; Wilkie, L.M. Teaching children to like and eat vegetables. *Appetite* **2015**, *93*, 75–84. [CrossRef] [PubMed]

39. Schwartz, C.; Chabanet, C.; Lange, C.; Issanchou, S.; Nicklaus, S. The role of taste in food acceptance at the beginning of complementary feeding. *Physiol. Behav.* **2011**, *104*, 646–652. [CrossRef] [PubMed]

40. Daniels, L.A.; Mallan, K.M.; Nicholson, J.M.; Thorpe, K.; Nambiar, S.; Mauch, C.E.; Magarey, A. An early feeding practices intervention for obesity prevention. *Pediatrics* **2015**, *136*, e40–e49. [CrossRef] [PubMed]

41. Northstone, K.; Emmett, P.M. Are dietary patterns stable throughout early and mid-childhood? A birth cohort study. *Br. J. Nutr.* **2008**, *100*, 1069–1076. [CrossRef] [PubMed]

42. Skinner, J.D.; Carruth, B.R.; Bounds, W.; Ziegler, P.J. Children's food preferences: A longitudinal analysis. *J. Am. Diet. Assoc.* **2002**, *102*, 1638–1647. [CrossRef]

43. Singer, M.R.; Moore, L.L.; Garrahie, E.J.; Ellison, R.C. The tracking of nutrient intake in young children: The Framingham Children's Study. *Am. J. Public Health* **1995**, *85*, 1673–1677. [CrossRef] [PubMed]

44. Kral, T.V.; Rauh, E.M. Eating behaviors of children in the context of their family environment. *Physiol. Behav.* **2010**, *100*, 567–573. [CrossRef] [PubMed]

45. Savage, J.S.; Fisher, J.O.; Birch, L.L. Parental influence on eating behavior: Conception to adolescence. *J. Law Med. Ethics* **2007**, *35*, 22–34. [CrossRef] [PubMed]

46. Mennella, J.A.; Kennedy, J.M.; Beauchamp, G.K. Vegetable acceptance by infants: Effects of formula flavors. *Early Hum. Dev.* **2006**, *82*, 463–468. [CrossRef] [PubMed]

17

Temporal Changes of Protein Composition in Breast Milk of Chinese Urban Mothers and Impact of Caesarean Section Delivery

Michael Affolter [1,*], Clara L. Garcia-Rodenas [1], Gerard Vinyes-Pares [2], Rosemarie Jenni [1], Iris Roggero [1], Ornella Avanti-Nigro [1], Carlos Antonio de Castro [1], Ai Zhao [3], Yumei Zhang [3], Peiyu Wang [4], Sagar K. Thakkar [1] and Laurent Favre [1]

[1] Nestlé Research Center, Nestec Ltd., Lausanne 1000, Switzerland; clara.garcia@rdls.nestle.com (C.L.G.-R.); rosemarie.jenni@rdls.nestle.com (R.J.); iris.roggero@rdls.nestle.com (I.R.); ornella.avanti-nigro@rdls.nestle.com (O.A.-N.); carlosantonio.decastro@rdls.nestle.com (C.A.d.C.); sagar.thakkar@rdls.nestle.com (S.K.T.); laurent.favre1@rdls.nestle.com (L.F.)
[2] Nestlé Research Center Beijing, Nestec Ltd., Beijing 100095, China; gerard.vinyespares@rd.nestle.com
[3] Department of Nutrition and Food Hygiene, School of Public Health, Peking University, Beijing 100191, China; xiaochaai@163.com (A.Z.); zhangyumei@hsc.pku.edu.cn (Y.Z.)
[4] Department of Social Medicine and Health Education, School of Public Health, Peking University, Beijing 100191, China; wpeiyu@bjmu.edu.cn
* Correspondence: michael.affolter@rdls.nestle.com

Abstract: Human breast milk (BM) protein composition may be impacted by lactation stage or factors related to geographical location. The present study aimed at assessing the temporal changes of BM major proteins over lactation stages and the impact of mode of delivery on immune factors, in a large cohort of urban mothers in China. 450 BM samples, collected in three Chinese cities, covering 8 months of lactation were analyzed for α-lactalbumin, lactoferrin, serum albumin, total caseins, immunoglobulins (IgA, IgM and IgG) and transforming growth factor (TGF) β1 and β2 content by microfluidic chip- or ELISA-based quantitative methods. Concentrations and changes over lactation were aligned with previous reports. α-lactalbumin, lactoferrin, IgA, IgM and TGF-β1 contents followed similar variations characterized by highest concentrations in early lactation that rapidly decreased before remaining stable up to end of lactation. TGF-β2 content displayed same early dynamics before increasing again. Total caseins followed a different pattern, showing initial increase before decreasing back to starting values. Serum albumin and IgG levels appeared stable throughout lactation. In conclusion, BM content in major proteins of urban mothers in China was comparable with previous studies carried out in other parts of the world and C-section delivery had only very limited impact on BM immune factors.

Keywords: breast milk; proteins; immune factors; Chinese mothers; CAESAREAN-section

1. Introduction

Evolution has shaped human breast milk (BM) composition to protect the infant against disease(s) and to supply their nutritional needs [1]. BM proteins are one of the major contributors to this dual role in early infancy. BM proteins are the primary source of amino acids required for body protein building and can facilitate nutrient digestion as well as increase their bioavailability. BM proteins can also act as immunologically active molecules able to confer passive protection against pathogens, to stimulate the infant's antimicrobial defences or to modulate the infant immune maturation and responses [2–4].

More than 2500 distinct protein sequences have been identified in BM [5]. The most abundant BM proteins include lactoferrin, α-lactalbumin, serum albumin and the β- and κ-casein fractions, collectively representing about 85% of total BM proteins [6]. Multiple biological activities have been proposed for lactoferrin, and possibly the best documented effect in the infants is protection against gastrointestinal infections [7]. Similarly, a multimeric α-lactalbumin-lipid complex (HAMLET) found in BM has potent pro-apoptotic effects on bacterial [8] and tumoral cells, while sparing healthy eukaryotic cells [9]. By contrast, serum albumin and caseins likely have a predominantly nutritional role as opposed to lactoferrin, and these proteins appear to be readily digested by the infant gastrointestinal proteases. Nevertheless, some biological activities have been proposed for the peptides produced during the digestion of these proteins [10]. For example, antibacterial activity has been found upon gastric digestion of β-casein in infants [11].

Immune factors are also important BM components, representing up to 10% of total proteins. Immunoglobulins (Ig) and members of the transforming growth factor (TGF)-β family are the most studied key partners of the immunological activity found in colostrum, transitional and mature milk, ensuring transfer of passive immunity from mother to offspring [12], as well as supporting the onset of gut homeostasis in the neonate [13–17]. IgA, or more precisely secretory IgA, is the major isotype found in BM, followed then by IgM and IgG. Its dynamic of secretion over lactation period has been investigated in several studies, showing high content in colostrum, followed by a rapid diminution during transition milk to then remain stable in mature milk [18,19]. The TGF-β family constitutes the most abundant cytokines of BM and consists of three isoforms, of which TGF-β2 predominates, followed by TGF-β1 [20]. Data on the changes of the secretion over lactation period of these two cytokines are more limited than for Igs, but tend to show overall similar patterns [21].

Infants born by Caesarean section (C-section) suffer from an associated increased risk of development later in life of immune-related diseases [22–24]. These alterations are commonly attributed to altered microbiota colonization patterns in those infants due to the absence of the initial inoculation of maternal vaginal and faecal microbiota [22]. However, potential impact of delivery mode on BM-related immune parameters may also be an important contributing factor. Indeed, data available from several studies indicate a delayed onset of lactation following C-section [25,26] preventing the new-born to gain prompt access to beneficial components of BM. In contrast, little is known about the impact of C-section delivery on BM composition and in particular on the milk immune factors. Current data from studies focusing on immunoglobulin content in colostrum samples do not allow us to draw a clear conclusion on a potential impact of the mode of delivery on the presence of these antibodies in the BM [4,27]. To our knowledge, no data are currently available on the effect of C-section delivery on major BM immune factors throughout transitional and mature milk.

Hence, the main objective of the present work was to assess the specific temporal changes of major proteins' content in BM across different stages of lactation, with a secondary interest in exploring the impact of the mode of delivery on BM immune factors. This work was performed in China, a country presenting one of the highest rates of C-section birth in the world [28], and is part of the larger Maternal Infant Nutrition Growth (MING) initiative, conducted in a large cohort of urban Chinese mothers [29].

2. Materials and Methods

2.1. Subjects

This study was part of MING, a cross-sectional study designed to investigate the dietary and nutritional status of pregnant women, lactating mothers, infants and young children up to three years of age living in urban areas of China. In addition, the BM composition of Chinese lactating mothers was characterized for major proteins and immune factors. The study was conducted between October 2011 and February 2012. A multi-stage BM sampling from lactating mothers in three cities (Beijing, Suzhou and Guangzhou) was performed for BM characterization. In each city, two hospitals with maternal and child care units were selected and, at each site, mothers at lactation period 0–240 days were randomly selected based on child registration information. Subjects included in the period 0–5 days were recruited at the hospital whereas the other subjects were requested by phone to join the study; if participation was dismissed a replacement was made. Response rate was 52%. Recruitment and BM sampling, as well as baseline data collection, were done on separate days.

A stratified BM sampling of 540 lactating mothers in six lactation periods of 0–4, 5–11 and 12–30 days, and 1–2, 2–4 and 4–8 months were obtained in MING study. Nevertheless, only 450 BM samples were analysed in the present study, as the 0–4 days stage could not be included due to the limited volume of BM collected during this period.

2.2. Inclusion and Exclusion Criteria

Eligibility criteria included women between 18 and 45 years of age with singleton pregnancy, apparently healthy, full-term infant and exclusively breastfeeding at least until 4 months post-partum. Exclusion criteria included gestational diabetes, hypertension, cardiac diseases, acute communicable diseases and postpartum depression. Lactating women who had nipple or lacteal gland diseases, who had been receiving hormonal therapy during the three months preceding recruitment, or who had insufficient skills to understand study questionnaires were also excluded.

2.3. Ethical and Legal Considerations

The study was conducted according to the guidelines in the Declaration of Helsinki. All of the procedures involving human subjects were approved by the Medical Ethics Research Board of Peking University (No. IRB00001052-11042, 15-11-2011). Written informed consent was obtained from all subjects participating in the study. The study was also registered in ClinicalTrials.gov with identifier NCT01971671.

2.4. Data Collection

All mothers completed a general questionnaire including socio-economic and lifestyle aspects. Self-reported weight during pre-pregnancy and at delivery, number of gestational weeks at delivery, and delivery method were also recorded. Additionally, a physical examination evaluated basic anthropometric parameters (height, weight, mid-arm circumference) blood pressure and haemoglobin.

Data collection was done through face-to-face interviews, on the day of BM sample collection. In addition, date of birth and gender information of the infant was collected after the data collection since the data was not included in the initial questionnaires. Subjects were contacted by phone and were asked to clarify these two aspects retrospectively.

2.5. Sample Characteristics

BM sampling was standardized for all subjects and an electric pump (Horigen HNR/X-2108ZB, Xinhe Electrical Apparatuses Co., Ltd., Beijing, China) was used to sample the BM. Samples were collected at the second feeding in the morning (9–11 a.m.) to avoid circadian influence on the outcomes. Single full breast was emptied and an aliquot of 40 mL BM for each time point was secured for characterization purposes. The rest of the BM was returned to the mother for feeding to the infant. Each sample was distributed in 5 mL freezing tubes, labelled with subject number, stored at $-80\,°C$ and then shipped to the Nestlé Research Centre (Lausanne, Switzerland) for analyses within 6 months of collection.

2.6. Milk Sample Processing before Analyses

Frozen BM samples were skimmed by thawing to 4 °C, high speed centrifugation ($2500\times g$ for 10 min at 4 °C) and collection of the liquid fraction below the lipid phase. Each skimmed BM sample was then aliquoted in separate microtubes (Eppendorf AG, Hamburg, Germany) and frozen again until use. This aliquoting approach was put in place to avoid thawing-freezing cycles between the different analytical runs for the BM immune factors of interest as one aliquot was then dedicated to each analysis.

2.7. Measurement of Major Breast Milk Proteins

The following major BM proteins were measured in all 450 BM samples: α-lactalbumin, serum albumin, lactoferrin and all caseins. Due to the large number of samples, a classical approach using, for example, gel electrophoresis or HPLC separation did not provide sufficient throughput and speed. Therefore, an innovative microfluidic chip based quantitative method was specifically implemented and validated for BM protein analysis. The method was established on a LabChip GX-II instrument (Perkin Elmer, Waltham, MA, USA) allowing high-throughput analysis in a 96-well format. The principle of this technique is based on traditional SDS-PAGE protein separation but the whole procedure (separation, staining and detection) is integrated and fully automated in a microfluidic system. Results are provided in digital format (no gel staining or scanning, etc.). The general approach of this method was described previously [30] for bovine milk protein analysis and needed some slight adaptations for the BM sample analysis as described below.

2.7.1. Sample Preparation

BM sample preparation was performed according to the LabChip (Perkin Elmer, Waltham, MA, USA) protocol. A simple 5-fold dilution of BM with water (Merck Lichrosolv quality) was found to be sufficient prior to protein denaturation and derivatization steps. In contrast to the immune factor analysis by ELISA, BM defatting was not required for the LabChip analysis thus avoiding potential protein losses. All sample preparation and processing steps were performed in 96-well format using electronic multichannel pipettes (Eppendorf Xplorer, Eppendorf AG, Hamburg, Germany). The HT Protein Express protein chip and reagent kit (Perkin Elmer, Waltham, MA, USA) was used for all analyses and highest purity reagents were required for all buffer preparations. Pure human milk proteins (α-lactalbumin, serum albumin, lactoferrin from Sigma, St. Louis, MO, USA) and bovine milk proteins (α-, β- and κ-casein from Sigma, as human proteins not available) were used as standards to generate individual calibration curves for each protein. The purity of each standard protein, according to the certificate of analysis, was used to calculate the true concentration of the protein standard in solution. Reported limit of detection of the LabChip system is 5 ng/μL according to the manufacturer. Calibration concentrations of the individual protein standards ranged from 25 to 750 ng/μL for serum albumin, from 50 to 1500 ng/μL for α-lactalbumin and lactoferrin, and from 100 to 3000 ng/μL for caseins. Note that as the individual casein proteins could not be fully resolved on the LabChip system, all casein peaks were integrated as one peak and thus one value for total casein concentration in BM was obtained (sum of α-, β- and κ-casein). In order to monitor system performance, a quality control sample (pooled BM from Lee Biosolutions Inc., Maryland Heights, MO, USA) was analyzed every 20th sample. All samples were analyzed in triplicates using a volume of 25 μL of BM.

2.7.2. Method Validation

The method was validated for the determination of the four different proteins in human milk. For each protein (α-, β- and κ-caseins measured as total casein) the linear response of the LabChip detector was checked over the concentration range expected to be present in human milk samples. Each protein was analyzed at 8 different levels in triplicate. A quadratic regression was performed and linearity was assessed from the r^2 and the plot of residuals.

To determine the trueness and precision of the method a milk sample was selected and spiked with the protein standards at 3 levels (the levels were adapted for each protein to cover the concentration range expected in milk). The non-spiked sample and the spiked samples were analyzed in duplicate on 6 different days. The spike experiments were used to determine recoveries, data from the duplicate analyses were used to determine repeatability (r) and data from the between day analyses were used to determine intermediate reproducibility (iR).

2.8. Measurement of Selected Breast Milk Immune Factors

Concentrations of IgA, IgG, IgM, TGF-β1 and TGF-β2 in BM samples were measured using selected commercial ELISA quantification kits that were specifically validated for their usage in milk matrix background. In more detail, IgA and IgG contents of BM were measured with Human IgA and IgG ELISA Kits from Bethyl Laboratories Inc., USA (Montgomery, TX, USA) (catalogue numbers E80-102 and E80-104, respectively), following manufacturer instructions and with milk samples tested at 1:20,000 and 1:1000 dilutions, respectively. Kit performance with such dilution factors were for IgA and IgG, respectively: average intra-plate repeatability 5% and 4.5%; average inter-plate repeatability 10.1% and 7.2%; average recovery 87% and 98%. IgM content was measured with the Human IgM Ready-SET-Go from Affimetrix eBioscience, USA (Santa Clara, CA, USA) (catalogue number 88-50620) following manufacturer instructions and with milk samples tested at 1:300 dilution. Kit performance with this dilution factor was: average intra-plate repeatability 3.8%; average inter-plate repeatability 4%; average recovery 90%. Finally, TGF-β1 and TGF-β2 contents were measured with Quantikine ELISA Human TGF-β1 and TGF-β2 Immunoassay Kits from R&D Systems, USA (Minneapolis, MN, USA) (catalogue numbers DB100B and DB250, respectively), following manufacturer instructions and with milk samples tested respectively at 1:5 and 1:4 dilutions on the top of the already 1:1.4 dilution of the original samples linked to the acidification and pH neutralization steps mandatory to activate latent TFG-βs from BM samples to their measured immune-reactive forms. Kit performance with such dilution factors were for TGF-β1 and TGF-β2 respectively: average intra-plate repeatability 4% and 9.3%; average inter-plate repeatability 6.1% and 10.8%; average recovery 84% and 92%.

2.9. Data Analysis

A multiple linear regression was applied to analyze the effect of lactation stage on the levels of the individual proteins. This model was adjusted for the effects of maternal age and BMI, infant gender, mode of delivery and geographical location.

A multiple regression model to explain the protein and immune parameter concentration was applied. The distribution of the residuals were checked via Box-Cox transformation method and a logarithmic transformation seemed to be adequate for all immune parameters. The following model was used:

$$\log(\text{concentration}) = \text{timeframe} + \text{sex} + \text{delivery} + \text{city} + \text{mother's age} + \text{mother's BMI} + \varepsilon$$

The above model was the general model that was used to test for the effect of stage of lactation (timeframe) on immune parameter concentration taking in to consideration other variables such as gender, mode of delivery (natural vs. C-section) and geographic location (city). The term ε refers to a residual error (observed value–predicted value). With this model, contrast estimates were calculated comparing the successive timeframes (5–11 days vs. 12–30 days, 12–30 days vs. 1–2 months, etc.) to observe at which timeframes there were significant changes in nutrient concentration.

The same stage of lactation model was used in the subgroup of mothers delivering by C-section and also for natural delivery. In this case the model become simpler:

$$\log(\text{concentration}) = \text{timeframe} + \text{sex} + \text{city} + \text{mother's age} + \text{mother's BMI} + \varepsilon$$

A similar model was used to assess the impact of mode of delivery with the difference of taking into account the interaction effect of time with the variable in question. The following model was used so that a comparison of the delivery modes can be made for each timeframe:

$$\log(\text{concentration}) = \text{timeframe} \times \text{delivery} + \text{sex} + \text{city} + \text{mother's age} + \text{mother's BMI} + \varepsilon$$

The same methods were used for the proteins, but a normality assumption is made and therefore no logarithmic transformation was performed on the 4 protein nutrients.

3. Results

3.1. Subject Characteristics

In this cross-sectional study, nine different proteins were quantified in 450 BM samples collected at different stages from early to late lactation (8 months) in apparently healthy Chinese women from three different cities (i.e., Beijing, Guangzhou, and Suzhou). Figure 1 displays the recruitment flowchart from eligibility to sample analysis.

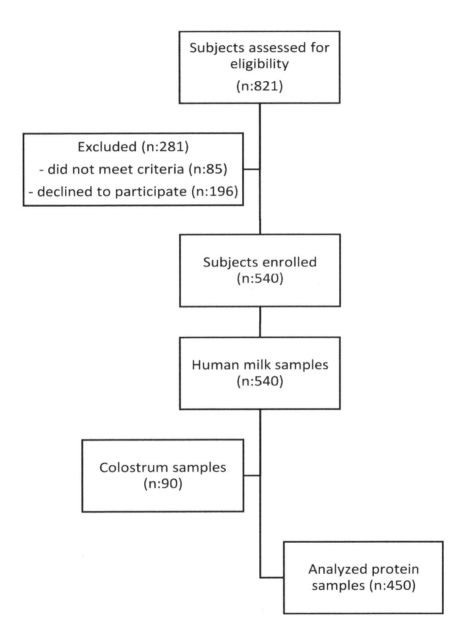

Figure 1. Study flow chart of subject recruitment.

Subject demographics and anthropometry are described in Table 1. Maternal age, weight, body mass index (BMI) and mode of delivery were significantly different among the lactation stage cohorts. No other significant differences were observed in maternal and infant characteristics analysed. Note that the significant differences were taken into consideration for the analyses of protein contents at the different lactation stages as the statistical model was adjusted for these potential confounding factors.

Table 1. Maternal and infant characteristics (adapted from [31]).

Study Population	5–11 Days (*n* = 90)	12–30 Days (*n* = 90)	1–2 Months (*n* = 90)	2–4 Months (*n* = 90)	4–8 Months (*n* = 90)
Mother					
Age (years), Mean (SD)	27 (4)	27 (3)	28 (4)	27 (4)	26 (4)
Height (cm), Mean (SD)	160 (4)	160 (5)	161 (5)	161 (5)	159 (5)
Weight (kg), Mean (SD)	60.7 (8.7)	60.8 (7.9)	61.9 (8.9)	58.4 (8.3)	56.2 (8.1)
BMI (kg/m^2), Mean (SD)	23.7 (3.3)	23.7 (2.8)	23.9 (3.1)	22.5 (2.9)	22.2 (3.1)
Gestational weight gain (kg), Mean (SD)	16.7 (7.4)	16.2 (6.0)	15.9 (5.7)	15.9 (5.9)	14.9 (7.6)
Postpartum weight loss (kg), Mean (SD)	9.1 (6.1)	8.6 (5.3)	9.8 (4.0)	10.0 (6.2)	10.6 (5.9)
Caesarean delivery, *N* (%)	39 (42)	43 (48)	53 (59)	35 (39)	35 (38)
Infant					
Males, *N* (%)	51 (57)	48 (53)	48 (53)	54 (60)	43 (48)
Gestational age at birth (weeks), Mean (SD)	39.3 (1.2)	39.2 (1.3)	39.2 (1.6)	39.4 (1.3)	39.5 (1.5)

3.2. Major Breast Milk Proteins

3.2.1. Analytical Method Performance

Each protein was quantified using an individual calibration curve (quadratic fitting, all $R^2 > 0.99$, LabChip GX-II software, v4.1, 2015), based on a dilution series of pure standard proteins. Figure 2A depicts a typical electropherogram trace of a BM sample measured with the LabChip GX II system. A calibration curve for α-lactalbumin is shown in Figure 2B which demonstrates the small variation of replicate measurements. Based on a simple 5-fold dilution of the BM samples, limit of detection was 50 ng/µL for α-lactalbumin and serum albumin, 100 ng/µL for caseins and 130 ng/µL for lactoferrin, respectively.

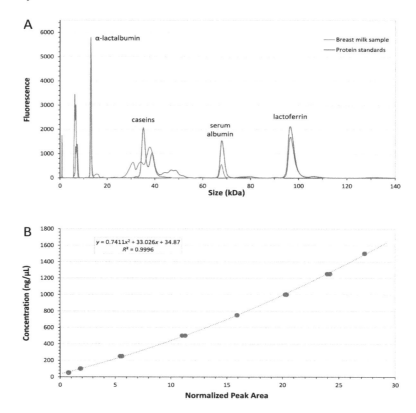

Figure 2. (**A**) Human breast milk protein separation on the LabChip GX II system. The electropherogram overlay depicts individual standard milk proteins (red) and a typical human breast milk sample trace (blue); (**B**) Calibration curve for α-lactalbumin (in duplicates, 50–1500 ng/µL, R^2 0.9996).

The method was fully validated. Recoveries of proteins, determined using spiking experiments (three spiking levels, analyzed in duplicate on six different days), were between 91.8% and 116.5%.

Relative repeatability (r%) for all proteins was <9.2% and relative intermediate reproducibility (iR%) was <26%. Measurement uncertainty was estimated using the simplified approach based on existing validation data proposed by Barwick [32]. The standard uncertainty (u) was determined at 11 ng/μL with relative standard uncertainty (u%) of 0.5%. Expanded uncertainty (U) was 19 ng/μL with relative expanded uncertainty (U%) of 1%.

3.2.2. Analysis of Major Breast Milk Proteins

The concentration of α-lactalbumin decreased from 3.27 to 2.28 g/L over the investigated lactation period (Table 2). With the exception of the two first stages, all subsequent stages showed a significant decrease ($p < 0.003$) in α-lactalbumin content, over time until eight months.

Table 2. Protein content of human breast milk from the different lactation stages (see also Figure S1).

Proteins	5–11 Days ($n = 90$)	12–30 Days ($n = 90$)	1–2 Months ($n = 90$)	2–4 Months ($n = 90$)	4–8 Months ($n = 90$)
Major breast milk proteins					
α-lactalbumin (g/L), Median (IQR)	3.27 (0.60)	3.16 (0.55)	2.84 [a] (0.55)	2.53 [a] (0.47)	2.28 [a] (0.63)
Lactoferrin (g/L), Median (IQR)	3.30 (2.11)	1.86 [a] (0.89)	1.24 [a] (0.53)	1.15 (0.46)	1.17 (0.47)
Serum albumin (g/L), Median (IQR)	0.48 (0.14)	0.48 (0.14)	0.42 (0.09)	0.44 (0.10)	0.42 (0.08)
Total caseins (g/L), Median (IQR)	5.84 (3.17)	6.57 [a] (2.15)	6.24 (2.25)	5.79 [a] (1.69)	5.60 (1.73)
Immune factors					
IgA (mg/L), Median (IQR)	1148 (1022)	615 [a] (494)	553 [a] (232)	557 (312)	564 (337)
IgM (mg/L), Median (IQR)	117 (168)	47 [a] (47)	35 [a] (31)	35 (29)	25 [a] (25)
IgG (mg/L), Median (IQR)	22 (13)	23 (12)	20 (14)	24 (15)	23 (14)
TGF-β1 (ng/L), Median (IQR)	1258 (1305)	685 [a] (482)	600 (356)	598 (379)	659 (410)
TGF-β2 (ng/L), Median (IQR)	5286 (10,444)	2322 [a] (3100)	1877 [a] (1890)	1920 [a] (2112)	2311 [b] (2868)

[a] $p < 0.05$ vs. previous stage; [b] $p < 0.05$ vs. previous 1–2 months stage.

The concentration of lactoferrin also decreased over full lactation period, from 3.30 to 1.17 g/L (Table 2). This decrease was constant during lactation until 1–2 months, with significant differences ($p < 0.000$) in lactoferrin content between the first three investigated stages, and then stabilizing until the eighth months.

The concentration of serum albumin during the lactation period ranged from 0.48 to 0.42 g/L (Table 2) and did not show any significant differences between stages.

The concentration of caseins during the lactation period followed a different pattern than the other proteins, showing a significant transient increase from 5.84 g/L at stage 1 to 6.57 g/L in Stage 2 and 6.24 g/L in Stage 3 before returning to starting values in later stages (Table 2).

3.3. Breast Milk Immune Factors

IgA and IgM contents reflected the temporal change pattern of most of the major BM proteins with significantly higher contents in early milk before rapidly decreasing over time, reaching a basal plateau after 1 month of infant's age (Table 2). IgG concentration did not follow the same pattern as it appeared stable throughout lactation (Table 2).

TGF-β1 and TGF-β2 BM contents proved to be also significantly higher in the very early milk (5–11 days period, Table 2). Then, while TGF-β1 concentration remained stable up to the end of the covered lactation period, TGF-β2 content continued to significantly decrease in the 1–2 months stage before significantly increasing again later back to 12–30 days levels.

Regarding impact of mode of delivery on immune factor contents in BM, even if occasional statistical significant differences or trends could be observed (see Figures 3 and 4), C-section delivery did not appear to consistently impact BM concentrations in immune factor.

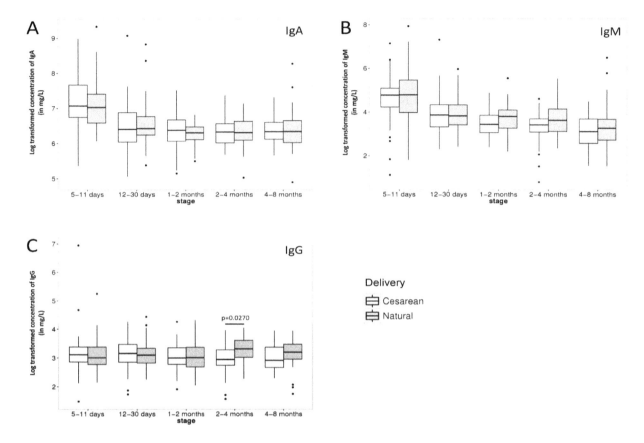

Figure 3. Comparison of (**A**) IgA; (**B**) IgM and (**C**) IgG immunoglobulin contents in breast milk from mothers delivering their infant either vaginally (Natural) or by Caesarean section for each lactation period of this study. Box plot represent medians with 25th and 75th percentile, min-max range and outliers. Statistical significance was set at $p < 0.05$ and significant p-values are indicated in the graphs.

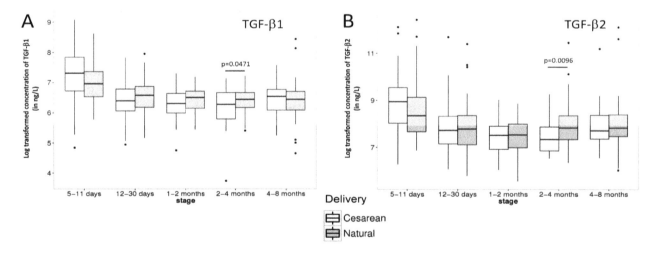

Figure 4. Comparison of (**A**) TGF-β1 and (**B**) TGF-β2 contents in breast milk from mothers delivering their infant either vaginally (Natural) or by Caesarean section for each lactation period of this study. Box plot represent medians with 25th and 75th percentile, min-max range and outliers. Statistical significance was set at $p < 0.05$ and significant p-values are indicated in the graphs.

4. Discussion

4.1. Major Breast Milk Proteins

Various separation techniques and approaches have been exploited to identify and quantify milk proteins. Traditionally, chromatographic or electrophoretic methods have been used to profile major BM proteins [33–35] whereas immuno-based approaches, i.e., ELISA or antibody arrays, were the method of choice for quantitative analysis of individual proteins [36–38]. More recently, targeted LC-MS techniques have been developed to separate and quantify specific milk proteins [39]. The low throughput nature of these methodologies is often the limiting factor for application to larger numbers of samples. In order to address the challenge to precisely quantify major BM proteins in a large number of individual samples, as in the case of the present study, an innovative microfluidic chip-based method was specifically implemented, validated and applied in a high-throughput approach.

Despite a small limitation in the quantification of individual caseins, we believe that the minimal sample preparation and the 96-well sample format ideally combines speed and robustness of the analysis process and thus paves the way for a new technological standard for the measurement of α-lactalbumin, lactoferrin, serum albumin and total caseins in future studies addressing BM protein composition.

α-lactalbumin was the most abundant whey protein in the Chinese mother's BM samples (Table 2), in agreement with previous data in the literature [19]. Even though its content decreased significantly over the first two months, it remained high in all lactation stages. The high levels of this protein in BM are likely key for the nutrition of the breast-fed infant. Contrary to other BM proteins, α-lactalbumin appears to be fully hydrolysed and absorbed in the infant intestine, thus to be a good source of nitrogen and indispensable amino acids [40]. This protein contributes as well to the balanced amino acid composition of BM and, in particular, to its high levels of tryptophan, which ultimately allows BM to cover the infant's amino acid requirements with limited amounts of protein [41]. High levels of tryptophan in this protein would be also associated with its protective effects against epileptic seizures in animal models [42]. Besides its nutritional role, the α-lactalbumin HAMLET complex found in BM has anti-tumoral [9] and bactericidal effects [8]. Furthermore, α-lactalbumin bears bioactive peptide sequences (e.g., mineral chelator or anti-microbial peptides) that may be released and transiently exert their activity (e.g., increased mineral absorption or prevention of infection) in the infant intestine. In line with this, Kelleher et al. [43] observed increased mineral absorption and Bruck et al. [44] inhibition of *E. coli*-induced diarrhoea in infant monkeys fed a formula supplemented with bovine α-lactalbumin.

The second most abundant whey protein in our samples was lactoferrin (Table 2) for which the observed concentration values and gradual decrease along lactation were similar to those previously reported [19,45]. The bioavailability of lactoferrin, thus its nutritional relevance as a source of amino acids and nitrogen to the infant, is not known. However, it has been found intact in infant faeces and resistant to digestion in an in vitro digestion model, which suggest that the nutritional role of lactoferrin may need reconsideration and further studies [40]. In contrast, multiple biological activities have been proposed for this protein [40] including infant protection against gastrointestinal infection and sepsis [7].

It is noteworthy that temporal changes trends of α-lactalbumin and lactoferrin along lactation are fully aligned with that of the total proteins measured in the same BM samples as previously reported [29].

Due to the complexity of the casein composition in BM and limitations in mass resolution of the new analytical method used in this study, caseins were not quantified individually but as total caseins (combining α-, β- and κ-casein concentrations, Table 2). This novel analytical approach, however, was potentially susceptible to introducing some bias in comparison to the more classical acid-precipitation based methodology. Interestingly, our results demonstrated that this was not the case as the increase of casein concentration at the beginning of lactation followed by a slight decrease at the later period was closely aligned with a previous report [46]. These results support the theory that casein and whey protein synthesis and/or secretion is regulated by different mechanisms in the mammary gland [47].

In contrast to the other major whey proteins, serum albumin concentration stayed mostly constant across the lactation stages. Comparison with literature data showed similar concentrations in our samples [19]. It is noteworthy that, contrary to other BM proteins that are synthesized by the mammary gland, serum albumin is transferred from the maternal blood [2]. To our knowledge, no specific biological activities have been attributed to this protein. It certainly contributes to the nutrition of the infant as it appears to be highly digestible [2].

4.2. Breast Milk Immune Factors

BM contents of immune factors at the different lactation stages (Table 2) were also in agreement with the previously published ranges [18,48–51], as well as with our own previous findings (unpublished data), indicating that BM from Chinese mothers does not differ from worldwide references in these bioactive components.

IgA and IgM BM contents were significantly high in early milk before rapidly decreasing over time, reaching a basal plateau after 1 month of infant's age, while IgG content was stable throughout lactation. These differences in production pattern between IgG and both other immunoglobulins resides in the fact that IgA and IgM are actively secreted in BM through the poly-immunoglobulin receptor expressed by mammary gland epithelial cells [12] while IgG is more passively appearing in BM through transudation from the systemic circulation, as already mentioned above for serum albumin.

While TGF-β1 contents of BM followed the same temporal changes that the majority of investigated proteins as previously described [21], variation of TGF-β2 concentration appeared to be slightly different, also with a strong decrease until the 1–2 months lactation stage but followed by an increase, reaching at 8 months the level observed in the second half of the first month of lactation (Table 2). Such type of fluctuating pattern of TGF-β2 BM content has already been observed in a previous study [49], however, to a smaller extent and at different time points. Whether this evolution of TGF-β2 has a physiological role for the infants remains to be determined. Indeed, studies mainly focusing on TFG-β1 and 2 demonstrated that milk-borne TGF-βs regulate inflammation [13], stimulation of IgA isotype switching in B cells [52], maintenance of intestinal epithelium barrier function [14], induction of oral tolerance [15], and consequently help to prevent allergic diseases [53,54].

It is noteworthy that C-section delivery did not appear to consistently impact BM content in the major immune factors measured in the present study. The high number of mothers participating in our study together with the high rate of C-section delivery thus allows increasing knowledge on the previously described limited impact of the mode of delivery on major immune BM proteins [4,27], while extending at the same time the former observations on colostrum to transitional and mature milk. Moreover, our data also tend to indicate that the increased risk of immune-related diseases associated with C-section delivery may not be associated with any alterations of major BM immune factors' composition. However, we cannot rule out a potential effect of the mode of delivery on the immune factor composition of the colostrum as our earliest milk samples were collected 5–11 days after delivery. In addition, the impact of delayed onset of lactation following C-section [25,26] on later infant health was not assessed in the present study and would deserve deeper investigation in order to further consolidate the above hypothesis.

The cross-sectional nature of our study limits the conclusions related to the stage-driven changes, which would have been best assessed by a longitudinal design. However, our statistical model adjusted for the maternal and infant baseline factors known or suspected to impact on milk nutrient composition [55]. Our results are also reinforced by the fact that they were remarkably consistent with those previously published.

5. Conclusions

This multi-centric cross-sectional study covering 8 months of lactation for 450 Chinese mothers demonstrated that their BM content in major proteins was comparable with previous studies carried out in other parts of the world, highlighting that key protein components of BM are conserved across geographic localization. Moreover, this study is to our knowledge the first one to address the effect of C-section delivery on major BM immune factors throughout transitional and mature milk, actually showing that C-section delivery had very limited impact on the maternal-to-offspring transmission of active immune competence.

Acknowledgments: The authors would like to thank the funding sources of this work and Nestec Ltd. for covering the costs for publishing open access. Special acknowledgment to all participants who volunteered for this study, Lawrence Li for project support and guidance, Celia Ning for project management, Qiaoji Li for clinical project management, Emilie Ba for data management and Yindong Zheng for statistical guidance. Special acknowledgment to Jiaji Wang at Guangzhou Medical University and Liqiang Qin at Soochow University School of Public Health and their teams as well as the project staff at Peking University School of Public Health, for their tasks in recruitment and data collection. A special thank goes to Alexandre Panchaud who initiated the LabChip method development.

Author Contributions: M.A., L.F. and C.G. interpreted the results, drafted, reviewed and revised the initial manuscript. R.J. performed the LabChip experiments and data analysis. I.R. and O.A.-N. measured the breast milk immune factors and processed the results. C.A.d.C. performed the statistical analysis of all data, drafted, reviewed and revised the manuscript. S.T. contributed to the study design, breast milk sampling protocol and interpretation of the results. G.V.-P. contributed to the study design, drafted and reviewed the manuscript. Y.Z. and P.W. were the PI of MING study. Y.Z. and A.Z. were responsible of data collection and quality control. All authors approved the final manuscript as submitted.

References

1. Vorbach, C.; Capecchi, M.R.; Penninger, J.M. Evolution of the mammary gland from the innate immune system? *Bioessays* **2006**, *28*, 606–616. [CrossRef] [PubMed]
2. Lonnerdal, B. Nutritional and physiologic significance of human milk proteins. *Am. J. Clin. Nutr.* **2003**, *77*, 1537S–1543S. [PubMed]
3. Lonnerdal, B. Bioactive proteins in breast milk. *J. Paediatr. Child. Health* **2013**, *49* (Suppl. 1), 1–7. [CrossRef] [PubMed]
4. Striker, G.A.; Casanova, L.D.; Nagao, A.T. Influence of type of delivery on A, G and M immunoglobulin concentration in maternal colostrum. *J. Pediatr.* **2004**, *80*, 123–128. [CrossRef]
5. Beck, K.L.; Weber, D.; Phinney, B.S.; Smilowitz, J.T.; Hinde, K.; Lonnerdal, B.; Korf, I.; Lemay, D.G. Comparative proteomics of human and macaque milk reveals species-specific nutrition during postnatal development. *J. Proteome Res.* **2015**, *14*, 2143–2157. [CrossRef] [PubMed]
6. Prentice, A. Constituents of human milk. *Food Nutr. Bull.* **1996**, *17*, 305–312.
7. Ochoa, T.J.; Pezo, A.; Cruz, K.; Chea-Woo, E.; Cleary, T.G. Clinical studies of lactoferrin in children. *Biochem. Cell Biol.* **2012**, *90*, 457–467. [CrossRef] [PubMed]
8. Hakansson, A.P.; Roche-Hakansson, H.; Mossberg, A.K.; Svanborg, C. Apoptosis-like death in bacteria induced by hamlet, a human milk lipid-protein complex. *PLoS ONE* **2011**, *6*, e17717. [CrossRef] [PubMed]
9. Hakansson, A.; Zhivotovsky, B.; Orrenius, S.; Sabharwal, H.; Svanborg, C. Apoptosis induced by a human milk protein. *Proc. Natl. Acad. Sci. USA* **1995**, *92*, 8064–8068. [CrossRef] [PubMed]

10. Wada, Y.; Lonnerdal, B. Bioactive peptides derived from human milk proteins—Mechanisms of action. *J. Nutr. Biochem.* **2014**, *25*, 503–514. [CrossRef] [PubMed]

11. Dallas, D.C.; Guerrero, A.; Khaldi, N.; Borghese, R.; Bhandari, A.; Underwood, M.A.; Lebrilla, C.B.; German, J.B.; Barile, D. A peptidomic analysis of human milk digestion in the infant stomach reveals protein-specific degradation patterns. *J. Nutr.* **2014**, *144*, 815–820. [CrossRef] [PubMed]

12. Brandtzaeg, P. The mucosal immune system and its integration with the mammary glands. *J. Pediatr.* **2010**, *156*, S8–S15. [CrossRef] [PubMed]

13. Kulkarni, A.B.; Karlsson, S. Transforming growth factor-beta 1 knockout mice. A mutation in one cytokine gene causes a dramatic inflammatory disease. *Am. J. Pathol.* **1993**, *143*, 3–9. [PubMed]

14. Planchon, S.M.; Martins, C.A.; Guerrant, R.L.; Roche, J.K. Regulation of intestinal epithelial barrier function by tgf-beta 1. Evidence for its role in abrogating the effect of a T cell cytokine. *J. Immunol.* **1994**, *153*, 5730–5739. [PubMed]

15. Gray, J.D.; Hirokawa, M.; Horwitz, D.A. The role of transforming growth factor beta in the generation of suppression: An interaction between CD8$^+$ T and NK cells. *J. Exp. Med.* **1994**, *180*, 1937–1942. [CrossRef] [PubMed]

16. Mathias, A.; Pais, B.; Favre, L.; Benyacoub, J.; Corthesy, B. Role of secretory IgA in the mucosal sensing of commensal bacteria. *Gut Microbes* **2014**, *5*, 688–695. [CrossRef] [PubMed]

17. Rogier, E.W.; Frantz, A.L.; Bruno, M.E.; Wedlund, L.; Cohen, D.A.; Stromberg, A.J.; Kaetzel, C.S. Secretory antibodies in breast milk promote long-term intestinal homeostasis by regulating the gut microbiota and host gene expression. *Proc. Natl. Acad. Sci. USA* **2014**, *111*, 3074–3079. [CrossRef] [PubMed]

18. Lonnerdal, B.; Forsum, E.; Hambraeus, L. A longitudinal study of the protein, nitrogen, and lactose contents of human milk from swedish well-nourished mothers. *Am. J. Clin. Nutr.* **1976**, *29*, 1127–1133. [PubMed]

19. Jensen, R.G. *Handbook of Milk Composition*; Academic Press: San Diego, CA, USA, 1995.

20. Saito, S.; Yoshida, M.; Ichijo, M.; Ishizaka, S.; Tsujii, T. Transforming growth factor-beta (TGF-β) in human milk. *Clin. Exp. Immunol.* **1993**, *94*, 220–224. [CrossRef] [PubMed]

21. Agarwal, S.; Karmaus, W.; Davis, S.; Gangur, V. Immune markers in breast milk and fetal and maternal body fluids: A systematic review of perinatal concentrations. *J. Hum. Lact.* **2011**, *27*, 171–186. [CrossRef] [PubMed]

22. Neu, J.; Rushing, J. Cesarean versus vaginal delivery: Long-term infant outcomes and the hygiene hypothesis. *Clin. Perinatol.* **2011**, *38*, 321–331. [CrossRef] [PubMed]

23. Penders, J.; Gerhold, K.; Thijs, C.; Zimmermann, K.; Wahn, U.; Lau, S.; Hamelmann, E. New insights into the hygiene hypothesis in allergic diseases: Mediation of sibling and birth mode effects by the gut microbiota. *Gut Microbes* **2014**, *5*, 239–244. [CrossRef] [PubMed]

24. Sevelsted, A.; Stokholm, J.; Bonnelykke, K.; Bisgaard, H. Cesarean section and chronic immune disorders. *Pediatrics* **2015**, *135*, e92–e98. [CrossRef] [PubMed]

25. Dewey, K.G.; Nommsen-Rivers, L.A.; Heinig, M.J.; Cohen, R.J. Risk factors for suboptimal infant breastfeeding behavior, delayed onset of lactation, and excess neonatal weight loss. *Pediatrics* **2003**, *112*, 607–619. [CrossRef] [PubMed]

26. Evans, K.C.; Evans, R.G.; Royal, R.; Esterman, A.J.; James, S.L. Effect of caesarean section on breast milk transfer to the normal term newborn over the first week of life. *Arch. Dis. Child Fetal Neonatal Ed.* **2003**, *88*, F380–F382. [CrossRef] [PubMed]

27. Kulski, J.K.; Smith, M.; Hartmann, P.E. Normal and caesarian section delivery and the initiation of lactation in women. *Aust. J. Exp. Biol. Med. Sci.* **1981**, *59*, 405–412. [CrossRef] [PubMed]

28. Hellerstein, S.; Feldman, S.; Duan, T. China's 50% caesarean delivery rate: Is it too high? *BJOG* **2015**, *122*, 160–164. [CrossRef] [PubMed]

29. Yang, T.; Zhang, Y.; Ning, Y.; You, L.; Ma, D.; Zheng, Y.; Yang, X.; Li, W.; Wang, J.; Wang, P. Breast milk macronutrient composition and the associated factors in urban chinese mothers. *Chin. Med. J.* **2014**, *127*, 1721–1725. [PubMed]

30. Anema, S.G. The use of "lab-on-a-chip" microfluidic sds electrophoresis technology for the separation and quantification of milk proteins. *Int. Dairy J.* **2009**, *19*, 198–204. [CrossRef]

31. Austin, S.; De Castro, C.; Bénet, T.; Hou, Y.; Sun, H.; Thakkar, S.; Vinyes-Pares, G.; Zhang, Y.; Wang, P. Temporal change of the content of 10 oligosaccharides in the milk of chinese urban mothers. *Nutrients* **2016**, *8*, 346. [CrossRef] [PubMed]

32. Barwick, V.J.; Ellison, S.L.; Lucking, C.L.; Burn, M.J. Experimental studies of uncertainties associated with chromatographic techniques. *J. Chromatogr. A* **2001**, *918*, 267–276. [CrossRef]
33. Velona, T.; Abbiati, L.; Beretta, B.; Gaiaschi, A.; Flauto, U.; Tagliabue, P.; Galli, C.L.; Restani, P. Protein profiles in breast milk from mothers delivering term and preterm babies. *Pediatr. Res.* **1999**, *45*, 658–663. [CrossRef] [PubMed]
34. Kunz, C.; Lonnerdal, B. Human-milk proteins: Analysis of casein and casein subunits by anion-exchange chromatography, gel electrophoresis, and specific staining methods. *Am. J. Clin. Nutr.* **1990**, *51*, 37–46. [PubMed]
35. Ferreira, I.M.P.L. Chromatographic separation and quantification of major human milk proteins. *J. Liq. Chromatogr. Relat. Technol.* **2007**, *30*, 499–507. [CrossRef]
36. Broadhurst, M.; Beddis, K.; Black, J.; Henderson, H.; Nair, A.; Wheeler, T. Effect of gestation length on the levels of five innate defence proteins in human milk. *Early Hum. Dev.* **2015**, *91*, 7–11. [CrossRef] [PubMed]
37. Mehta, R.; Petrova, A. Biologically active breast milk proteins in association with very preterm delivery and stage of lactation. *J. Perinatol.* **2011**, *31*, 58–62. [CrossRef] [PubMed]
38. Collado, M.C.; Santaella, M.; Mira-Pascual, L.; Martinez-Arias, E.; Khodayar-Pardo, P.; Ros, G.; Martinez-Costa, C. Longitudinal study of cytokine expression, lipid profile and neuronal growth factors in human breast milk from term and preterm deliveries. *Nutrients* **2015**, *7*, 8577–8591. [CrossRef] [PubMed]
39. Altendorfer, I.; König, S.; Braukmann, A.; Saenger, T.; Bleck, E.; Vordenbäumen, S.; Kubiak, A.; Schneider, M.; Jose, J. Quantification of αs1-casein in breast milk using a targeted mass spectrometry-based approach. *J. Pharm. Biomed. Anal.* **2015**, *103*, 52–58. [CrossRef] [PubMed]
40. Lonnerdal, B. Infant formula and infant nutrition: Bioactive proteins of human milk and implications for composition of infant formulas. *Am. J. Clin. Nutr.* **2014**, *99*, 712S–717S. [CrossRef]
41. Lonnerdal, B.; Lien, E.L. Nutritional and physiologic significance of alpha-lactalbumin in infants. *Nutr. Rev.* **2003**, *61*, 295–305. [CrossRef] [PubMed]
42. Russo, E.; Scicchitano, F.; Citraro, R.; Aiello, R.; Camastra, C.; Mainardi, P.; Chimirri, S.; Perucca, E.; Donato, G.; De Sarro, G. Protective activity of alpha-lactoalbumin (ALAC), a whey protein rich in tryptophan, in rodent models of epileptogenesis. *Neuroscience* **2012**, *226*, 282–288. [CrossRef] [PubMed]
43. Kelleher, S.L.; Chatterton, D.; Nielsen, K.; Lonnerdal, B. Glycomacropeptide and alpha-lactalbumin supplementation of infant formula affects growth and nutritional status in infant rhesus monkeys. *Am. J. Clin. Nutr.* **2003**, *77*, 1261–1268. [PubMed]
44. Bruck, W.M.; Kelleher, S.L.; Gibson, G.R.; Nielsen, K.E.; Chatterton, D.E.; Lonnerdal, B. Rrna probes used to quantify the effects of glycomacropeptide and alpha-lactalbumin supplementation on the predominant groups of intestinal bacteria of infant rhesus monkeys challenged with enteropathogenic *Escherichia coli*. *J. Pediatr. Gastroenterol. Nutr.* **2003**, *37*, 273–280. [CrossRef] [PubMed]
45. Rai, D.; Adelman, A.S.; Zhuang, W.; Rai, G.P.; Boettcher, J.; Lonnerdal, B. Longitudinal changes in lactoferrin concentrations in human milk: A global systematic review. *Crit. Rev. Food Sci. Nutr.* **2014**, *54*, 1539–1547. [CrossRef] [PubMed]
46. Kunz, C.; Lonnerdal, B. Re-evaluation of the whey protein/casein ratio of human milk. *Acta Paediatr.* **1992**, *81*, 107–112. [CrossRef] [PubMed]
47. Lonnerdal, B.; Adkins, Y. Developmental changes in breast milk protein composition during lactation. In *Development of the Gastrointestinal Tract*; Sanderson, R., Walker, W., Eds.; B.C. Decker Inc.: Hamilton, ON, Canada, 1999; pp. 227–244.
48. Goldman, A.S.; Garza, C.; Nichols, B.L.; Goldblum, R.M. Immunologic factors in human milk during the first year of lactation. *J. Pediatr.* **1982**, *100*, 563–567. [CrossRef]
49. Hawkes, J.S.; Bryan, D.L.; James, M.J.; Gibson, R.A. Cytokines (IL-1β, IL-6, TNF-α, TGF-β1, and TGF-β2) and prostaglandin E2 in human milk during the first three months postpartum. *Pediatr. Res.* **1999**, *46*, 194–199. [CrossRef] [PubMed]
50. Oddy, W.H.; Halonen, M.; Martinez, F.D.; Lohman, I.C.; Stern, D.A.; Kurzius-Spencer, M.; Guerra, S.; Wright, A.L. Tgf-beta in human milk is associated with wheeze in infancy. *J. Allergy Clin. Immunol.* **2003**, *112*, 723–728. [CrossRef]
51. Urwin, H.J.; Zhang, J.; Gao, Y.; Wang, C.; Li, L.; Song, P.; Man, Q.; Meng, L.; Froyland, L.; Miles, E.A.; et al. Immune factors and fatty acid composition in human milk from river/lake, coastal and inland regions of China. *Br. J. Nutr.* **2013**, *109*, 1949–1961. [CrossRef] [PubMed]

52. Van, V.P.; Punnonen, J.; de Vries, J.E. Transforming growth factor-beta directs iga switching in human B cells. *J. Immunol.* **1992**, *148*, 2062–2067.

53. Kalliomaki, M.; Ouwehand, A.; Arvilommi, H.; Kero, P.; Isolauri, E. Transforming growth factor-beta in breast milk: A potential regulator of atopic disease at an early age. *J. Allergy Clin. Immunol.* **1999**, *104*, 1251–1257. [CrossRef]

54. Penttila, I.A. Milk-derived transforming growth factor-beta and the infant immune response. *J. Pediatr.* **2010**, *156*, S21–S25. [CrossRef] [PubMed]

55. Stam, J.; Sauer, P.J.; Boehm, G. Can we define an infant's need from the composition of human milk? *Am. J. Clin. Nutr.* **2013**, *98*, 521S–528S. [CrossRef] [PubMed]

Permissions

All chapters in this book were first published by MDPI; hereby published with permission under the Creative Commons Attribution License or equivalent. Every chapter published in this book has been scrutinized by our experts. Their significance has been extensively debated. The topics covered herein carry significant findings which will fuel the growth of the discipline. They may even be implemented as practical applications or may be referred to as a beginning point for another development.

The contributors of this book come from diverse backgrounds, making this book a truly international effort. This book will bring forth new frontiers with its revolutionizing research information and detailed analysis of the nascent developments around the world.

We would like to thank all the contributing authors for lending their expertise to make the book truly unique. They have played a crucial role in the development of this book. Without their invaluable contributions this book wouldn't have been possible. They have made vital efforts to compile up to date information on the varied aspects of this subject to make this book a valuable addition to the collection of many professionals and students.

This book was conceptualized with the vision of imparting up-to-date information and advanced data in this field. To ensure the same, a matchless editorial board was set up. Every individual on the board went through rigorous rounds of assessment to prove their worth. After which they invested a large part of their time researching and compiling the most relevant data for our readers.

The editorial board has been involved in producing this book since its inception. They have spent rigorous hours researching and exploring the diverse topics which have resulted in the successful publishing of this book. They have passed on their knowledge of decades through this book. To expedite this challenging task, the publisher supported the team at every step. A small team of assistant editors was also appointed to further simplify the editing procedure and attain best results for the readers.

Apart from the editorial board, the designing team has also invested a significant amount of their time in understanding the subject and creating the most relevant covers. They scrutinized every image to scout for the most suitable representation of the subject and create an appropriate cover for the book.

The publishing team has been an ardent support to the editorial, designing and production team. Their endless efforts to recruit the best for this project, has resulted in the accomplishment of this book. They are a veteran in the field of academics and their pool of knowledge is as vast as their experience in printing. Their expertise and guidance has proved useful at every step. Their uncompromising quality standards have made this book an exceptional effort. Their encouragement from time to time has been an inspiration for everyone.

The publisher and the editorial board hope that this book will prove to be a valuable piece of knowledge for researchers, students, practitioners and scholars across the globe.

List of Contributors

Dana F.J. Yumani, Alexandra K. Calor and Mirjam. M. van Weissenbruch
Amsterdam UMC, Department of Pediatrics, VU University Medical Center, 1081 HV Amsterdam, The Netherlands

Ingmar Fortmann, Janina Marißen, Bastian Siller, Juliane Spiegler, Alexander Humberg, Kathrin Hanke, Kirstin Faust, Leila Eyvazzadeh, Kim Brenner, Egbert Herting and Wolfgang Göpel
Department of Pediatrics, University of Lübeck, 23562 Lübeck, Germany

Claudia Roll
Department of Pediatrics, Vestische Children's Hospital Datteln, 45711 Datteln, Germany

Sabine Pirr and Dorothee Viemann
Department of Neonatology, Hannover Medical School, 30159 Hannover, Germany

Dimitra Stavropoulou
Center for Pediatrics and Adolescent Medicine, Medical Center and Medical Faculty, University of Freiburg, 79098 Freiburg, Germany

Philipp Henneke
Center for Pediatrics and Adolescent Medicine, Medical Center and Medical Faculty, University of Freiburg, 79098 Freiburg, Germany
Institute for Immunodeficiency, Medical Center and Medical Faculty, University of Freiburg, 79098 Freiburg, Germany

Birte Tröger and Thorsten Körner
Children's Hospital Links der Weser Bremen, 28277 Bremen, Germany

Anja Stein
Department of Neonatology and General Pediatrics, University of Essen, 45147 Essen, Germany

Christoph Derouet and Michael Zemlin
Department of Neonatology and General Pediatrics, Saar University of Homburg, 66424 Homburg, Germany

Christian Wieg
Children's Hospital Ascha enburg-Alzenau, 63739 Ascha enburg, Germany

Jan Rupp
German Center for Infection Research (DZIF), Partner Site Hamburg-Lübeck-Borstel-Riems, 38124 Braunschweig, Germany
Department of Infectious Diseases and Medical Microbiology, University of Lübeck, 23562 Lübeck, Germany

Christoph Härtel and Julia Pagel
Department of Pediatrics, University of Lübeck, 23562 Lübeck, Germany
German Center for Infection Research (DZIF), Partner Site Hamburg-Lübeck-Borstel-Riems, 38124 Braunschweig, Germany

Clara L. Garcia-Rodenas, Michael Affolter, Leonidas G. Karagounis, Rosemarie Jenni, Iris Roggero, Ornella Avanti-Nigro, Carlos Antonio de Castro, Sagar K. Thakkar and Laurent Favre
Nestlé Research Center, Nestec Ltd., Lausanne 1000, Switzerland

Yumei Zhang
Department of Nutrition and Food Hygiene, School of Public Health, Peking University, Beijing 100191, China

Elin Östman, Anna Forslund, Eden Tareke and Inger Björck
Food for Health Science Centre, Lund University, 221 00 Lund, Sweden

Kevin B. Hadley, Sheila Gautier and Norman Salem Jr.
DSM Nutritional Products, 6480 Dobbin Road, Columbia, MD 21045, USA

Alan S. Ryan
Clinical Research Consulting, 9809 Halston Manor, Boynton Beach, FL 33473, USA

Stewart Forsyth
School of Medicine, Dentistry & Nursing, University of Dundee, Ninewells Hospital and Medical School, Dundee, UK

Jian Zhao, Yun Zhao, Colin W. Binns and Andy H. Lee
School of Public Health, Curtin University, Perth 6102, Australia

Melissa Thoene
Newborn Intensive Care Unit, Nebraska Medicine, 981200 Nebraska Medical Center, Omaha, NE 68198, USA

Elizabeth Lyden
College of Public Health, University of Nebraska Medical Center, 984375 Nebraska Medical Center, Omaha, NE 68198-4375, USA

Kara Weishaar, Elizabeth Elliott, Ruomei Wu, Katelyn White, Hayley Timm and Ann Anderson-Berry
Department of Pediatrics, University of Nebraska Medical Center, 981205 Nebraska Medical Center, Omaha, NE 68198-1205, USA

Arianna Aceti
Neonatology and Neonatal Intensive Care Unit, Department of Medical and Surgical Sciences (DIMEC), University of Bologna, S.Orsola-Malpighi Hospital, Bologna 40138, Italy
Task Force on Probiotics of the Italian Society of Neonatology, Milan 20126, Italy

Davide Gori and Maria Pia Fantini
Task Force on Probiotics of the Italian Society of Neonatology, Milan 20126, Italy
Department of Biomedical and Neuromotor Sciences (DIBINEM), University of Bologna, Bologna 40138, Italy

Giovanni Barone
Task Force on Probiotics of the Italian Society of Neonatology, Milan 20126, Italy
Neonatal Unit, Catholic University, Rome 00168, Italy

Maria Luisa Callegari and Lorenzo Morelli
Task Force on Probiotics of the Italian Society of Neonatology, Milan 20126, Italy
Institute of Microbiology, UCSC, Piacenza 29122, Italy

Flavia Indrio
Task Force on Probiotics of the Italian Society of Neonatology, Milan 20126, Italy
Department of Pediatrics, Aldo Moro University, Bari 70124, Italy
Study Group of Neonatal Gastroenterology and Nutrition of the Italian Society of Neonatology, Milan 20126, Italy

Luca Maggio
Task Force on Probiotics of the Italian Society of Neonatology, Milan 20126, Italy
Neonatal Unit, Catholic University, Rome 00168, Italy
Study Group of Neonatal Gastroenterology and Nutrition of the Italian Society of Neonatology, Milan 20126, Italy

Fabio Meneghin
Task Force on Probiotics of the Italian Society of Neonatology, Milan 20126, Italy
Division of Neonatology, Children Hospital V. Buzzi, ICP, Milan 20154, Italy

Gianvincenzo Zuccotti
Task Force on Probiotics of the Italian Society of Neonatology, Milan 20126, Italy
Department of Pediatrics, Children Hospital V. Buzzi, University of Milan, Milan 20154, Italy

Luigi Corvaglia
Neonatology and Neonatal Intensive Care Unit, Department of Medical and Surgical Sciences (DIMEC), University of Bologna, S.Orsola-Malpighi Hospital, Bologna 40138, Italy
Task Force on Probiotics of the Italian Society of Neonatology, Milan 20126, Italy
Study Group of Neonatal Gastroenterology and Nutrition of the Italian Society of Neonatology, Milan 20126, Italy

Francesca Giuffrida, Cristina Cruz-Hernandez, Emmanuelle Bertschy, Patric Fontannaz, Isabelle Masserey Elmelegy, Isabelle Tavazzi, Cynthia Marmet, Belén Sanchez-Bridge, Sagar K. Thakkar and Carlos Antonio De Castro
Nestlé Research Center, Nestec Ltd., Vers-chez-les-Blanc, 1000 Lausanne 26, Switzerland

Peiyu Wang
Department of Social Medicine and Health Education, School of Public Health, Peking University Health Science Center, Beijing 100191, China

Maria Lorella Giannì, Nadia Liotto, Paola Roggero, Laura Morlacchi, Pasqua Piemontese, Camilla Menis and Fabio Mosca
Fondazione I.R.C.C.S. Ca Granda Ospedale Maggiore Policlinico, Neonatal Intensive Care Unit, Department of Clinical Science and Community Health, University of Milan, Via Commenda 12, 20122 Milano, Italy

Dario Consonni
Fondazione IRCCS Ca' Granda Ospedale Maggiore Policlinico, Epidemiology Unit, Via San Barnaba 8, 20122 Milan, Italy

Anita Jorgensen and Jillian Sherriff
School of Public Health, Curtin University, Perth 6102, Australia

Peter O'Leary
Faculty of Health Sciences, Curtin University, Perth 6102, Australia

Ian James
Institute for Immunology & Infectious Diseases, Murdoch University, Murdoch 6150, Australia

Sheila Skeaff
Department of Human Nutrition, University of Otago, Dunedin 9054, New Zealand

Corrine Hanson
College of Allied Health Professions, University of Nebraska Medical Center, Medical Nutrition Education, 984045 Nebraska Medical Center, Omaha, NE 68198-4045, USA

Jeremy Furtado
Department of Nutrition, Harvard School of Public Health, 655 Huntington Avenue, Boston, MA 02215, USA

Matthew Van Ormer and Ann Anderson-Berry
Pediatrics, University of Nebraska Medical Center, 981205 Nebraska Medical Center, Omaha, NE 68198-1205, USA

Heather C. Hamner, Cria G. Perrine and Kelley S. Scanlon
National Center for Chronic Disease Prevention and Health Promotion, Centers for Disease Control and Prevention (CDC), Atlanta, GA 30341, USA

Viola Christmann, Charlotte J. W. Gradussen, Michelle N. Körnmann and Arno F. J. van Heijst
Department of Paediatrics, Subdivision of Neonatology, Radboudumc Amalia Children's Hospital, Radboud University Medical Center, Nijmegen 6500HB, The Netherlands

Nel Roeleveld
Department for Health Evidence, Radboud Institute for Health Science, Radboud University Medical Center, Nijmegen 6500HB, The Netherlands
Department of Paediatrics, Radboudumc Amalia Children's Hospital, Radboud University Medical Center, Nijmegen 6500HB, The Netherlands

Johannes B. van Goudoever
Department of Paediatrics, VU university medical center Amsterdam, Amsterdam 1081HV, The Netherlands
Department of Paediatrics, Emma Children's Hospital-AMC Amsterdam, Amsterdam 1105AZ, The Netherlands

Juan Francisco Haro-Vicente and Maria Jose Bernal-Cava
Department of Research and Development, Hero Group, Alcantarilla, Murcia 30820, Spain

Amparo Lopez-Fernandez and Gaspar Ros-Berruezo
Department of Food Science and Nutrition, University of Murcia, Campus de Espinardo, Espinardo, Murcia 30071, Spain

Stefan Bodenstab and Luis Manuel Sanchez-Siles
Department of Research and Development, Hero Group, Lenzburg 5600, Switzerland

Valentina De Cosmi
Valentina De Cosmi Pediatric Intensive Care Unit, Fondazione IRCCS Cà Granda Ospedale Maggiore Policlinico, Branch of Medical Statistics, Biometry, and Epidemiology "G. A. Maccacaro", Department of Clinical Sciences and Community Health, University of Milan, 20122 Milan, Italy

Silvia Scaglioni
Silvia Scaglioni Fondazione De Marchi Department of Pediatrics, Fondazione IRCCS Cà Granda Ospedale Maggiore Policlinico, 20122 Milan, Italy

Carlo Agostoni
Carlo Agostoni Pediatric Intermediate Care Unit, Fondazione IRCCS Cà Granda Ospedale Maggiore Policlinico, Department of Clinical Sciences and Community Health, University of Milan, 20122 Milan, Italy

Gerard Vinyes-Pares
Nestlé Research Center Beijing, Nestec Ltd., Beijing 100095, China
Nestlé Health Sciences, Nestec Ltd., Epalinges 1066, Switzerland
Nestlé Research Center Beijing, Building E-F, No. 5 Dijin Road, Haidian District, Beijing 100091, China

Ai Zhao and Yumei Zhang
Department of Nutrition and Food Hygiene, School of Public Health, Peking University, Beijing 100191, China

Index

Printed in the USA
CPSIA information can be obtained
at www.ICGtesting.com
JSHW051407091023
49903JS00006B/320